TEXTBOOK OF
Psoriasis

TEXTBOOK OF

Psoriasis

Edited by P.C.M. van de Kerkhof
DEPARTMENT OF DERMATOLOGY
UNIVERSITY HOSPITAL NIJMEGEN
THE NETHERLANDS

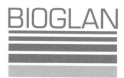

Provided as an educational service to dermatology by
Bioglan Laboratories Limited

Blackwell
Science

© 1999 by
Blackwell Science Ltd
Editorial Offices:
Osney Mead, Oxford OX2 0EL
25 John Street, London WC1N 2BL
23 Ainslie Place, Edinburgh
  EH3 6AJ
350 Main Street, Malden
  MA 02148 5018, USA
54 University Street, Carlton
  Victoria 3053, Australia
10, rue Casimir Delavigne
  75006 Paris, France

Other Editorial Offices:
Blackwell Wissenschafts-Verlag
  GmbH
Kurfürstendamm 57
10707 Berlin, Germany

Blackwell Science KK
MG Kodenmacho Building
7–10 Kodenmacho Nihombashi
Chuo-ku, Tokyo 104, Japan

First published 1999
Reprinted with amendments 2000

Set by
Sparks Computer Solutions Ltd,
Oxford, UK
Printed and bound in Great Britain
by MPG Books Ltd, Bodmin,
Cornwall

The Blackwell Science logo is a
trade mark of Blackwell Science
Ltd, registered at the United
Kingdom Trade Marks Registry

A catalogue record for this title is
available from the British Library

ISBN 0-632-05166-3

Library of Congress
Cataloging-in-publication Data

Textbook of psoriasis / edited by
P.C.M. van de Kerkhof
    p.   cm.
  Includes bibliographical
references and index
  ISBN 0-632-05166-3
  1. Psoriasis. I. Kerkhof, Petrus
Cornelis Maria van de, 1952– .
II. Title: Psoriasis
  [DNLM: 1. Psoriasis.
WR 205 T3553 1999]
RL321.T49 1999
616.5'26—dc21
DNLM/DLC
for Library of Congress   99-20850
                                     CIP

DISTRIBUTORS

Marston Book Services Ltd
PO Box 269
Abingdon, Oxon OX14 4YN
(*Orders*: Tel: 01235 465500
            Fax: 01235 465555)

USA
Blackwell Science, Inc.
Commerce Place
350 Main Street
Malden, MA 02148 5018
(*Orders*: Tel: 800 759 6102
                 781 388 8250
            Fax: 781 388 8255)

Canada
Login Brothers Book Company
324 Saulteaux Crescent
Winnipeg, Manitoba R3J 3T2
(*Orders*: Tel: 204 837 2987)

Australia
Blackwell Science Pty Ltd
54 University Street
Carlton, Victoria 3053
(*Orders*: Tel: 3 9347 0300
            Fax: 3 9347 5001)

For further information on
Blackwell Science, visit our
website:
www.blackwell-science.com

Contents

List of Colour Plates

Plates 1.1–2.1 appear between pages 36 and 37, and Plates 11.1–12.3 appear between pages 196 and 197

Contributors

B. Bonnekoh, *Otto van Guericke University, Department of Dermatology, Leipziggerstraße 44, 39120 Magdeburg, Germany.*

J.D. Bos, *Academisch Medisch Centrum Amsterdam, Department of Dermatology, Postbus 22660, 1100 DD Amsterdam, The Netherlands.*

M.A. de Rie, *Academisch Medisch Centrum Amsterdam, Department of Dermatology, Postbus 22660, 1100 DD Amsterdam, The Netherlands.*

K. Fogh, *Marselisborg Hospital, Department of Dermatology, University of Aarhus, 8000 Aarhus, Denmark.*

G. Folchetti, *Hôpital Saint Marguerite, Service de Dermatologie, Boîte Postale 29, 13009 Marseille, France.*

M.J.A.M. Franssen, *St Maartensklinik, Afdelim Rheumatologie, Postbus 9011, 6500 GM Nijmegen, The Netherlands.*

M.J.P. Gerritsen, *Univerity Hospital of Nijmegen, Department of Dermatology, P.O. Box 9101, 6500 HB Nijmegen, The Netherlands.*

H.P.M. Gollnick, *Otto van Guericke University, Department of Dermatology, Leipziggerstraße 44, 39120 Magdeburg, Germany.*

J.J. Grob, *Hôpital Saint Marguerite, Service de Dermatologie, Boîte Postale 29, 13009 Marseille, France.*

F.H.J. van den Hoogen, *Academisch Ziekenhuis Nijmegen, Postbus 9101, 6500 HB Nijmegen, The Netherlands.*

J. Hughes, *The Royal Free Hospital, Department of Dermatology, Pond Street, London NW3 2QG, UK.*

S. Kang, *University of Michigan, Department of Dermatology, Taubman Center 1910, 48109-0314 Ann Arbor, Michigan, USA.*

P.C.M. van de Kerkhof, *University Hospital of Nijmegen, Department of Dermatology, P.O. Box 9101, 6500 HB Nijmegen, The Netherlands.*

K. Kragballe, *Marselisborg Hospital, Department of Dermatology, University of Aarhus, 8000 Aarhus, Denmark.*

J. Krutmann, *Heinrich-Heine University of Düsseldorf, Department of Dermatology, Mooren straße 5, 40225 Dusseldorf, Germany*

L.B.A. van de Putte, *Academisch Ziekenhuis Nijmegen, Afdeling Rheumatologie, Postbus 9101, 6500 HB Nijmegen, The Netherlands.*

M.H.A. Rustin, *The Royal Free Hospital, Department of Dermatology, Pond Street, London NW3 2QG, UK.*

J.A. Savin, *The Royal Infirmary of Edinburgh, Department of Dermatology, 1 Lauriston Place, Edinburgh EH3 9YW, UK.*

H. Traupe, *University of Münster, Department of Dermatology, Von Esmarchstraße 56, 48149 Münster, Germany.*

J.J. Voorhees, *University of Michigan, Department of Dermatology, Taubman Center 1910, 48109-0314 Ann Arbor, Michigan, USA.*

H. Zachariae, *Marselisborg Hospital, Department of Dermatology, University of Aarhus, 8000 Aarhus C, Denmark.*

Preface

Questions on the management of psoriasis need up-to-date answers. What are triggering factors? What is the inheritance? What are the causes of the disease? Which treatments are available?

During the last decade, our insight into the pathogenesis has increased and new treatments are available. In particular, developments in research on molecular genetics, inflammatory mechanisms and immunology have changed our understanding of psoriasis. New therapeutic possibilities have been introduced for the patient of today. These include new classes of drugs such as vitamin D_3 analogues, new retinoids and cyclosporin. New therapeutic principles have been introduced for the patient of tomorrow. These include immunomodulatory drugs and modulators of signal transduction.

In many countries standardized operating procedures for treatment of diseases are requested by healthcare authorities. This implies that protocol development for existing treatments is indispensable nowadays. Therefore this textbook on psoriasis focuses on guidelines of available treatments and will inform the reader on the cutting edge of development in our insight in pathogenesis and modern treatment options for patients with psoriasis.

This textbook has been written by a team of experts in the field. The book is a result of a group rather than the sum of individual chapters.

The first part of the book is on clinical presentations involving the clinical morphology of the skin, an account on psoriatic arthropathy and a critical account on psychosocial aspects.

The second part of the book is on aetiology and pathogenesis. Epidemiology and genetics are of major importance with respect to management of diseases. Information on genetic counselling is provided for consultation purposes. The pathogenesis of psoriasis includes various aspects including inflammation control, epidermal proliferation, keratinization, endocrine factors and immune mechanisms. In the last decade our insight into the immunopathogenesis has expanded resulting in new possibilities to treat psoriasis with immunomodulatory approaches.

Part 3 provides information on the available treatments. Modes of action, efficacy, side-effects and guidelines are discussed.

Knowledge about clinical presentations, aetiology and treatment are essential for adequate management of patients with psoriasis. Every patient has his or her distinctive form of psoriasis; therefore the management of psoriasis has to be individualized.

Peter C.M. van de Kerkhof

Part 1
Clinical Presentations

This part aims to provide a comprehensive presentation of the clinical aspects which are relevant to dermatologists, residents, general practitioners and insurance, as well as occupational healthcare workers.

In Chapter 1 the various cutaneous manifestations, eliciting factors, spontaneous course and the histopathology will be described in particular with regard to differential diagnosis.

In Chapter 2 the diagnosis, spontaneous course and the treatment of psoriatic arthropathy will be presented.

In Chapter 3 the psychosocial aspects will be described, focusing in particular on the impact of psychological stress as elicitor of first signs and relapses of psoriasis.

Chapter 1: Clinical Features

P.C.M. van de Kerkhof

1.1 Introduction

1.1.1 History

Hippocrates (460–377 BC) provided detailed descriptions of many skin disorders. He grouped together dry, scaly eruptions under 'lopoi' (λοποσ = epidermis). This group probably included psoriasis and leprosy.

Also in the old testament both conditions were grouped together, with the result that many psoriatics were rejected by the community (Pusey 1933).

Galen was the first who used the word 'psoriasis'. Under this name he described a skin disorder, characterized by a scaliness of the eyelids, the corners of the eyes and scrotum. The clinical picture of this disorder, which itched, is in fact more compatible with eczema although it was designated by Galen as 'psoriasis' (Pusey 1933).

The confusion between psoriasis and leprosy remained for many centuries (Wahba *et al.* 1980). From 1000 to 1400 AD the prevalence of psoriasis was very high. Many psoriatic patients, diagnosed as leprosy, received the same brutal treatment as leprosy patients; they were isolated from the community, the church declared them officially dead and in 1313 Philip the Fair even ordered them to be burned at the stake. It was not until the 19th century that psoriasis was recognized as an entity apart from leprosy.

Robert Willan (1809) was the first to give an accurate description of psoriasis (Willan 1809). However, it would still take 30 years to break with a history of more than two millennia; in 1941, Hebra definitively separated the clinical picture of psoriasis from that of leprosy.

An extensive description of the clinical appearance of psoriatic skin manifestations is presented in this chapter.

1.1.2 Cutaneous manifestations

Psoriasis is a rather common disease. About 2% of the world's population is affected. As the disease is generally chronic and persistent in nature, and because patients with psoriasis have a similar life expectancy to individuals without the disease, the prevalence of psoriasis increases with age (Bonifati *et al.* 1998).

Sharply demarcated erythematosquamous lesions are the most important hallmark of the psoriatic lesion. However, within the spectrum of cutaneous manifestations of psoriasis different expressions are seen. Individual lesions may vary in size from pinpoint to large plaques, or even erythroderma (erythrodermic psoriasis). If the clinical picture is dominated by small lesions, it is described as guttate psoriasis. If coin-sized (nummular) or palm-sized plaques predominate, the term chronic plaque psoriasis is used. If the inflammatory processes dominate, pustules may be the most important sign and this manifestation is designated as pustular psoriasis. These lesions may be generalized (generalized pustular psoriasis) or localized (persistent pustulosis of palms and soles and acrodermatitis continua Hallopeau).

A major question remains to be answered: 'Are these manifestations of psoriasis different expressions of one single disease or are they different disease entities? From a morphological point of view the diseases should be regarded as different phenotypical expressions of one single disease.

1 The clinical appearance in all expressions share the erythematosquamous appearance as the most common feature. The spongiform pustule (as micropustule in the erythematosquamous variants and as macropustule in the pustular variants) is the common pathognomonic characteristic.

2 At the same moment different manifestations may coexist.

3 At different times in a patients life different manifestations may appear.

4 In one single family different members may show different manifestations.

Therefore, from an epidemiological and clinical point of view psoriasis may be characterized as a three-dimensional spectrum, whose extremes are the classical manifestations of 'guttate', 'chronic plaque', 'erythrodermic' and 'pustular' psoriasis. This is illustrated in Fig. 1.1.

The variability in the expression of psoriasis is also apparent from the life of the individual lesions. Lesions are initiated, grow and regress. Lesions may be fairly constant over many years. However, in some patients a considerable variability is recorded. It is then important to search for triggering factors.

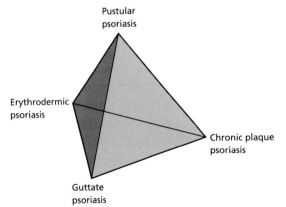

Pustular psoriasis

Erythrodermic psoriasis

Chronic plaque psoriasis

Guttate psoriasis

Fig. 1.1 Spectrum of manifestations.

The response to skin injury may differ considerably between different patients, some having a positive response with appearance of a lesion at sites following trauma (positive Koebner phenomenon) and others not. The Koebner phenomenon is an all-or-none phenomenon (Eyre & Krueger 1982).

Although different manifestations may be regarded as expressions of one single disease, the question arises to what extent genetic factors may predispose to some preferential manifestations.

From studies on the association with HLA subtypes we know that HLA Cw6 type is associated with an early onset of psoriasis (Brenner *et al.* 1978). In pustular psoriasis no association with HLA A13 and A17 was found in contrast to the erythematosquamous variants (Svejgaard *et al.* 1974) and in patients suffering from palmoplantar pustulosis, an increased frequency of HAL B8 was found (Ward & Barnes 1978).

1.1.3 Extracutaneous manifestations

Common extracutaneous manifestations of psoriasis are:
1   *nails*—both the nail bed and nail matrix are involved;
2   *mucosal membranes*—the oral mucosa may be involved in pustular psoriasis;
3   *joints*—psoriatic arthropathy may occur in psoriatic patients. The reader is referred to Chapter 2 for further details.

1.2 Erythematosquamous manifestations of psoriasis

1.2.1 Clinical presentations

The lesion

Static picture. The macromorphological appearance of the psoriatic lesion is highly characteristic (Plate 1.1 [Plates 1.1–1.22 fall between pp 52 and 53]). The outline of the lesion is mostly polycyclic, indicating that the lesion is constituted from several smaller units.

A further characteristic is the sharp demarcation of the lesion without any gradual change to normal skin. Occasionally, a white blanching ring is seen around the psoriatic lesion, which was described for the first time by Woronoff (1926). Scaling, erythema and induration constitute the macromorphological elements of the psoriatic lesion. The scaling has a typical silvery aspect. The psoriasis-specific characteristics of the silvery scaling can be studied using a curette. A characteristic coherence is observed, as if scratching on a wax candle (*'signe de la tache de bougie'*). By repeated scratching the Auspitz phenomenon can be shown: a last membrane is removed and a wet surface with characteristic pinpoint bleedings is observed. The *signe de la tache de bougie* is equivalent to the parakeratosis, and the Auspitz phenomenon is

equivalent to the upward proliferation of dermal papillae with vasodilatation. The grattage method is of special diagnostic value if erythema alone is
observed without any apparent scaling (as is the case in partially treated patients).

The degree of scaling may differ considerably between patients. Sometimes erythema is the dominating feature such as in early, exanthematic forms
of psoriasis. Sometimes the scaling and induration are the dominating features.

1   Rupoid psoriasis or psoriasis ostracea: this rare manifestation is characterized by limpet-like lesions (Plate 1.2). The lesions are cone-shaped and
demonstrate horizontal rather than vertical lamellations.

2   Inveterate or elephantine psoriasis: this form is more common than the
former and is characterized by a massive, thickened horny layer (Plate 1.3).

The subjective sensation of a psoriatic lesion can be painful if the lesion is
dry and cracked. Itch is experienced in early exacerbating lesions. In cases
with a strong psychological component the lesions may itch severely. However, itch and pain are not psoriasis-characteristic symptoms.

Dynamics. Lesions grow and regress. The dynamic cycle may be relatively
short, such as in guttate psoriasis (weeks to months) or very chronic such as
in chronic plaque psoriasis (months to years). Systemic triggering factors dic-
tate the morphological aspects of the eruption as a whole and will be discussed later. Local factors will be discussed in this section together with the
morphological aspects of growth and regression of the lesion.

External triggering factors are of utmost importance in the pathogenesis
of the psoriatic lesion. The artificial production of the psoriatic lesion from
the symptomless skin (Fig. 1.2) was described for the first time by Heinrich
Koebner (1878). Figure 1.2 is an artistic representation of his experiments
on the elicitation of psoriatic lesions by a trauma. Dermal trauma alone (such
as the intradermal injection of chymotrypsin) does not result in a clinical
lesion (Farber *et al.* 1965).

The epidermis must be damaged in order to induce a clinical lesion. Another intriguing observation was that pretreatment with xylocaine significantly reduced the number of positive responses. This effect was ascribed to
the vasoconstrictory action of the substance.

Several authors have demonstrated that pressure on the skin or temporary obliteration of the vessels prevented the 'Koebner phenomenon'. These
clinical observations indicate the importance of the vascular compartment in
the initiation of the psoriatic lesion. Between trauma and the appearance of
the psoriatic lesion a time lag exists of 1–4 weeks. This indicates that after the
eliciting trauma a complex cascade of metabolic events occurs. In a prospective study Eyre and Krueger (1982) reported on a positive Koebner phenomenon in 25% of the patients. Although some authors are of the opinion that
a positive Koebner phenomenon is observed more often in patients with

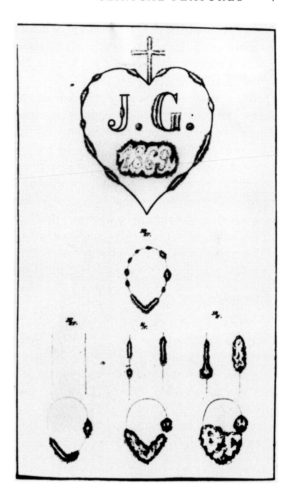

Fig. 1.2 Koebner phenomenon, an original illustration. (From Weyl 1883.)

eruptive, florid or progressive psoriasis (Pedace *et al.* 1969), such statements are not based on solid statistical analysis of data. Indeed, Illig and Holz were unable to show a significant difference between guttate, chronic plaque and unstable psoriasis (Illig & Holz 1966). Eyre and Krueger (1982) reported that the Koebner-negative patients had a more mild course as compared to the Koebner positive patients. The Koebner phenomenon is an all-or-none phenomenon. All uninvolved skin sites respond to injury with a psoriatic plaque and all clinically involved sites heal leaving psoriatic skin *or* none of the injured sites of the uninvolved skin respond with a psoriatic lesion whereas all injured lesions heal leaving clinically normal skin (Eyre & Kreuger 1982).

The inverse relationship of the all-or-none phenomenon indicates that endogenous factors govern the development or clearing of psoriasis after injury. Endogenous factors that might be of significance will be discussed later.

The clinician should be aware of the possibility of local triggering factors in case a patient responds insufficiently to treatments. Local triggering factors which may be relevant are: contact dermatitis and certain eczemas, irritant dermatitis, impetigo contagiosa, herpes zoster, mycotic infection, mechanical trauma and sunburn.

Growth and regression of lesions show a psoriasis-specific pattern. Lesions start with small, pinpoint papules, which early in the evolution show scaling (Plate 1.4). The initial papules grow to larger elements and coalesce resulting in a polycyclic outline. Lesions may grow by centrifugal expansion from guttate (drop-like), to nummular (coin-sized), palm-sized and even larger. They sometimes resolve in the centre, whilst expanding in the periphery (Plate 1.5). The lesion involutes starting in the centre, resulting in annular psoriasis. The persistence of the lesions in the margin zone is typical during antipsoriatic treatment. In contrast to lichen planus, which resolves leaving hyperpigmentation, hypopigmentation is associated with clearing of the psoriatic plaque: 'psoriatic leucoderma'.

The eruption

The objective of this section is to describe the skin manifestations as a whole. Systemic triggering factors regulate the dynamics and the extent of the eruption. In this section we will present systemic triggering factors, erythematosquamous manifestations with different size of the lesion and manifestations with a special localization.

Systemic factors. Systemic factors are those which affect not only some single lesions, but rather affect the eruption as a whole, for example:
- infection;
- endocrine factors;
- hypocalcaemia;
- psychogenic factors;
- drugs.

Infections which trigger psoriasis are usually focal and not septic. Provoking infections could be traced in 44% of a mixed series of psoriatic patients (Nörholm-Pedersen 1952). In younger patients focal infections seem to be very frequent. In these children the clinical picture is mostly that of a guttate psoriasis. The site of infection is mostly the upper respiratory tract (Holzmann *et al.* 1974). Guttate psoriasis proved to be encountered mostly in association with a focal infection, an association that is of pathogenetic relevance (Holzmann *et al.* 1974). Although clinical praxis literature describes a link between dental infections and aggravation of psoriasis, data to support this association are sparse.

Endocrine factors may be of relevance in the pathogenesis of psoriasis. Serum levels of dehydroepiandrosterone, aldosterone and somatotropic hormone proved to be abnormal in psoriatic patients as compared to normal controls (Weber *et al.* 1981; Holzmann *et al.* 1974; van de Kerkhof 1982).

However, psoriatic patients do not show pathological values of these parameters. Many cases start in puberty and sometimes in the menopause. Pregnancy may change the course of the disease, 50% of the patients reported improvement and 74% of the patients did not indicate that their psoriasis was adversely affected by the pregnancy (Farber *et al.* 1968) Systemic treatment with corticosteroids usually will result in a relapse after discontinuation.

Hypocalcaemia has been reported to be a triggering factor in two patients suffering from chronic plaque psoriasis (Cornbleet 1956). Hypocalcaemia has been reported to be a triggering factor in generalized pustular psoriasis (p. 18).

Psychogenic stress has been reported to be a triggering factor in patients with psoriasis. The relationship between psychogenic factors and psoriasis will be presented in Part 3.

Drugs may elicit psoriasis in predisposed subjects or aggravate psoriasis in patients with manifestations of the disease. Several drugs have been incriminated in case reports as inducing psoriasis. The relationship with aggravation of the disease is well established for the following drugs:

1   antimalarials (Cornbleet 1956);
2   lithium (White & Colonel 1982);
3   β-adrenergic antagonists (Söndergaard *et al.* 1976);
4   systemic corticosteroids;
5   indometacin (Katayama and Kawada 1981).

The age of onset. At present the diagnosis of 'minimal expression of psoriasis' or latent psoriasis remains impossible. There is no diagnostic laboratory test to certify that a subject has the psoriatic predisposition or not. The diagnosis of 'minimal psoriasis' is a rather variable exercise when various departments for dermatology are compared. Sometimes a few pits and some scaling of the elbows, knees or scalp will suffice for the diagnosis psoriasis, whereas in other centres the complete signs of psoriasis are required for the diagnosis. As psoriasis is in part genetically determined, this implies that there are many people with latent psoriasis. So far there is no way to estimate the size of this population as there is no diagnostic test to trace a genetic predisposition for the disease. The age of onset varies considerably between different patients. A very extensive investigation has been undertaken by Farber and Nall who studied the natural history of 5600 psoriatics (Farber and Nall 1974).

The mean age of onset for the total sample was 27.8 ± 0.38 (SEM) years. For the males this figure was 29.2 ± 0.58 and for the females 26.6 ± 0.49. Ten per cent of the whole group had an onset before the age of 10, 35% before 20 years and 58% before the age of 30. Based on epidemiological investigations one can conclude the earlier the psoriasis starts, the worse the prognosis.

Manifestations with different sizes of individual lesions. The manifestations that will be described are: guttate, chronic plaque and erythrodermic psoriasis. 'Restless' psoriasis is the unstable form of plaque psoriasis.

Guttate psoriasis is characterized by erythematosquamous papules distributed as 'droplets' over the whole body surface (Plate 1.6). The trunk is the site which is most commonly affected, whereas the palms and soles are usually spared. It is the presenting manifestation in 14–17% of all patients (Camp 1993). It is especially common in children (44–95%). In a total sample of psoriatic patients the frequency was only 1.9% (Camp 1993). The exanthematic appearance suggests a systemic factor in the initiation of this eruption. In many patients the eruption is preceded by a focal infection, most commonly of the upper respiratory tract. The prognosis of this manifestation is excellent in children, spontaneous remissions occurring in the course of weeks or months. In adults the prognosis is worse (Lomholt 1963).

Chronic plaque psoriasis is by far the most common manifestation. It is characterized by sharply defined erythematosquamous plaques, usually distributed fairly symmetrically (Plate 1.7). This distribution is compatible with the fact that both external and internal triggering factors are involved. The size of the lesions varies from coin-sized to palm-sized and larger than palm-sized. The term nummular psoriasis is used if coin-sized lesions predominate. If larger than palm-sized lesions predominate, the term geographical psoriasis is the term of choice (Plate 1.8). Table 1.1 shows the frequencies of the different localizations (van de Kerkhof *et al.*, 1998).

The most frequent site of involvement is the scalp, whereas the face is relatively spared from psoriasis. The relative frequency of plaque psoriasis approaches 90% in adults. In epidemiological surveys complete remissions up to 5 years or more have been reported in about 10% of all patients.

Unstable psoriasis is the transition phase of chronic plaque psoriasis to a more extensive involvement. Due to triggering factors, a patient with chronic plaque psoriasis may develop unstable psoriasis. It is of therapeutic relevance that a lowered erythema threshold exists to irritants. Indeed, personal experience strongly supports that patients with unstable psoriasis have a rela-

Location	% of responders
Scalp	79.7
Elbows	77.8
Legs	73.7
Knees	56.6
Arms	54.2
Trunk	52.6
Lower part of the body	46.8
Base of the back	38.0
Other	37.7
Soles of feet	12.9

Table 1.1 Location of psoriasis (n = 784 responders).

tively low erythema threshold following UVB radiation and dithranol application.

Erythrodermic psoriasis is the manifestation where the characteristic psoriatic lesions have been replaced by totally generalized erythema and scaling. This reaction pattern is not unique for psoriasis but may also occur in pityriasis rubra pilaris, atopic dermatitis, reticulosis and as a reaction to drugs. Serious systemic dysregulation may occur including hypo- and hyperthermia, protein loss and imbalance of salt–water metabolism. Dehydration, renal failure and cardiac failure may result. In cases of erythrodermic psoriasis the skin as a whole is involved; however, a few areas of clinically uninvolved skin are seen where the sharp demarcation might suggest psoriasis. Sometimes the typical changes of the nails suggest psoriasis, but mostly these are engulfed by the gross nail deformations which occur in erythroderma. Previous history with involvement of typical sites, minor signs of psoriasis and histology are of help in the diagnosis of erythrodermic psoriasis. Erythrodermic psoriasis may occur at any age. This manifestation may occur *de novo* via a restless psoriasis or in the course of pustular psoriasis. The clearing time varies between 3 weeks and 2 months on a conservative therapy.

Manifestations with a special localization. As has been shown in Table 1.1 the *scalp* is the most common localization in psoriasis. If there is a marked seborrhoea the characteristic features may be less clear cut at this site. Sometimes the whole scalp is involved, sometimes the lesions are more localized. The lesions may advance over the hair margin on the facial skin (Plate 1.9). The scales sometimes have an asbestos-like appearance and are attached for some distance to the scalp hair (pityriasis amiantacea). Eventually hair growth may be impaired with a telogen effluvium (Schoorl *et al.* 1992). In some patients cicatricial alopecia may develop (van de Kerkhof and Chang 1992).

Involvement of *palms and soles* has been reported in up to 12% of the patients. The lesions are characterized by their sharp demarcation, scaling and fissuring (Plate 1.10). The lesions may be palm-sized or distributed as smaller units over palms and soles. If fissuring is prominent the differentiation from eczema hyperkeratoticum may be difficult. In some patients the correlation between this localization and friction or orthoergic dermatitis may be difficult.

In the *sacral region* indurated and inveterated plaques may occur.

Flexural psoriasis is estimated at 2–6% in psoriatic patients.

Possible localizations are the axillae, groins, submammary region, perianal region and the retroauricular folds (Plates 1.11 and 1.12). It is possible that psoriasis inversa is the Koebner response to a preceding infective or seborrhoeic dermatosis. It is advisable in any patient with flexural psoriasis to exclude a mycotic infection or erythrasma.

The diagnosis of *napkin psoriasis* is rather difficult and should be differentiated from napkin dermatitis or seborrhoeic dermatitis. Sharp demarcation of plaques and silvery scaling might be helpful, but often this diagnosis re-mains very uncertain.

Mucosal membranes may be involved in psoriasis. Involvement of the oral cavity is discussed in relation to pustular psoriasis. However, oral lesions char-acterized by erythematous areas with a histological picture compatible with psoriasis have been described (Rozell *et al.* 1997). Localization at the genita-lia has been reported in 2% of the patients (Plate 1.13). It is likely that previ-ous *Candida* infections have triggered this condition. Therefore swabs for *Candida* culture are indicated in psoriasis of the genital region. Ocular in-volvement has been reported in 10% of psoriatic patients. Blepharitis and keratitis are the established features of ocular psoriasis (Lomato *et al.* 1982).

1.2.2 Histological appearance

The psoriatic plaque

The fully developed psoriatic plaque consists of 'hot spots' and 'cold spots'(Griffin *et al.* 1988). In general the margin of the psoriatic plaque shows the highest density of the hot spots. The histopathological picture of a 'cold spot' is that of an aspecific dermatitis, with epidermal acanthosis, parakera-tosis and a largely mononuclear inflammatory infiltrate, partly showing epidermotropism. The 'hot spots' show a more acute and more psoriasis-specific pattern (Plate 1.14). As the margin zone shows the highest density of hot spots, it is important to take the biopsy from the margin zone of a psori-atic plaque or from an early psoriatic papule. The characteristics of these active sites of the psoriatic lesion are:

1 regular elongation of the rete ridges with thickening in their lower por-tions;
2 long oedematous and often club-shaped papillae;
3 thinning of the suprapapillary plate;
4 focal absence of the granular layer;
5 focal parakeratosis;
6 micropustules of Kogoj (Plate 1.15);
7 microabscesses of Munro (Plate 1.16).

The epidermis is characterized by a psoriasis-specific architecture with elon-gated rete ridges which are slender at their upper portion and thicker in their lower portion. The number of mitoses is increased and remarkably this in-crease is not restricted to the basal cell layer but rather involves the first few suprabasal cell layers. Some spongiosis may be present, although this is by no means a characteristic of the psoriatic lesion. Changes in the keratinizing zone have a more focal pattern in both the horizontal and vertical axes, and this organization is psoriasis specific.

The parakeratotic foci coincide with the focal absence of stratum granu-losum (Pinkus & Mehregan 1981). In the massive stratum corneum of palms and soles the psoriatic process is also arranged focally which implies that the underlying process in not only restricted in size but is also restricted in duration. At the macro level the same 'staccato' is presented by the tones of the 'pits of nail'.

A third psoriasis-specific pattern is the exocytosis of polymorphonuclear leucocytes into the skin as micropustules of Kogoj (Plate 1.15). These pustules are spongiform with eosinophilic strands as remnants of keratinocytes intermingled with polymorphonuclear leucocytes. These pustules invade into the stratum corneum to form the microabscesses of Munro (Plate 1.16). These microabscesses are characterized by remnants of polymorphonuclear leucocytes.

In one series it was shown that these microabscesses were invariably surrounded by a parakeratotic halo. Although the occurrence of micropustules and microabscesses are highly characteristic for psoriasis (Lever & Schaumburg-Lever 1983), the occurrence of this phenomenon is rather low (van de Kerkhof *et al.* 1996a). The dermis is characterized by elongation of the dermal papillae, which comprise tortuous capillaries. The capillaries protrude just beneath the stratum corneum, leaving only a small suprapapillary plate of epithelial cells (Plate 1.17). This represents the micromorphology of the Auspitz phenomenon.

In the dermis the density of the inflammatory infiltrate differs, depending from the focal maturation of the lesion (cold spots vs. hot spots). The inflammatory infiltrate comprises T lymphocytes, monocytes, macrophages, polymorphonuclear leucocytes and mast cells.

The incipient psoriatic lesion

Pinpoint lesions and the margin of spreading psoriatic lesions comprise a relatively early stage of the psoriatic lesion. For a review on this subject the reader is referred to van de Kerkhof *et al.* 1996. Incipient psoriatic lesions are characterized by a mixed inflammatory infiltrate with some epidermotropism of T lymphocytes, mast cells and monocytes/macrophages. Various investigators have studied which cell types are the first invaders. The large body of evidence is that the T lymphocyte is the first invader. The increase of epidermal thickness follows the inflammatory changes.

Psoriatic erythroderma

Erythroderma may be the result of various dermatoses. The characteristic histopathological sign of psoriasis was observed in 88% of 45 cases of psoriatic erythroderma (Tomasini *et al.* 1997).

1.3 Pustular manifestations of psoriasis

1.3.1 Clinical presentations

Pustular psoriasis comprised those forms of psoriasis in which macroscopic pustules appear. Two main types can be distinguished: localized and generalized forms. The localized forms can be divided in pustulosis palmoplantaris and acrodermatitis continua of Hallopeau (ACH); the generalized forms are classified as the acute generalized pustular psoriasis of von Zumbusch, impetigo herpetiformis, annular pustular psoriasis, juvenile and infantile pustular psoriasis and localized forms (not acral or palmoplantar) (Baker 1985; Tay & Tham 1997). Pustular manifestations have recently been reviewed in greater detail by Kuijpers (1998).

Localized forms of pustular psoriasis

Pustulosis palmoplantaris (PPP) is a common condition in which erythematous, scaly plaques with sterile pustules develop on the palms and soles (Plate 1.18). It is a disease of adults and it seldom occurs in children. The onset of this manifestation occurs mostly between 20 and 60 years. In 12% the onset is before the age of 60. There is a predominance of females, only 10–30% being males. A positive family history of psoriasis is reported in 10–25% of the cases. The lesions are often symmetrical, especially on the feet. The pustules are most prominent on the thenar, hypothenar, and on the soles and sides of the heels. The pustules may vary in size from 1 mm to 1 cm. They are yellow when fresh, but later become yellow–brown and even dark brown. Typically, pustules at all stages of evolution are apparent (Plate 1.18).

The differential diagnoses includes tinea and vesicular eczema. The term pustular bacterid, as introduced by Andrews and Machacek (1935), describes an acute monomorphic sterile pustular eruption of hands and feet, which in most cases simply represents an acute exanthematous variant of PPP. The lesions are in general not provoked by a remote form of bacterial infection. The relationship of PPP to psoriasis is controversial (van de Kerkhof et al. 1996b). Sometimes the presence of typical psoriasis elsewhere, or a personal or strong family history of psoriasis or subsequent development of psoriasis vulgaris, established the relationship. However, typical PPP often occurs in the absence of such evidence. Signs of psoriasis elsewhere on the body occur in 2% (Ashurst 1964) to 19% (Enfors and Molin 1971) of all cases. The reason for this confusion in the epidemiology is the difficulty in the interpretation of minimal psoriasis (a few pits in the nails, some scaling on the scalp, etc.). Furthermore, HLA associations of plaque psoriasis are different from PPP, indicating that PPP is genetically distinct from psoriasis vulgaris. The course is mostly persistent (Everall 1957). Enfors and Molin reported in their follow-up study that only about 28% of the patients were healed on re-examination 10 years or more after onset (Enfors and Molin 1971).

In ACH chronic, sterile pustules are located on the tips of fingers and toes (Plate 1.19). ACH is a rare disorder. The skin of the distal phalanx becomes red and scaly and pustules develop. The nail plate may be completely destroyed and bony changes may occur with osteolysis of the tuft of the distal phalanx.

Often the lesions are painful, disabling the patient considerably. ACH may evolve into generalized pustular psoriasis, especially in the elderly (Baker and Ryan 1968). The tongue may become involved with fissuring or may adapt the pattern of the annulus migrans (O'Keefe *et al.* 1973).

Generalized forms of pustular psoriasis

A few studies on large series of patients with generalized pustular psoriasis (GPP)have been reported. By far the largest study was by Baker and Ryan (1968), who reported on 104 patients with GPP, 24 of these were their own patients. In these patients information was obtained through questionnaires sent to dermatologists in the UK.

In this series the male/female ratio was the same as for psoriasis in general. Baker and Ryan described two subgroups in the 104 cases of GPP. The first subgroup, 52 out of 104 patients, had an early onset of psoriasis, with a typical psoriatic morphology during many years, a long prepustular phase and the generalized pustular flare was frequently provoked. The second subgroup, 27 out of 104 patients, was characterized by late onset of the disease, with atypical prepustular morphological features during a few months and a rapid spontaneous progression to GPP. In 10 patients the disease began as a persistent pustulosis of palms and soles, in eight as ACH, in seven as a flexural dermatosis with psoriasiform changes and in the remaining patients no classification of the prepustular phase was possible. It is possible that GPP with the atypical prephase may form a special subclass.

Baker and Ryan further divided their patients into four categories, depending on the clinical pattern: the Zumbusch pattern, the annular pattern, the exanthematic type and the localized pattern. Besides the classification of Baker and Ryan, a slightly different classification is proposed by Zelickson and Muller, based on 63 cases seen in a 29-year period (Zelickson & Muller 1991). The patients were classified in four categories based on the dynamics of onset and clinical pattern of their disease, i.e. acute GPP von Zumbusch type, subacute annular GPP, chronic acral GPP and mixed GPP. The prevalence of GPP in Japan was 7.46/million, indicating the rarity of the disease (Ohkawara *et al.* 1996). The first clinical description of *acute generalized pustular psoriasis* (GPP) was published by von Zumbusch (1910). The clinical picture of acute GPP von Zumbusch type consists of erythema and pustulation in the form of isolated pustules or lakes of pus involving particularly the flexures and genital regions, but also resulting in generalized erythroderma. In the acute pustular phase the skin is painful (Plate 1.20a). In a later phase pustulation fades away and generalized desquamation follows. The skin manifestations are accompanied by high fever and severe malaise. Hypoalbuminaemia may be profound, perhaps because of a sudden loss of plasmaprotein. The acute phase is a life-threatening situation. In the original case, von Zumbusch (1910) describes nine such episodes followed over a period of 10 years (von Zumbusch 1910). Mucosal membrane abnormalities may accompany the lesions of the skin. The buccal mucosa and tongue can be involved with frank pustules or an acute geographical tongue (Hubler 1984). Geographic tongue was seen in 17% of patients with GPP, the prevalence in the normal population is 2%.

A subdivision of patients with GPP of the von Zumbusch type is by the presence or absence of a preceding history of psoriasis vulgaris. In the study of Ohkawara *et al.* (1996) 143 of 208 cases (69%) with acute GPP of the von Zumbusch type had no history of ordinary psoriasis. The patient groups differ in incidence of HLA antigens, age of onset, the precipitating factors and the distribution of skin lesions (Ohkawara *et al.* 1996). In the study of Zelickson and Muller, 11 of 35 patients(31%) with acute GPP had no history of psoriasis vulgaris before the flare (Zelickson & Muller 1991).

Impetigo herpetiformis is a form of GPP occurring during pregnancy. Essentially, the histological and clinical features are as in GPP, with a predilection for flexural areas. No consensus has been reached whether impetigo herpetiformis is a separate entity or a variant of pustular psoriasis (Lotem *et al.* 1989).

Annular pustular psoriasis presents as a subacute or chronic form of generalized pustular psoriasis. Lesions begin as discrete areas of erythema which become raised and oedematous (Degos *et al.* 1966). The lesions spread centrifugally, with pustules at the edge, and a central healing of the lesion (Plate 1.20b). General discomfort and fever may occur.

Juvenile and infantile pustular psoriasis is very rare (fewer than 100 cases have been reported), and has often a benign course (Zelickson & Muller 1991; van de Kerkhof 1985). Circinate and annular forms are common. Systemic symptoms are often absent and spontaneous remissions occur.

A more appropriate term for *the localized forms of GPP* is 'psoriasis with pustules'.

One or more plaques of psoriasis vulgaris may develop pustules following prolonged irritant topical therapy. Resolution is usually prompt with bland topical treatment.

It is general agreed that GPP of the Zumbusch type carries some risk of death (Ryan & Baker 1971). In total 34 patients of the 106 with GPP (Ryan & Baker 1971) died, 26 of these deaths being attributed to the disease or its therapy. Uncontrolled disease accounted for eight deaths; in 12 systemic steroids were blamed and in six methotrexate was held responsible. Those patients with a previous history of ACH have an especially bad prognosis. The long-term course of GPP is variable, periods with an erythematosquamous manifestation often occurring.

Erythroderma occurs in two-thirds of the patients with GPP. It has been reported as an invariable complication in those patients with an onset of ACH or flexural psoriasiform changes (Baker and Ryan 1968). Renal and liver toxicity have been reported, possibly due to oligaemia, psoriatic toxicity or drugs (Warren *et al.* 1974). Amyloidosis is a rare complication. David *et al.* (1982) described a patient with this complication and reviewed the literature.

Exanthematic pustular psoriasis (Roujeau *et al.* 1991) may occur in association with various medications, it usually has a rather benign course.

Association of GPP with a clinically manifest arthritis was 32% in the series of Baker and Ryan (1968). It is seen in all subgroups of GPP except in the exanthematic group.

1.3.2 Histopathology

The histological picture of pustular psoriasis differs from psoriasis vulgaris in that the spongiform pustule occurs as a macropustule and is the characteristic lesion (McKee 1996). As the spongiform pustule increases in size, the epidermal cells die, with resulting central cavation. At the edges a shell of thinned epidermal cells remains, which causes the spongiform appearance. Eventually polymorphonucleocytes (PMN) accumulate into the horny layer and intraepidermal large accumulations of PMN are seen, which is a 'macro' of the microabscess of Munro (see Plate 1.16). Otherwise the epidermal and dermal features are similar to those of psoriasis vulgaris.

1.3.3 Genetics and triggering factors

Genetics and epidemiology of pustular psoriasis

HLA association with pustular psoriasis differs from psoriasis vulgaris, indicating that pustular psoriasis is genetically distinct from psoriasis vulgaris. In pustular psoriasis no association with HLA A13 and A17 was found, in contrast to increased expression in psoriasis vulgaris. HLA typing was performed on 93 unrelated patients with palmoplantar pustulosis, revealing an increased frequency of HLA B8. The incidence of HLA B13 or B17 was not significantly increased (Ward & Barnes 1978). Pustular psoriasis may arise at any age. Pustular psoriasis may present at early childhood (Zelickson & Muller 1991).

Triggering factors

Provocative factors for development of GPP as described by Baker and Ryan in their review of 104 cases included pregnancy, infections, hypocalcaemia, local irritants, and reduction or withdrawal of corticosteroid therapy. The *pregnancy*-induced forms of GPP were later described as impetigo herpetiformis (Bajaj *et al.* 1977). In the latter half of pregnancy the levels of progesterone are increased. The outbreak of GPP following the administration of this hormone has been described (Murphy & Stolman 1979). Following the induction of ovulation by clomiphencitrate in a patient with GPP severe recurrent attacks were shown in conjunction with increased urinary excretion of progesterone metabolites. The exanthematous forms of GPP occurring after *infection* were later described as acute generalized exanthematous pustulosis (Murphy & Stolman 1979). Infections, especially of the upper respiratory tract, may trigger GPP. Baker and Ryan stated that in three of the five exanthematic cases and in 11 of the others with GPP, an infection had provoked the disease. In the Baker and Ryan series, in only five of 57 patients with GPP *hypocalcaemia* was reported, which was transient in four patients. None of the 104 patients was known to have hypocalcaemia before the GPP episodes. Therefore, hypocalcaemia might well be a secondary phenomenon. On the other hand, hypocalcaemia precipitating GPP was reported in a patient with surgical hypoparathyroidism (Stewart *et al.* 1984). In 21 of 37 patients with GPP, who were treated with *corticosteroids systematically* before the onset of the first attack of GPP, this was provoked by the therapy.

Pustulosis occurred for the first time within a few days or weeks of reduction or complete withdrawal of steroids (Baker & Ryan 1968). Of these 21 patients, 17 had preceding a psoriasis of the ordinary pattern. Strong *irritants*, local therapy with dithranol or phototherapy, may precipitate GPP.

1.4 Psoriasis of the nails

1.4.1 Epidemiology

The frequency of psoriasis of the nails varies considerably between different authors, ranging from 10 to 55% (Calvert *et al.* 1963; de Jong & van de Kerkhof 1996). The finger nails are more often involved than the toe nails. In psoriatic arthritis a frequency as high as 85% is found.

An interview with 1728 patients with psoriasis concerning nail abnormalities revealed that 51.8% of patients suffered from pain caused by the nail changes and between 47 and 59% of the patients were restricted in their daily activities for reason of nail changes (de Jong & van de Kerkhof 1996).

1.4.2 Clinical picture

Nail changes (Plate 1.21) can be grouped according to their origin, either the nail matrix or the nail plate. Although the nail changes are characteristic of psoriasis, they are not disease specific.

Pitting of the nails, characterized by sharply punched-out pinhead-sized pits, is a frequently occurring characteristic sign of psoriasis originating from involvement of the matrix.

The nail pits correspond to small parakeratotic foci in the matrix. A change originating from the nail bed and hyponychium is *subungual parakeratosis* which can be seen frequently under the free edge of the nail. This macromorphological equivalent of parakeratosis of the hyponychium has a yellowish, greasy appearance. The *"öl-fleckphenomenon"* is a yellowish-brown, rounded discoloration under the nail plate, which may be tender. This frequently encountered abnormality of the nail bed results from accumulation of serous exudate as part of the psoriatic process. A sign which is seen less frequently is *splinter haemorrhage* and results from increased capillary fragility. *Distal onycholysis* is a frequently occurring nail change. It is characterized by the appearance of a space between the nail plate and hyponychium. If this space moves more proximally, *total onycholysis* may occur.

1.5 Associated dermatoses

Psoriasis may be complicated by other dermatoses or alternatively other dermatoses might trigger psoriasis. It is not always possible to separate both principles.

1.5.1 Skin cancer

Two decades ago, Kocsard reported that psoriasis is practically non-existent in patients with solar keratoses and sun-related skin cancers (Kocsard 1976). Further, psoriatic patients showed a remarkably low incidence of these latter conditions. In contrast, many studies have demonstrated an increased occurrence of squamous cell carcinomas in patients who have been treated in the past with X-rays or arsenic (Stern *et al.* 1984; Mali-Gerrits *et al.* 1991; Stern & Laid 1994; Sai Siong Wong *et al.* 1998). High-dose PUVA and cyclosporin are other treatments which increase the risk for squamous cell carcinomas (Halprin *et al.* 1982; Stern *et al.* 1984; McKenna *et al.* 1996; van de Kerkhof & de Rooij 1997).

1.5.2 Allergic contact dermatitis

Positive patch tests were observed in 25 out of 32 patients who had psoriasis on atypical localizations and/or showed therapy resistance of these lesions (Steigleder & Orfanos 1967). In 15 of these patients it was likely that the lesions had been provoked by delayed-type hypersensitivity. In case of stubborn lesions on atypical localizations but especially on the hands (occupational factors!) or external auditory canal (prolonged use of sensitizers such as neomycin and vioform) patch testing is mandatory.

1.5.3 Lichen simplex chronicus

The coexistence with psoriasis is frequent (Plate 1.22). The relationship is bidirectional. If a psoriatic lesion itches, the lesion may become complicated by lichen simplex (= neurodermatitis) and the surface takes on a glistening appearance. The rubbing resulting from the itching, on the other hand, may worsen psoriasis, the patient enters a vicious circle, and the resistance to therapy of such a lesion can be a real problem. The combination of psoriasis and neurodermatitis is designated as neurodermatitis psoriasiformis or psoriasis neurodermiformis.

1.5.4 Infections

Quantitative data regarding bacteriological and mycological investigations have been reviewed before (von Seneczko & Ruszczak 1982). Psoriatic patients do not run an increased risk for pyogenic infections; however, lymphangitis and lymphadenitis may occur in patients with palmoplantar pustulosis. It is advisable to investigate material from psoriatic plaques by serial cultures before an operation is carried out. In patients with palmoplantar lesions, flexural or genital localizations one should search for a complicating candida infection. Dermatophytic infections are seldomly found in psoriatic lesions. Perhaps the increased cell turnover of the psoriatic epidermis is responsible for this negative association. In contrast, candida species and not dermatophytes are frequently occurring in the parakeratotic material under the nail plates (von Seneczko and Ruszczak 1982). The preferential growth of candida species and not dermatophytes in psoriatic material is intriguing.

1.5.5 Inflammatory linear verrucous epidermal naevus

Inflammatory linear verrucous epidermal naevus (ILVEN) has been suggested to be a separate disease entity. However, the distinction between linear psoriasis and ILVEN is not sharp (de Jong *et al.* 1991). The remarkable treatment resistance of ILVEN, perhaps, is the most marked difference with true linear psoriasis (Rulo & van de Kerkhof 1991).

1.5.6 Other dermatoses

Several reports have claimed the association between a skin condition and psoriasis. In this respect three associations are of practical importance.
1   The relationship between psoriasis and pemphigoid has been reported. However the cases described suggest that PUVA, Goeckerman therapy or dithranol had triggered pemphigoid. Indeed, it is well established that intensified exposure to sunlight may trigger pemphigoid.

2 Wahba *et al.* (1980) reported the total absence of psoriasis in 309 leprosy patients. This supports the hypothesis that psoriasis results from an immuno-logical dysregulation.

3 The co-occurrence of psoriasis and vitiligo has been reported and indi-cates that psoriasis has no preference for depigmented or dark skin (Koransky & Roenigk 1982).

1.6 Associated internal diseases

Psoriasis is not restricted to the skin. Extracutaneous involvement has been described, including involvement of the nails and mucosal membranes. Pso-riatic arthropathy is described in Chapter 2. A few internal diseases have been claimed to be associated with psoriasis.

1.6.1 Human immunodeficiency virus-associated psoriasis

In human immunodeficiency virus (HIV)-positive patients psoriasis may be triggered and severe psoriasis or psoriatic arthropathy has been reported (Duvic 1990; Tourne *et al.* 1997).

1.6.2 Crohn's disease and ulcerative colitis

Psoriasis, peripheral arthropathy, sacroiliitis and ankylosing spondylitis are associated with Crohn's disease and ulcerative colitis. This is probably due to the fact that all these disorders are genetically linked with HLA B27. The association between these gut diseases and psoriasis has been described by Yates *et al.* (1982).

1.6.3 Dermatogenic enteropathy

Malabsorption due to dysfunctioning of the small bowel has been reported in patients with extensive psoriasis and erythrodermic psoriasis (Shuster *et al.* 1967). In localized psoriasis the reports are less convincing (Preger *et al.* 1970). It is of interest that increased enterocyte cell turnover in the small intestine of psoriatic patients has been reported (Hendel 1982).

1.6.4 Liver impairment

Fatty metamorphosis, periportal inflammation and focal necrosis of the liver have been reported more frequently in psoriatic patients compared to the non-psoriatic population (Zachariae & Sogaard 1983). However, hepatic fi-brosis and cirrhosis of the liver were not more common amongst psoriatics.

Although it has been suggested that psoriatics have a more substantial alco-hol intake, this could not be confirmed by a comparative analysis (Grunnet 1974).

1.6.5 Diabetes and hyperlipoproteinaemia

In a questionnaire survey, under 144 patients, 2% of the responders, stated that they had diabetes (Farber *et al.* 1968). In contrast to the normal, frequency of diabetes type IV hyperlipoproteinaemia occurred more frequently in the psoriatic population (Pfahl *et al.* 1975).

1.6.6 Occlusive vascular disease

Increased frequencies of vascular diseases such as thrombophlebitis, myocardial infarction, pulmonary embolism and cerebrovascular accident has been reported in the psoriatic population. The risk for occlusive vascular disease in this population is increased 2.6-fold and the risk for venous occlusion 1.6-fold (McDonald & Calabresi 1978).

1.6.7 Amyloidosis

In total 14 cases with amyloidosis and psoriasis have been reported: twelve patients with psoriatic arthropathy and two with pustular psoriasis without arthropathy (David *et al.* 1982). The risk for amyloidosis does not therefore seem to be increased in the psoriatic population.

1.6.8 Gout

Elevated serum levels of uric acid can be found in 30–50% of psoriatic patients (Luudquist *et al.* 1982). The association between psoriasis and gout seems to be well established.

1.7 Differential diagnosis

The diagnosis of psoriasis is usually made simply by the clinical appearance. However, the macromorphology of several skin disorders may sometimes resemble psoriasis. In case of doubt the histopathological appearance of skin biopsy from lesional skin may be helpful.

1.7.1 Seborrhoeic dermatitis

Seborrhoeic dermatitis is characterized by yellowish scaling and erythema localized on the face, the scalp, the presternal, interscapular and flexural areas. Seborrhoeic dermatitis is often elicited or aggravated by *Pityrosporon* overgrowth.

In psoriasis, facial involvement in general is restricted to the hairline. In contrast, seborrhoeic dermatitis usually affects the furrows of the face.

1.7.2 Eczema of palms and soles

In cases of acute eczema with vesiculation, erythema and scaling, the differential diagnosis with psoriasis is simple, as vesiculation is not a feature of psoriasis. Hyperkeratotic eczema of palms and soles is more problematic. The designation hyperkeratotic eczema of palms and soles is not a specific diagnosis. It is used to describe several conditions:

1   chronic palmoplantar eczema (allergic contact dermatitis, irritant dermatitis);
2   a dermatitis of palms and soles that is not eczema and not psoriasis;
3   the 'common manifestation' of a chronic dermatitis of palms and soles.

It is important to restrict the diagnosis palmoplantar psoriasis to patients with sharply demarcated erythematosquamous plaques. Patients with chronic hyperkeratotis and erythema of palms and soles should have biopsies in order to determine the histopathological appearance.

1.7.3 Syphilis

Secondary syphilis may be difficult to differentiate from psoriasis guttata. In syphilis the face, the palms and soles may be involved. Serology and histopathological investigation of skin biopsies are indicated in case of doubt.

1.7.4 Candidiasis

Candidiasis should be differentiated from flexural psoriasis. In candidiasis colarette scaling *and* pustules in the margin are the characteristics, and this combination is not present in psoriasis. Direct preparation with potassium hydroxide and cultures are informative.

1.7.5 Pityriasis lichenoides chronica

Pityriasis lichenoides chronica is characterized by brownish papules and central scales. Again histology is diagnostic.

1.7.6 Hypertrophic lichen planus

This condition may mimic psoriasis. However, the violaceous colour, the adherent scaling and the postinflammatory hyperpigmentaion are characteristic of hypertrophic lichen planus. Histology is helpful.

1.7.7 Pityriasis rubra pilaris

Pityriasis rubra pilaris may resemble the clinical appearance of psoriasis. However, the follicular arrangement of papules, 'islands' of unaffected skin surrounded by involved skin and yellowish palmoplantar hyperkeratosis may be diagnostic. Histological investigation of a hyperkeratotic papule is usually diagnostic.

1.7.8 Dermatophytic infections

In case of solitary lesions, with colarette scaling and elevated margins dermatophytic infections have to be considered. Direct preparation with potassium hydroxide and cultures are helpful.

1.7.9 (Pre)malignancies

Mycosis fungoides and premycotic eruptions may mimic closely the appearance of psoriasis. Suspicion should arise if the lesions show increased infiltration, are heavily pruritic and are not sharply demarcated. In case of doubt multiple biopsies are needed for differential diagnoses.

Bowen's disease is characterized by sharply demarcated erythematosquamous lesion showing remarkable therapy resistance. Histology is diagnostic.

1.7.10 Pustular eruptions

The differential diagnosis of GPP includes the subcorneal pustular dermatosis of Sneddon–Wilkinson, in which the subcorneal pustules are located subcorneal. This disorder has a predilection for the flexures. It consists of annular and gyrated lesions. In both pustular psoriasis and subcorneal pustular dermatosis the characteristic feature is the accumulation of PMN in the upper part of the epidermis. Several authors believe that the clinical and histological criteria of Sneddon and Wilkinson for the diagnosis of subcorneal pustular dermatosis (i.e. the histology of a subcorneal pustule and the response to dapsone) are not specific enough to merit subcorneal pustular dermatosis a unique disease which can be differentiated from pustular psoriasis (Sanchez & Ackerman 1979; Sanchez *et al.* 1981). Furthermore, acute generalized exanthematous pustulosis must be differentiated from GPP. This condition may result from medications (Feind-Koopmans *et al.* 1996). It differs from GPP in the mild general symptoms and the fact that the skin lesions are usually self-limiting, with short duration.

Reiter's disease, characterized by urethritis and arthritis, 'overlaps' with pustular psoriasis. However, in Reiter's disease skin lesions occur preferentially at the soles, extensor surfaces of the legs, dorsal aspects of the hands, the fingers, nails and scalp. The lesions are thicker and more 'yellowish'. The course is self-limiting in weeks or months.

References

Andrews, G.C. & Machacek, G.F. (1935) Pustular bacterids of the hands and feet. *Arch Dermatol. Syphilology* **32**, 837–847.

Ashurst, P.J.C. (1964) Relapsing pustular eruptions of the hands and feet. *Archives of Dermatology* **76**, 169–179.

Bajaj, A.K., Swarup, V., Gupta, O.P. & Gupta, S.C. (1977) Impetigo herpetiformis. *Dermatologica* **155**, 292–295.

Baker, H. (1985) Generalized pustular psoriasis. In: *Psoriasis* (eds Roenigk, H.H. & Maibach, H.I.), pp. 15–33. Marcel Dekker, New York.

Baker, H. & Ryan, T.J. (1968) Generalized pustular psoriasis. A clinical and epidemiological study of 104 cases. *British Journal of Dermatology* **80**, 771–793.

Bonifati, C., Carducci, M., Mussi, A., D'Auria, L. & Ameglio, F. (1998) Recognition and treatment of psoriasis; special considerations in elderly patients. *Drug Therapy* **12**, 177–190.

Brenner, W., Gschnait, F. & Mayr, W.R. (1978) HLA B13, B17, B37 and Cw6 in 'psoriasis vulgaris': association with the age of onset. *Archives of Dermatolological Research* **262**, 337–339.

Calvert, H.I., Smith, M.A. & Well, R.S. (1963) Psoriasis and the nails. *British Journal of Dermatology* **75**, 415–418.

Camp, R.D.R. (1993) Psoriasis. In: *Textbook of Dermatology* (eds Champion, R.G., Burton, J.L. & Ebbing F.J.G.), 5th edn., pp. 1391–1458. Blackwell Scientific Publications, Oxford.

Cornbleet, T. (1956) Action of synthetic antimaterial drugs in psoriasis. *Journal of Investigations Dermatology* **26**, 435–436.

David, M., Abraham, D., Weinberger, A. & Feuerman, E.J. (1982) Generalised pustular psoriasis, psoriatic arthritis and nephrotic syndrome associated with systemic amyloidosis. *Dermatologica* **165**, 168–171.

de Jong, E.M.G.J., Rulo, H.F.C. & van de Kerkhof, P.C.M. (1991) Inflammatory linear verrucous epidermal naevus (ILVEN) versus linear psoriasis. A clinical, histological and immunohistochemical study. *Acta Dermato-Venereologica* **71**, 343–346.

de Jong, E.M.G.J. & van de Kerkhof, P.C.M. (1996) Co-existence of palmoplantar lichen planus and lupus erythematosus with response to treatment using acitretin. *British Journal of Dermatology* **134**, 538–541.

Degos, R., Civatte, J. & Arrouy, M. (1966) Psoriasis et psoriasis pustuleux a type d'érytheme annulaire centrifuge (3 cas). *Bulletin de la Societe Francaise de Dermatologie et de Syphiligraphie* **73**, 356–358.

Duvic, M. (1990) Immunology of AIDS related to psoriasis. *Journal of Investigations Dermatology* **95** (Suppl.), 385–405.

Enfors, W. & Molin, L. (1971) Pustulosis palmaris at plantaris. *Acta Dermato-Venereologica* **51**, 289–294.

Everall, J. (1957) Intractable pustular eruptions of the hands and feet. *British Journal of Dermatology* **69**, 269–272.

Eyre, R.W. & Krueger, G.P. (1982) Response to injury of skin involved and uninvolved with psoriasis, and its relation to disease activity: Koebner reactions. *British Journal of Dermatology* **106**, 153–159.

Farber, E.M., Bright, R.D. & Nall, M.D. (1968) Psoriasis, a questionnaire survey of 2144 patients. *Archives of Dermatology* **98**, 248–259.

Farber, W.M. & Nall, M.L. (1974) The natural history of psoriasis in 5600 patients. *Dermatologica* **148**, 1–18.

Farber, E.M., Roth. R.J., Aschheim, E., Eddy, D. & Epinette, W.V.V. (1965) Role of trauma in isomorphic response in psoriasis. *Archives of Dermatology* **91**, 246–251.

Feind-Koopmans, A., van der Valk, P.G.M., Steijlen, P.M. & van de Kerkhof, P.C.M. (1996) Toxic pustuloderma associated with clemastine therapy. *Clinical Experimental Dermatology* **21**, 293–295.

Griffin, Th.D., Van Lattanand, A. & Scott, E.J. (1988) Clinical and histological heterogenity of psoriatic plaques. *Archives of Dermatology* **124**, 216–220.

Grunnet, E. (1974) Alcohol consumption in psoriasis. *Dermatologica* **149**, 136–139.

Halprin, K.M., Comerford, M. & Tailor, R. (1982) Cancer in patients with psoriasis. *Journal of the American Academy of Dermatology* **7**, 633–638.

Hendel, L. (1982) Epithelial cell turnover in the small intestine of psoriatics. *Psoriasis: Proceedings of the Third International Symposium* (eds Farber, E.M. Cox, A.J.), pp. 331–332. Grune and Stratton, New York.

Holzmann, H., Fränz. J., Morsches, B. & Bröckelschen, H.U. (1976) Dehydroepiandrosterone and psoriasis. *Proceedings of the Second International Symposium in 'Psoriasis'* (eds Farber, E.M.& Cox, A.J.), pp. 81–90. York Medical Books, New York.

Holzmann, H., Krupp, R., Hoede, N. & Morsches, B. (1974) Exo and endogenous provocation of psoriasis. *Archiv fur Dermatologische Forschung* **249**, 1–12.

Hubler,W.R. Jr (1984) Lingual lesions of generalized pustular psoriasis. Report of five cases and a review of the literature. *Journal of the American Academy of Dermatology* **11**, 1069–1076.

Illig, L. & Holz, U. (1966) Die Blutgefässreaction bei der Psoriasis vulgaris; das experimentelle Koebner Phenomenon. *Archif für Klinische und Experimentelle Dermatologie* **226**, 239–264.

Katayama, H. & Kawada, A. (1981) Exacerbations of psoriasis induced by indomethacin. *Journal of Dermatology Tokyo* **8**, 323–327.

Kocsard, E. (1976) The rate of solar keratoses in psoriatic patients. *Australian Journal of Dermatology* **17**, 65–73.

Koebner, H. (1878) Klinische experimentelle und therapeutische Mitteilungen über Psoriasis. *Berliner Klinische Wochenschrift* **21**, 631–632.

Koransky, J.S. & Roenigk, H.H. (1982) Vitiligo and psoriasis. *Journal of the American Academy of Dermatology* **7**, 183–189.

Kuypers, A.L.A. (1998) Severe forms of psoriasis. Clinical and experimental studies. Thesis, Nijmegen University.

Lever, W.F. & Schaumburg-Lever, G. (1983) Psoriasis. In: *Histopathology of the Skin*, 6th edn. pp. 139–146. J.B. Lippincott, Philadelphia.

Lomato, M., Ranieri, J. & Coviello. C. (1982) Results of ocular examination in psoriasis. In: *Psoriasis: Proceedings of the Third International Symposium* (eds Farber, E.M., Cox, A.J.), pp. 341–342. Grune and Stratton, New York.

Lomholt, G. (1963). *Psoriasis, prevalence, spontaneous course and genetics*. Thesis, Copenhagen.

Lotem, M., Katzenelson, V., Rotem, A., Hod, M. & Sandbank, M. (1989) Impetigo herpetiformis: a variant of pustular psoriasis or a separate entity? *Journal of the American Academy of Dermatology* **20**, 338–341.

Luudquist, C.D., Aronson, I.K., Henderson, T.W., Skosey, J.L. & Salomon, L.M. (1982) Psoriasis and normouricemic gout. *Dermatology* **164**, 104–108.

Mali-Gerrits, M.G., Gaasbeek, D., Boezeman, J. & Van de Kerkhof, P.C.M. (1991) Psoriasis therapy and the risk of skin cancers. *Clinical Experimental Dermatology* **16**, 85–89.

McDonald, C. & Calabresi, P. (1978) Psoriasis and occlusive vascular disease. *British Journal of Dermatology* **99**, 469–475.

McKee, P.H. (1996) Inflammatory dermatoses. In: *Pathology of the Skin with Clinical Correlations* (ed. McKee, P.H.), pp. 8.1–8.8. Mosby-Wolfe, London.

McKenna, K.E., Pattersson, C.C. & Handley, J. (1996) Cutaneous neoplasia following PUVA therapy for psoriasis. *British Journal of Dermatology* **134**, 639–642.

Murphy, F.R. & Stolman, L.P. (1979) Generalised pustular psoriasis. *Archives of Dermatology* **115**, 1215–1216.

Nörholm-Pedersen, A. (1952) Infections and psoriasis. *Acta Dermato-Venereologica* **32**, 159–167.

O'Keefe, E., Braverman, I.M. & Cohen, I. (1973) Annulus migrans. Identical lesions in pustular psoriasis, Reiter's syndrome, and geographic tongue. *Archives* **107**, 240–244.

Ohkawara, A., Yasuda, H., Kobayashi, H., Inaba, Y., Ogawa, H., Hashimoto, I. & Imamura, S. (1996) Generalized pustular psoriasis in Japan: two distinct groups formed by differences in symptoms and genetic background. *Acta Dermato-Venereologica* **76**, 68–71.

Pedace, J., Muller, A. & Winkelmann, R.K. (1969) Biology of psoriasis; experimental study of Koebner phenomenon. *Acta Dermato-Venerologica* **49**, 390–400. Stockholm.

Pfahl, F., Rouffy, J., Puissant, A. & Dubberat, B. (1975) Hyperlipoproteinemies et psoriasis. *Annales de Dermatologies et de Syphiligraphie* **103**, 588–590.

Pinkus, H. & Mehregan, A.H. (1981) Psoriasis. In: *A Guide to Dermatohistopathology*, 2nd edn, pp. 101–104. Appleton, Century-Crofts, New York.

Preger, L., Maibach, H.I., Osborne, R.B., Shapiro, H.A. & Lee, J.C. (1970) On the question of psoriatic arthropathy. *Archives of Dermatology* **102**, 151–153.

Pusey, W.A. (1933). *The History of Dermatology*. Charles C. Thomas, Springfield, Illinois.

Roujeau, J.C., Bioulac-Sage, P. *et al.* (1991) Acute generalized exanthematous pustulosis. Analysis of 63 cases. *Archives of Dermatology* **127**, 1333–1338.

Rozell, B., Grever, A.C. & Macusson, J.A. (1997) Oral psoriasis: Report on a case without epidermal involvement. *Acta Dermato-Venereologica* **77**, 399–400. Stockholm.

Rulo, H.F.G. & van de Kerkhof, P.C.M. (1991) Treatment of inflammatory linear verrucous epidermal naevus. *Dermatologica* **182**, 112–114.

Ryan, T.J. & Baker, H. (1971) The prognosis of generalised pustular psoriasis. *British Journal of Dermatology* **85**, 407–411.

Sai Siong Wong, Kong Chong Tan & Chee Leok Goh. (1998) Cutaneous manifestations of chronic arsenicism. *Journal of the American Academy of Dermatology* **38**, 179–185.

Sanchez, N.P. & Ackerman, A.B. (1979) Subcorneal pustular dermatosis: a variant of pustular psoriasis. *Acta Dermato-Venereologica* **59** (Suppl.), 147–151. Stockholm.

Sanchez, N.P., Perry, H.O. & Muller, S.A. (1981) On the relationship between subcorneal pustular dermatosis and pustular psoriasis. *American Journal of Dermatopathology* **3**, 385–386.

Shuster, S., Watson, A.J. & Marks, J. (1967) Small intestine in psoriasis. *British Medical Journal* **3**, 458–460.

Söndergaard, J., Wadskov, S., Aerenlund-Jansen, H. & Mikkelsen, H.I. (1976) Aggravation of psoriasis and occurrence of psoriasiform cutaneous eruptions induced by practolol. *Acta Dermato-Venereologica* **56**, 239–243.

Steigleder, G.K. & Orfanos, C. (1967) Provozierte Psoriasis. *Hautarzt* **18**, 508–513.

Stern, R.S. & Laid, N. (1994) The carcinogenic risk of treatment of severe psoriasis with PUVA. *Cancer* **73**, 2759–2764.

Stern, R.S., Laid, N. & Melski, J. (1984) Cutaneous squamous cell carcinoma in patients treated with PUVA. *New England Journal of Medicine* **310**, 1156–1161.

Stewart, A.F., Battaglini-Sabetta, J. & Millstone, L. (1984) Hypocalcemia-induced pustular psoriasis of von Zumbusch. New experience with an old syndrome. *Annals of Internal Medicine* **100**, 677–680.

Svejgaard, E., Nielsen, L.S., Hjortskøj, A & Zachariae, H. (1974) HLA in psoriasis vulgaris and in pustular psoriasis-population and family studies. *British Journal of Dermatology* **91**, 145–153.

Tay, Y.K. & Tham, S.N. (1997) The profile and outcome of pustular psoriasis in Singapore: a report of 28 cases. *International Journal of Dermatology* **136**, 266–271.

Tomasini, C., Aloi, F., Solaroli, C. & Pippione, M. (1997) Psoriatic erythroderma: a histopathological study of forty five patients. *Dermatology* **194**, 102–106.

Tourne, L., van Durez, P., Vooren, J.P., Farber, C.M., Liesnard, C., Heenen, M. & Parent, D. (1997) Alleviation of HIV-associated psoriasis and psoriatic arthritis with cyclosporine. *Journal of the American Academy of Dermatology* **37**, 501–502.

van de Kerkhof, P.C.M. (1982) Plasma aldosterone and cortisol levels in psoriasis and atopic dermatitis. *British Journal of Dermatology* **106**, 423–428.

van de Kerkhof, P.C.M. (1985) Generalised pustular psoriasis in a child. *Dermatologica* **170**, 244–248.

van de Kerkhof, P.C.M. & Chang, A. (1992) Scarring alopecia and psoriasis. *British Journal of Dermatology* **126**, 524–525.

van de Kerkhof, P.C.M. & de Rooij, M.J.M. (1997) Multiple squamous cell carcinomas in a psoriatic patient following high-dose photochemotherapy and cyclosporin treatment: response to long-term acitretin maintenance. *British Journal of Dermatology* **136**, 275–278.

van de Kerkhof, P.C.M., Gerritsen, M.J. & de Jong, E.G.J.M. (1996a) Transition from symptomless to lesional psoriatic skin. *Clinical Experimental Dermatology* **21**, 325–329.

van de Kerkhof, P.C.M., Kuijpers, A.L.A. & Feind-Koopmans, A.G. (1996b) On the nosology of palmoplantar psoriasis. *Journal of the European Academy of Dermatology* **7**, 182–196.

van de Kerkhof, P.C.M., Steegers-Theunissen, R.P.M. & Kuipers, M.V. (1988) Evaluation of topical drug treatment in psoriasis. *Dermatology* **197**, 31–36.

van Schoorl, W.J., Baar, H.J. & van de Kerkhof, P.C.M. (1992) The hair root pattern in psoriasis of the scalp. *Acta Dermato-Venereologica* **72**, 141–142.

von Seneczko, F. & Ruszczak, Z. (1982) Bacterien und Pilzflora der Haut bei Psoriasiskranken. *Dermatologische Monatschrift* **168**, 65–74.

von Zumbusch, L.R. (1910) Psoriasis und pustuloses Exanthem. *Archives of Dermatolology and Syphilology* **1910** (99), 335–346.

Wahba, A., Dorfman, M. & Sheskin, J. (1980) Psoriasis and other common dermatoses in leprosy. *International Journal of Dermatology* **19**, 93–95.

Ward, J.M. & Barnes, R.M. (1978) HLA antigens in persistent palmoplantar pustulosis and its relationship to psoriasis. *British Journal of Dermatology* **99**, 477–483.

Warren, D.J., Winney, R.J. & Beveridge, G.W. (1974) Oligaemia, renal failure and jaundice associated with acute pustular psoriasis. *British Medical Journal* **25**, 406–408.

Weber, G., Neidkort, M., Schmidt, A. & Geiger, A. (1981) The correlation of growth hormone and clinical picture of psoriasis. *Arch Dermatol. Forschung* **270**, 129–140.

Weyl, A. (1883) Psoriasis: In: *Handbuch der Hautkrankheiten* (ed. Ziemssen, H.), p. 500. Von Vogel, Leipzig.

White, G.W. & Colonel, M.C. (1982) Palmoplantar pustular psoriasis provoked by lithium therapy. *Journal of the American Association of Dermatology* **7**, 660–662.

Willan, R. (1809). *On Cutaneous Diseases*, Vol. 1, p. 115. Kimber and Conrad, Philadelphia.

Woronoff, D.L. (1926) Die peripheren Veränderungen der Haut um die Effloreszenzen der Psoriasis Vulgaris und Syphilis Corymbosa. *Dermatologischen Wochenschrift* **82**, 249–257.

Yates, V.M., Watkinson, G. & Kelman, A. (1982) Further evidence for an association between psoriasis, Crohns disease and ulcerative colitis. *British Journal of Dermatology* **106**, 323–330.

Zachariae, H. & Sogaard, H. (1983) Liver biopsy in psoriasis, a controlled study. *Dermatologica* **146**, 149–155.

Zelickson, B.D. & Muller, S.A. (1991) Generalized pustular psoriasis in childhood. Report

of thirteen cases. *Journal of the American Academy of Dermatology* **24**, 186–194.
Zelickson, B.D. & Muller, S.A. (1991) Generalized pustular psoriasis. A review of 63 cases. *Archives of Dermatology* **127**, 1339–1345.

Chapter 2: Psoriatic Arthropathy

M.J.A.M. Franssen, F.H.J. van den Hoogen and
L.B.A. van de Putte

2.1 Historical background

The term 'psoriasis arthritique' was first used by the French physician, Pierre
Bazin in 1860. The condition was studied in detail by Charles Bourdillon in
1888 in his thesis 'Psoriasis et Arthropathies'. Although in the past psoriasis
associated with arthritis has been known under different terms, currently
the terms psoriatic arthritis (PsA) and psoriatic arthropathy are in common
use. In the first half of the 20th century two opposing concepts of PsA emerged:
one held that the association of arthritis and psoriasis was a distinct clinical
entity, the other that this association was a coincident occurrence of rheumatoid arthritis (RA) and psoriasis. However, clinical and epidemiological
studies established the distinction between RA and PsA. This resulted in including PsA as a distinct clinical entity in a classification of rheumatic diseases in 1964 by the American Rheumatism Association (Blumberg *et al.* 1964).

The recognition of overlapping clinical features, including sacroiliitis, a
seronegative anodular asymmetric peripheral oligoarthritis, hyperkerototic
skin lesions, enthesitis, iridocyclitis, mucocutaneous ulceration and familial
aggregation culminated in the concept of the seronegative spondyloarthropathies (Wright & Moll 1976). Psoriatic arthritis, ankylosing spondylitis, the arthritis of inflammatory bowel disease and Reiter's disease are
considered to be part of this concept. The high prevalence of HLA B27 in the
seronegative spondyloarthropathies consolidated this concept and provided
confirmation of PsA as an arthropathy separate from RA (Brewerton *et al.*
1973).

The recent finding that human immunodeficiency virus (HIV)-infected
individuals may experience a remission of RA while pre-existing psoriasis
and psoriatic arthritis deteriorate rapidly in this condition further supports
the distinction between PsA and RA (Arnett *et al.* 1991).

2.2 Epidemiology

Population-based incidence studies of PsA are not available. Several prevalence surveys have reported widely different prevalence rates. This is largely
based on the elusive nature of psoriatic skin lesions, which are often minimal, hidden or periodical. Although in one survey studying inpatient
populations with severe psoriasis up to 39% of patients with psoriasis had

inflammatory arthritis (Leonard *et al.* 1978), the occurrence of arthritis in psoriasis is generally estimated to be approximately 7% (Blumberg *et al.* 1964). Since the prevalence of psoriasis is found to be 1–3%, the prevalence of PsA can be calculated to be approximately 0.2%. A recent review of population-based figures of PsA showed estimates varying from 0.02 to 0.1% (O'Neill & Silman 1994).

The male/female ratio is approximately equal for PsA, although there are differences between subgroups: distal arthritis and spinal disease is predominantly seen in males, whereas symmetrical polyarthritis mainly occurs in females (Gladman *et al.* 1987). Juvenile PsA is a rare disease that is more frequent in girls. The peak age of onset of PsA is similar to that of RA, i.e. within the third and fourth decades (Roberts *et al.* 1976).

PsA has been described in other than caucasian races, but little is known about racial or ethnic differences in the prevalence and manifestations of PsA.

2.3 Definition

Although ample clinical and epidemiological evidence supports the concept of PsA being a separate disorder as well as its classification as a spondylarthropathy, validated diagnostic or classification criteria are lacking.

This is mainly due to the polymorphic manifestations of PsA. In 1973 Moll and Wright proposed the following definition of PsA: an inflammatory arthritis associated with psoriasis of skin or nails and usually a negative serological test for rheumatoid factor and absence of nodules (Moll & Wright 1973a). The inflammatory arthritis can involve peripheral and/or axial joints.

2.4 Etiology and pathogenesis

Psoriasis and PsA are associated with certain HLA types, but environmental factors are likely to have a role in its pathogenesis.

Evidence for a heritable factor in PsA is derived from the increased occurrence (8.3%) of PsA in first-degree relatives of patients with PsA, whereas none of the spouse controls did so (Moll & Wright 1973b). There is no evidence that inheritance is sex-linked or sex-limited. The genetic factors involved in the aetiology of PsA appear to be manifold. Increased frequencies of HLA A26, B38 and DR4 are reported in patients with PsA in general. Moreover, HLA associations are found with subdivisions of PsA: HLA B27 is especially found in spondylitis and sacroiliitis (Woodrow & Ilchsyn 1985) and HLA Cw6 is associated with oligoarthritis (Lopez-Larrea *et al.* 1990).

A recent study showed an association between HLA B27, B39 and DQw3 with progression of PsA, whereas HLA DR7 was associated with a less progressive disease course (Gladman & Farewell 1995).

Although little is known about environmental factors in the pathogenesis of PsA, some evidence exists that infections and trauma might be involved.

Streptococcal infections of the upper respiratory tract are a known triggering factor for some forms of psoriasis and it is assumed that these infections could elicit an autoimmune reaction in genetically predisposed individuals (Krueger & Duvic 1994). Prolonged exposure to bacteria or bacterial products entrapped in cutaneous lesions of psoriasis may cause arthritis in the same way as in the development of reactive arthritis (Veys & Mielants 1994). Another association between infection and psoriasis or PsA stems from the observation that HIV-1 infection deteriorates pre-existing psoriasis and PsA (Arnett *et al.* 1991) and that (reactive) arthritis can be the presenting symptom of HIV infection (Cuellar *et al.* 1994). Injuries of the skin cause a Koebner reaction in approximately 25% of psoriasis patients. With regard to PsA, it has been proposed that arthritis might be caused by activated inflammatory cells, directed towards injured joints after a minor or major trauma.

The synovial membrane in the psoriatic joint cannot be distinguished by histological or immunohistological methods from that in RA. The inflammatory cell infiltrate of the affected joint in PsA primarily consists of macrophages, T lymphocytes and occasional B cells. Most of the T lymphocytes within the synovial membrane are $CD4^+$ and are in an activated state (Smith *et al.* 1992). However, for unknown reasons, T lymphocytes in the synovial fluid are predominantly of the $CD8^+$ subset (Cantagrel *et al.* 1988).

Some evidence exists that in early PsA the synovial fluid contains more $CD4^+$ cells as compared to established PsA (Nilsson & Biberfeld 1984). Monocytes and mature activated macrophages are increased in the synovium and appear to produce interleukin 1 (IL-1), tumour necrosis factor α (TNF-α) and IL-6. There is ample evidence that immune complexes are deposited in the synovium of PsA and the complement system locally activated.

2.5 Clinical features

The initial description of PsA was a combination of psoriasis and arthritis of the distal interphalangeal joints. Since then, several subsets of PsA have been described. In 1973, Moll and Wright, on the basis of clinical observations, classified PsA into the following subsets (Moll & Wright 1973a) (Table 2.1).

Classification of psoriatic arthritis
1 Distal interphalangeal arthritis
2 Symmetrical polyarthritis
3 Mono- or asymmetrical oligoarthritis
4 Spinal disease
5 Arthritis mutilans

Table 2.1 Subgroups of psoriatic arthritis (Moll & Wright 1973a).

1 *Distal interphalangeal arthritis.* This arthritis may be symmetrical or asymmetrical in distribution and is almost always associated with psoriatic changes in the associated nail (Plate 2.1 facing p. 52). It is considered the most classical form of PsA and occurs in up to 50% of cases, and may be part of all other subsets.

2 *Symmetrical polyarthritis.* This form of arthritis occurs in about 25% of cases and has a distribution that is often indistinguishable from RA. Several features can help to differentiate between PsA and RA. Rheumatoid factor is usually not present in PsA and in general PsA follows a milder disease course with less discomfort than RA. Furthermore, extra-articular manifestations, such as nodules, vasculitis, pulmonary or renal involvement that may complicate RA, are seldomly observed in PsA.

3 *Mono- or asymmetrical oligoarthritis.* This is the most common form of PsA and occurs in approximately 70% of cases. Usually a large joint, such as the knee or elbow, is involved together with one or two interphalangeal or metatarsophalangeal joints and a dactylitic toe or digit.

4 *Spinal involvement.* The prevalence of spinal involvement is reported to be 5% of arthritic cases. Since sacroiliitis and spondylitis may have an asymptomatic course, the prevalence is probably much higher. The lumbar spine is more frequently affected than the thoracic and cervical spine. The radiological features of spinal involvement are typical non-marginal, unilateral or asymmetrical syndesmophytes. Sacroiliitis occurs in 50% of cases with spinal involvement: it is mostly unilateral, and when bilateral is clinically indistinguishable from ankylosing spondylitis. However, a less disabling disease course, atypical spinal involvement and a lower prevalence of HLA B27 (50% vs. 90%) differentiate between this subset and ankylosing spondylitis.

5 *Arthritis mutilans.* This is a rare subset occurring in fewer than 1% of cases. It is the result of destructive osteolytic changes of the phalanges and metacarpals and is often referred to as pencil-in-cup or opera-glass deformities.

There is no association between type or extent of psoriasis and subset of articular involvement. In 75% of the cases psoriasis precedes the onset of arthritis, in 15% of cases the onset of joint and skin disease is synchronous, and in 10% arthritis precedes psoriasis. Onychopathy is more frequently present in psoriasis patients with arthritis (63%) than in those without (37%), and is nearly always associated with arthritis of the distal interphalangeal joints.

Osteoarticular manifestations, including synovitis, sternoclavicular hyperostosis and recurrent aseptic osteomyelitis are associated with palmoplantar pustulosis. An acronym, the SAPHO syndrome (synovitis, acne, pustulosis, hyperostosis and osteitis) is proposed for this group of disorders. It is still debated as to whether the SAPHO syndrome is part of the PsA spectrum.

Enthesopathies are inflammatory changes at the attachment of tendon to bone. The most common enthesopathy found in PsA is at the insertion of the

Achilles tendon into the calcaneum, and at musculotendinous insertions around the symphysis pubis and pelvis. Enthesopathies predominantly occur in patients with spinal involvement; it is even stated that spondylitis may be regarded as multiple enthesitic sites in the spine (Helliwell & Wright 1998).

Ocular inflammation is a common feature of PsA: it is found in almost 30% of patients. Both conjunctivitis and iritis are found in a considerable percentage (20% and 7%, respectively).

2.6 Laboratory investigations

No laboratory feature is characteristic for PsA. In the classic definition of PsA, a seronegative arthritis was obligatory. In view of the fact that prevalence of rheumatoid factor in the general population is between 5 and 15% (depending on age), the presence of rheumatoid factor does not exclude the diagnosis. In a study of 220 PsA patients, rheumatoid factor was found to be present in 7% (Gladman *et al.* 1987). However, when rheumatoid factor is detected in psoriatic patients with arthritis, one must also consider a coincident combination of psoriasis and RA.

HLA typing is of little clinical use in the diagnosis of PsA. The presence of HLA B27 can at the most be helpful in cases of diagnostic doubt but its predictive value is virtually none (Khan & Khan 1990).

As in RA, elevated C-reactive protein (CRP) levels and erythrocyte sedimentation rate (ESR) reflect the degree of joint inflammation. However, if only the spinal joints are involved, this relationship between CRP, ESR and disease activity is not observed. Reduced levels of haemoglobin can be found in PsA patients; this is mostly due to the anaemia that often develops in patients with active chronic disease and resolves following remission.

2.7 Imaging techniques

2.7.1 Plain radiographs

Radiological manifestations of PsA can be demonstrated in joints and musculotendinous insertions to bone (Resnick & Niwayama 1988). Plain radiographs of hands and feet show the most characteristic deformities: marginal erosions with adjacent proliferation of bone, joint space narrowing and periostitis (Rahman *et al.* 1998).

Advanced disease may result in complete joint destruction which can lead to (sub)luxation, and in osteolysis of the terminal phalanges, resulting in the pencil-in-cup appearance (Fig. 2.1). Ankylosis of the affected joints may also occur, leading to contractures. At sites of musculotendinous attachments, proliferative new bone formation might develop, especially around the calcaneum and the pelvis. The large joints in PsA (knee, hip, shoulder) show similar changes as can be observed in RA.

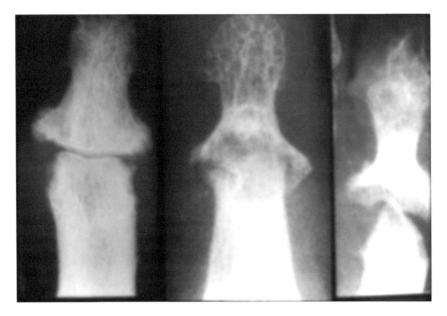

Fig. 2.1 Psoriatic arthritis: progressive joint changes (roentgenograms). Reprinted from the Clinical Slide Collection on the Rheumatic Diseases, copyright 1991, 1995, 1997. Used by permission of the American College of Rheumatology.

Several radiological features of spinal involvement in PsA can be observed, as follows.

1 Sacroiliitis, manifested by erosions, sclerosis, joint-space widening and eventually joint-space narrowing and ankylosis. Sacroiliitis is usually asymmetrical, but bilateral involvement may occur.

2 Paravertebral ossifications, so-called paramarginal syndesmophytes, of the lower thoracic and upper lumbar spine. In contrast to ankylosing spondylitis these syndesmophytes are mostly asymmetric.

3 Ossification of the anterior longitudinal ligament of the cervical spine, often accompanied by syndesmophytes. Erosive involvement of the ondontoid process may result in atlantoaxial subluxation, similar to RA.

2.7.2 Isotope scintigraphy

This technique has no clearly defined role in imaging PsA. Scintigraphy with bone-seeking radioisotopes accumulate in bone by a process not directly related to inflammation or joint damage. It is even suggested that the scintigraphic changes observed in PsA might result from the enhanced turnover of collagen or from diffuse osteopathy.

2.7.3 Computed tomography and magnetic resonance imaging

Computed tomography (CT) is considerably more sensitive than plain radiography in the demonstration of sacroiliitis and has replaced conventional tomography. Magnetic resonance imaging (MRI) can be of potential benefit to assess active joint inflammation and early cartilage damage. However, the exact role of CT and MRI in the management of PsA has yet to be established.

2.8 Differential diagnosis

2.8.1 Rheumatoid arthritis

Psoriatic arthritis differs from RA in its clinical presentation, which in PsA is often asymmetrical, and the presence of distal interphalangeal joint and spinal involvement. Since one of the subsets of PsA has an articular distribution pattern indistinguishable from RA, a meticulous search for psoriatic skin and nail lesions should be performed in patients with seronegative RA.

2.8.2 Osteoarthrosis

Ostearthrosis of the distal interphalangeal joints may be accompanied by osteophytic outgrowths (Heberden nodes). These might be confused with arthritis of these joints as can be observed in PsA. The presence of psoriatic changes in the associated nail helps to differentiate between these conditions.

2.8.3 Reactive arthritis

Since PsA and reactive arthritis are part of the group of the seronegative spondylarthropathies, they share common features and distinction between both conditions can be difficult. Oligoarthritis preceded by an infection of the gastrointestinal or urogenital tract, favours a diagnosis of reactive arthritis.

2.8.4 Ankylosing spondylitis

Spinal involvement in PsA concerns mostly an asymmetric sacroiliitis and fewer syndesmophytes as compared with ankylosing spondylitis. The syndesmophytes in PsA are also somewhat different in shape (Table 2.2).

Differential diagnosis of psoriatic arthritis
1 Rheumatoid arthritis
2 Osteoarthrosis
3 Reactive arthritis
4 Ankylosing spondylitis

Table 2.2 Differential diagnosis to be considered in arthritis accompanying psoriasis.

2.9 Disease course and prognosis

The concept of PsA being a mild disease with episodic arthritis and no significant residual damage has recently been challenged when it was shown that many patients with PsA suffer from joint damage and deformities resulting in marked limitation of functional capacity. In 11% of arthritic patients significant disability was found and in 16% of patients destructive lesions in more than five joints could be demonstrated. Prognostic markers for severe disease were younger age at onset of arthritis, a high number of actively inflamed joints and many previous antirheumatic drugs (Gladman *et al.* 1995). The HLA antigens B27, B39 and DQw3 are also predictive of a poor outcome (Gladman & Farewell 1995). No increase in mortality has been observed in PsA.

2.10 Management and treatment

The ultimate goal of treatment of patients with PsA is to induce remission, which unfortunately can seldom be achieved. The main goals therefore are to alleviate symptoms such as pain and stiffness by controlling disease activity and hence slow the rate of joint damage, and to maintain function for essential activities of daily living. To satisfy these goals pharmacological, rehabilitative and surgical reconstructive therapies are available (Table 2.3).

Pharmacological therapy aims at inhibiting mediators of inflammation. At present three groups of drugs are involved, as follows.

2.10.1 Non-steroidal anti-inflammatory drugs

In general these drugs are effective in the management of PsA, especially the

Table 2.3 Currently available treatments for psoriatic arthritis.

Drug treatment in psoriatic arthritis
1 Non-steroidal anti-inflammatory drugs
2 Disease modifying agents
antimalarials
gold
sulfasalazine
methotrexate
cyclosporin A
azathioprine
combination
methotrexate & cyclosporin A
3 Corticosteroids
systemic
intraarticular

oligoarticular form of PsA. These drugs have an anti-inflammatory and anal-gesic effect by interfering with prostaglandin production.

Non-steroidal anti-inflammatory drugs (NSAIDs) should be given at full doses for at least 4 weeks. Sometimes it is necessary to try several NSAIDs to achieve relief of symptoms. There is no conclusive evidence that the under-lying skin involvement will improve or deteriorate during treatment with NSAIDs. Gastrointestinal side-effects may necessitate concomitant gastroprotective therapy in patients at risk.

2.10.2 Disease-modifying agents

When NSAIDs fail, disease modifying agents, usually referred to as disease-modifying antirheumatic drugs (DMARDs) or slow-acting antirheumatic drugs (SAARDs) can be required. These drugs have been shown to be effective not only in RA, but also in PsA. Several SAARDs are currently available and are briefly discussed.

Antimalarials

With the use of hydroxychloroquine, control of articular involvement can be obtained. The previously presumed likelihood of psoriasis exacerbation dur-ing treatment with hydroxychloroquine has been refuted in recent studies. However, the availability of more effective agents has pushed hydroxy-chloroquine somewhat to the background (Gladman *et al.* 1992).

Gold therapy

Gold compounds, either orally or intramuscularly administered, have been shown to be effective in PsA (Dorwart *et al.* 1978). The oral preparation ap-pears to be less effective than parenteral gold. The polyarticular pattern of joint involvement appears to respond the best. Side-effects of gold therapy are similar to those observed in patients with RA and include skin rash and proteinuria. Some patients experience a worsening of psoriasis during gold therapy.

Sulfasalazine

Recent evidence has been obtained that sulfasalazine is effective for the treat-ment of both skin and articular involvement in psoriasis (Farr *et al.* 1990; Clegg *et al.* 1996). Use of sulfasalazine is limited by gastrointestinal side-effects, occurring in approximately 40% of patients. Potential haematological and hepatotoxic side-effects necessitate close control of patients while on treat-ment with sulfasalazine, especially in the first year.

Methotrexate

Methotrexate has long been recognized as an effective treatment for both psoriasis and PsA. In general, efficacy can be obtained in 60% of patients (Cuellar & Espinoza 1997). Therefore methotrexate has become the drug of choice for many patients with PsA unresponsive to NSAIDs. The most common side-effects are gastrointestinal discomfort and an increase in liver enzymes.

The incidence of side-effects can be decreased by concomitant administration of folic acid. Serious side-effects, although rarely occurring, include pneumonitis, pancytopenia and cirrhosis. The latter usually occurs after long-term treatment in susceptible patients. Careful monitoring of patients on methotrexate therapy is mandatory.

Cyclosporin A

Severe psoriasis and related arthritis can be successfully treated with cyclosporin A (Mahrle *et al.* 1996; Olivieri *et al.* 1997). The clinical response of both skin and joint disease is dose related. Its use is limited by side-effects such as nephrotoxicity and hypertension. Relapse upon discontinuation of cyclosporin A is reported and when remission is achieved, the drug should be tapered rather than abruptly stopped.

Azathioprine

Azathioprine has been shown to induce clinical response in PsA, with regard to both skin and joint disease (LeQuintec *et al.* 1990). The use of azathioprine is nowadays restricted to those patients who do not respond to other SAARDs.

Combination therapy

Combination therapy, as used in RA, is increasingly being explored in PsA. Combinations of methotrexate and sulfasalazine, and methotrexate and cyclosporin A are currently under investigation.

Corticosteroids

The high relapse rate of skin disease upon dicontinuation hampers the use of corticosteroids in PsA. However, corticosteroids can be used to bridge the period that SAARDs are not yet effective. Intra-articular administered corticosteroids are of benefit in patients with mono- or oligoarticular involvement.

Physiotherapy and occupational therapy are often necessary to preserve maximal physical activities. Physiotherapeutic modalities include hydrotherapy, application of local heat, cryotherapy in the form of cold packs, and balneotherapy. Many orthotic devices are available to improve ambulation and functional capacity.

Surgical treatment is indicated for patients in whom significant joint damage has occurred. Synovectomy may be used in persistent synovitis and major reconstructive surgery, including arthrodesis and joint arthroplasty, may be performed in selected cases.

2.11 Summary

PsA can be defined as a rheumatoid factor-negative inflammatory arthritis associated with psoriasis of skin or nails. It gradually emerged as a disease *sui generis* based on clinical and epidemiological data. The cause of PsA is unknown, but heritable and environmental factors appear to be involved in its pathogenesis. The heterogeneous clinical features and the relapsing and remitting nature of both psoriasis and arthritis hamper the construction of diagnostic criteria. PsA is subdivided into several clinical subsets that helps the differentiation with other chronic inflammatory arthritides. Clearly defined prognostic factors are not available, but younger age at onset of arthritis, polyarticular disease and the presence of HLA B27, B39 and DQw3 have all been associated with a worse prognosis. Several drugs are available that can delay or stop joint damage, but in some cases persistent synovitis or joint damage may necessitate surgical intervention.

References

Arnett, F.C., Reveille, J.D. & Duvic, M. (1991) Psoriasis and psoriatic arthritis associated with human immunodeficiency virus infection. *Rheumatic Diseases Clinics of North America* **17**, 59–78.

Blumberg, B.S., Bunim, J.J., Calkins, E., Pirani, C.L. & Zvaifler, N.J. (1964) ARA nomenclature and classification of arthritis and rheumatism (tentative). *Arthritis and Rheumatism* **7**, 93–97.

Brewerton, D.A., Caffrey, M., Hart, F.D., James, D.C.O., Nicholls, A. & Sturrock, R.D. (1973) Ankylosing Spondylitis and HLA-B27. *Lancet* **i**, 904–907.

Cantagrel, A., Roubinet, F., Lassoued, S. *et al.* (1988) The transsynovial lymphocyte ratio. Characterization of blood and synovial fluid lymphocytes from patients with arthritic diseases. *Journal of Rheumatology* **15**, 899–904.

Clegg, D.O., Reda, D.J., Mejias, E. *et al.* (1996) Comparison of sulfasalazine and placebo in the treatment of psoriatic arthritis. A department of veterans affairs cooperative study. *Arthritis and Rheumatism* **39**, 2013–2020.

Cuellar, M.L. & Espinoza, L.R. (1997) Methotrexate use in psoriasis and psoriatic arthritis. *Rheumatic Diseases Clinics of North America* **23**, 797–809.

Cuellar, M.L., Silveira, L.H. & Espinoza, L.R. (1994) Recent developments in psoriatic arthritis. *Current Opinions in Rheumatology* **6**, 378–384.

Dorwart, B., Gall, E.P., Schumacher, H.R. & Krauser, R.E. (1978) Chrysotherapy in psoriatic arthropathy. *Arthritis and Rheumatism* **21**, 513–515.

Farr, M., Kitas, G.D., Waterhouse, L., Jubb, R., Felix-Davies, D.D. & Bacon, P.P. (1990) Sulphasalazine in psoriatic arthritis. A double-blind placebo-controlled study. *British*

Journal of Rheumatology **29**, 46–49.

Gladman, D.D., Blake, R., Brubacher, B. & Farewell, V.T. (1992) Chloroquine therapy in psoriatic arthritis. *Journal of Rheumatology* **19**, 1724–1726.

Gladman, D.D. & Farewell, V.T. (1995) The role of HLA antigens as indicators of disease progression in psoriatic arthritis. *Arthritis and Rheumatism* **38**, 845–850.

Gladman, D.D., Farewell, V.T. & Nadeau, C. (1995) Clinical indicators of progression in psoriatic arthritis, multivariate relative risk model. *Journal of Rheumatism* **22**, 675–679.

Gladman, D.D., Shuckett, R., Russell, M.L., Thorne, J.C. & Schachter, R.K. (1987) Psoriatic arthritis, an analysis of 220 patients. *Quarterly Journal of Medicine* **62**, 127–141.

Helliwell, P.S. & Wright, V. (1998) Psoriatic arthritis, clinical features. In: *Rheumatology* (eds Klippel, J.H. & Dieppe, P.A.), pp. 621.1–621.8. Mosby, London.

Khan, A.K. & Khan, M.K. (1990) HLA-B27 as an aid to diagnosis of ankylosing spondylitis. *Spine: State of the Art Review* **4**, 617–625.

Krueger, G.G. & Duvic, M. (1994) Epidemiology of psoriasis: clinical issues. *Journal of Investigations in Dermatology* **102**, 14S–18S.

Leonard, D.G., O'Duffy, J.D. & Rogers, R.S. (1978) Prospective analysis of psoriatic arthritis in patients hospitalised for psoriasis. *Mayo Clinic Proceedings* **53**, 511–518.

LeQuintec, J.L., Menkes, C.J. & Amor, B. (1990) Rheumatisme psoriatique grave. Traitement par l'azathioprine. *Revue de Rhumatisme* **57**, 815–819.

Lopez-Larrea, C., Torre-Alonso, J.C., Rodriguez-Perez, A. & Coto, E. (1990) HLA antigens in psoriatic arthritis subtypes of a Spanish population. *Annals of Rheumatic Disease* **49**, 318–319.

Mahrle, G., Schulze, H.J., Bräutigam, M. *et al.* (1996) Anti-inflammatory efficacy of low-dose cyclosporin A in psoriatic arthritis. A prospective multicentre study. *British Journal of Dermatology* **135**, 752–757.

Moll, J.M.H. & Wright, V. (1973a) Psoriatic arthritis. Seminars. *Arthritis and Rheumatism* **3**, 55–78.

Moll, J.M.H. & Wright, V. (1973b) Familial occurrence of psoriatic arthritis. *Annals of Rheumatic Disease* **32**, 181–201.

Nilsson, E. & Biberfeld, G. (1984) Differences in the distribution of synovial T lymphocyte subpopulations between patients with acute and chronic exudative synovitis. *Clinical Experimental Rheumatology* **2**, 57–62.

O'Neill, T. & Silman, A.J. (1994) Psoriatic arthritis. Historical background and epidemiology. In: *Psoriatic Arthritis* (eds Wright, V. & Helliwell, P.S.), pp. 263–267. Baillieres Clinics in Rheumatology vol. **8**.

Olivieri, I., Salvarani, C., Cantini, F. *et al.* (1977) Therapy with cyclosporine in psoriatic arthritis. *Seminars in Arthritis and Rheumatism* **27**, 36–43.

Rahman, P., Gladman, D.D., Cook, R.J., Zhou, Y., Young, G. & Salonen, D. (1998) Radiological assessment in psoriatic arthritis. *British Journal of Rheumatology* **37**, 760–765.

Resnick, D. & Niwayama, G. (1988) Psoriatic arthritis. In: *Diagnosis of Bone and Joint Disorders* (eds Resnick, D. & Niwayama, G.), 3rd edn, pp. 1171–1198. W.B. Saunders, Philadelphia.

Roberts, M.E.T., Wright, V., Hill, A.G.S. & Mehra, A.C. (1976) Psoriatic arthritis: follow up study. *Annals of Rheumatic Diseases* **35**, 206–212.

Smith, M.D., O'Donell, J., Highton, J., Palmer, D.G., Rozenbilds, M. & Roberts Thompson, P.J. (1992) Immunohistochemical analysis of synovial membranes from inflammatory and non-inflammatory arthritides: scarcity of CD5 positive B cells and IL2 receptor bearing T cells. *Pathology* **24**, 19–26.

Veys, E.M. & Mielants, H. (1994) Current concepts in psoriatic arthritis. *Dermatology* **189** (Suppl. 2), 35–41.

Woodrow, J.C. & Ilchsyn, A. (1985) HLA antigens in psoriasis and psoriatic arthritis. *Journal of Medical Genetics* **22**, 492–495.

Wright, V. & Moll, J.M.H. (1976). *Seronegative Polyarthritis*, pp. 169–235. North Holland, Amsterdam.

Chapter 3: Psychosocial Aspects

J.A. Savin

3.1 Introduction

No one now doubts that psoriasis can damage the quality of life of those who have it. The writings of John Updike, Vladimir Nabokov and Dennis Potter, all psoriatics themselves, make this clear (Meulenberg 1997); and over the last few years much time has been spent looking into this side of the disease.

A 'quality of life industry' has sprung up, and patients' views on the impact of psoriasis on their activities and feelings are now being sounded out with the aid of an ever-increasing array of questionnaires. Each must be shown to be valid, reliable and responsive to any change in a patient's condition. Some workers have occasionally seemed to be more interested in this technical side of the questionnaires than in the meaning of the answers to them. Others have teetered on the edge of proving the obvious while trying to show that answers to their questionnaire truly reflect changes in disease severity, for example that patients' quality-of-life scores improve when their psoriasis clears (Kurwa & Finlay 1995). Too many reports are written in an opaque jargon that hides meaning; but, despite this, good quality-of-life studies give a patient-based view of the condition that can be of use in assessing the value of new treatments and the burden psoriasis imposes on the community.

More controversial is the idea that psoriasis can be triggered by sudden stress, though many anecdotes can be quoted in support of it. As long ago as 1825, Alibert reported the case of a valet who had developed acute guttate psoriasis after seeing his master led to the guillotine (Lomholt 1963); and, more recently, the psoriasis of five patients was accepted as having been influenced by terrorism in Northern Ireland (Beare *et al.* 1978). But, however numerous, case reports of this type can never rule out the possibility of coincidence.

Studies of larger series are needed to confirm that the association between the start of psoriasis and preceding stressful events is genuine, and several exist, although the design of some is open to criticism.

Other topics touched on in this chapter include the lack of evidence for a specific 'psoriatic personality type', and the relatively minor impact that psychological treatments have on the physical side of psoriasis.

3.2 Quality of life in psoriasis (Finlay 1997)

Psoriasis ruins the lives of some of those who suffer from it, but the problems it creates do not necessarily tally with the extent and severity of the eruption as judged by an outside observer (Root *et al.* 1994). The burden of illness cannot be described fully by such simple physical measures. Quality-of-life measures present a different, patient-based view of the condition, and offer a reasonable way of gauging the value of treatments used for it. However, there is no precise definition of quality of life: in the case of psoriasis, investigators have been interested in its effects, and those of treatments for it, on patients' daily lives and life satisfaction.

3.2.1 Questionnaires and their uses

Questionnaires of many types can be used to estimate quality of life, but the temptation to ask a single patient to complete more than one or two should usually be resisted as this leads to waning interest and less accurate replies. Questionnaires and structured interviews can also sow ideas in patients'minds that they would not have thought of themselves.

General-health questionnaires

These enquire into the overall effects of ill health, conventionally divided into psychological, social and physical domains. Their use allows the problems of people with psoriasis to be compared with those of patients with other conditions, and with healthy controls.

For example, use of the Sickness Impact Profile showed that a group of hospital-treated patients with psoriasis suffered less disability than those with cardiac failure but at least as much as those with angina or hypertension (Finlay *et al.* 1990). The physical effects of the psoriasis were only moderate but its psychosocial effects were profound. The condition had a massive effect on sleep and the ability to cope with domestic and recreational activities, and with work. Nevertheless, in another study (Finlay & Coles 1995), a majority of patients with severe psoriasis felt it would be worse to have diabetes, asthma or bronchitis.

Another questionnaire has recently been used to study a group of 435 patients with psoriasis in general practice. They saw themselves as less healthy than a normal population (O'Neill & Kelly 1996). The most severe problems were in manual workers, whose skin condition affected their physical, mental and social activities.

Skin-disease questionnaires

Questionnaires specific to psoriasis include the Psoriasis Disability Index and the Psoriasis Life Stress Inventory. Using them, some have shown that the impact of psoriasis tends to decrease with increasing age (Gupta & Gupta 1995; McKenna & Stern 1997).

Other questionnaires can be used to score the impact of skin diseases of any type (Morgan *et al.* 1997). Each has its own value. Questionnaires dealing only with psoriasis may be the most suitable for evaluating psoriasis treatments. Dermatology-specific questionnaires are useful for comparing the quality of life of those with a variety of skin diseases.

3.2.2 Utility measures

Utility measures estimate the value patients put on their health and so can also be used to compare different diseases. They can be expressed in various ways: for example patients can be asked how much money they would pay for a cure of their psoriasis, or how much time they would be prepared to devote each day to a successful treatment for it. In one study, for example, one-half of a group of patients with severe psoriasis were prepared to spend 2 or 3 h a day on treatment if this would ensure that they had a normal skin for the rest of the day (Finlay & Coles 1995).

3.3 Some psychosocial effects of psoriasis

3.3.1 Stress

The stresses caused by psoriasis have been divided into two groups (Fortune *et al.* 1997). In the first, stress is caused by anticipating other peoples' possible reactions, and this can lead to the avoidance of worrying situations such as going to public places. Secondly, stress can arise from patients' beliefs about, or the actual experience of, being evaluated by others on the basis of the skin condition, for example dealing with people who seem to avoid contact with the lesions of psoriasis.

3.3.2 Work

Severe psoriasis can make it impossible for patients to work. In one study (Finlay & Coles 1995), some 60% of patients with severe psoriasis, who were currently working, had lost an average of 26 days from work during the preceding year; and of the 180 not working, 33.9% attributed this to their psoriasis. Men experience more work-related stress than women (Gupta & Gupta 1995).

3.3.3 Itching and depression

Despite a general impression to the contrary, psoriasis is often itchy. In one study, 67% of 82 inpatients with psoriasis reported moderate or severe itching (Gupta *et al.* 1988). Sometimes this even interferes with sleep (Savin *et al.* 1990). Psoriatics' self-ratings for itching correlate well with their scores on the Carroll Rating for Depression; however, the same is also true for atopic eczema, and chronic urticaria (Gupta *et al.* 1994). Depression seems to modulate the perception of itching.

3.3.4 Sexual activity

In one series of patients (Jobling 1976), 84% said that the worst thing about having psoriasis was the difficulty it created in establishing social contact and relationships. In another study, 50% of 104 hospital patients with psoriasis felt that the condition had inhibited their sexual relationships (Ramsay & Reagan 1988).

Psoriatic patients whose sexual activity had declined since the onset of their psoriasis were compared with those who had not experienced this change (Gupta & Gupta 1997). The first group had more joint pains, more itching, and marginally more severe psoriasis in the groins. They were also more depressed and tended to drink more alcohol.

Psoriatics, particularly female ones, have difficulty in starting sexual relationships (van Dorssen *et al.* 1992). Sexual responsiveness does not correlate with the extent of the skin disease or its location on the genital areas, but rather with self-esteem.

3.3.5 Drinking, smoking and eating

Alcoholism, cirrhosis of the liver, and, in women at least, cancer of the lung, were all associated significantly with psoriasis in one massive Swedish population study (Lindegard 1986). Few clinical dermatologists will be surprised by this.

Many psoriatics know that alcohol worsens their skin disease, but, despite this, psoriatics drink more alcohol than controls—both before they develop the disorder (Poikolainen *et al.* 1990) and afterwards. In women, at least, the heavier the drinking, the more extensive the psoriasis tends to be (Poikolainen *et al.* 1994). A high alcohol intake therefore is a risk factor for psoriasis, and, conversely, the stress of having psoriasis can lead to relief drinking and neglected treatment.

Smoking is also commoner in psoriatics than controls, both before and after the onset of the disease (Mills *et al.* 1992). Of course, smoking and drinking alcohol are often linked, but, after controlling for alcohol intake, smoking seems still to be a risk factor for the development of psoriasis (Naldi *et al.* 1992).

The dietary aspects of psoriasis have been less well researched, but the high alcohol intake of psoriatics may be accompanied by an excessive intake of high-fat foods and saturated fats (Zamboni *et al.* 1989), with a high body mass index, and a low consumption of carrots, tomatoes and fresh fruit (Naldi *et al.* 1996). It is not clear whether or not these findings are due to 'comfort eating' as a response to the stress of the condition.

3.3.6 Stigmatization and suicidal ideas

Most people with psoriasis have ordinary and natural characteristics: those with different and less desirable attributes risk being seen as abnormal, or even tainted, and may be disqualified from full social acceptance.

Feelings of being an outcast are a serious problem for many patients with psoriasis. In one study (Ginsberg & Link 1993), 19% had been through episodes of gross rejection which led them to feel stigmatized. A questionnaire designed for patients with psoriasis (Ginsberg & Link 1989) revealed that stigmatization has six components: anticipation of rejection, feelings of being flawed, sensitivity to the attitudes of others, guilt and shame, secretiveness, and, somewhat paradoxically, the possession of positive attitudes to the disease. Older people, females, and those with a long history of psoriasis are especially liable to feel stigmatized (Schmid-Ott *et al.* 1996). Bleeding from the skin is the strongest predictor of stigma feelings and of despair (Ginsberg & Link 1989).

A proportion of patients, ranging from 4.3% (Schmid-Ott *et al.* 1996) to 9.7% (Gupta *et al.* 1993), have had suicidal thoughts. These are most common in patients with high depression scores and those who think they have bad psoriasis

3.4 The effects of stress on psoriasis

Many patients are sure that stress triggered their psoriasis originally and still exacerbates it (Savin 1970; Jobling 1976). Scientific publications on the subject continue to proliferate, adding to an already vast literature, most of which supports the existence of this association. Yet an aura of doubt lingers on— for a variety of reasons.

3.4.1 Stress and life events

The concept of stress is not a simple one and the terms in which it is discussed have sometimes been used rather vaguely. At one time, a specific stress response was thought to follow a variety of external influences (stressors), but in reality each type of stress may well provoke its own pattern of response. For example, fear of losing a spouse leads to anxiety, whereas the actual loss of one causes depression. For this reason, many investigators prefer to record damaging life events rather than to speculate about the presence of stress itself. These life events can be quantified and ranked, for example on one Social Adjustment Scale, the death of a spouse earns 100 points and retirement only 45. Events like these can cause major upheavals in people's lives, overtaxing their ability to adapt and so contributing to the onset of diseases of various types. Vulnerability to these life events, and to the stresses they generate, depends on many factors, of which genetic ones are clearly important in psoriasis.

3.4.2 Study design

Simply asking patients with psoriasis about such events is not enough: the questions have to be devised carefully, as those with other skin conditions might well put them down to stress if asked the right leading questions.

Controls are clearly needed. Patients' recollections of these life events can then be matched against those given by a control group of patients with conditions thought not to be related to stress. But, even then, there are still problems: many patients with psoriasis have heard that there is a widely accepted relationship to stress and may 'remember' stressful events because that is precisely what doctors expect of them (Shuster 1979), but not of others, with conditions like upper respiratory tract infections and skin tumours, who have been part of some control series (Seville 1977; Seville 1978). Prospective studies lessen some of these difficulties.

3.4.3 Some recent findings

A recent study, that tried to avoid the methodological studies of its predecessors (Al'abadie *et al.* 1994), concluded that stressful life events were more likely to be associated with the onset of psoriasis, and with its exacerbations, than was the case with the conditions of two groups of control patients. Family upsets, such as bereavements, were the most commonly related events, followed by work or school pressures, and financial worries. The incubation period between event and onset tended to be longer than between event and exacerbation, but the more stressful life events did not have a shorter incubation time, which was usually under 4 weeks.

Some argue that a barrage of minor daily annoyances may well be more important than these major life events. Certainly in one study (Mazzetti *et al.* 1994), in which a stress factor was found in nearly 90% of patients with a relapse of their psoriasis, most of the stressful events were very minor. The authors felt that the meaning of the event to the patient was more important than its apparent severity as seen by others.

Another approach to the same problem was to divide patients with psoriasis into those under high or under low stress (Harvima *et al.* 1996); actively spreading psoriasis was then found to be associated with stressful life events for men but not for women.

3.4.4 Stress reactors

People with psoriasis can also be divided into those who say that psychosocial stresses worsen their psoriasis and those who deny this. Some workers have not been able to find other differences between these groups; however, stress reactors may have the more disfiguring disease (Gupta *et al.* 1989), perhaps starting more often on the head (Leuteritz & Shimshoni 1982), and early-onset psoriasis may especially be triggered by stress (Gupta *et al.* 1996).

3.4.5 Mechanisms

The mechanisms connecting psychological factors with psoriatic lesions remain largely unknown, and cannot be fully explained just in terms of alterations of neuropeptides in the skin (Pincelli *et al.* 1994), although stress does increase the neuropeptide content of psoriatic lesions, with a concomitant decrease in the activity of enzymes that degrade neuropeptides, especially mast-cell chymase (Harvima *et al.* 1993). In addition, the concentration in the blood of certain neuromediators, especially β-endorphin, changes during exacerbations (Misery 1997).

3.5 Patients' views about psoriasis and its treatment

Misconceptions about psoriasis are common (Savin 1970) and may make medical advice seem unreasonable. For example, topical treatment seems illogical to patients who think that psoriasis is emotional in origin. Many patients see psoriasis as a vicious circle, for example having psoriasis makes them worried or depressed, which then worsens the skin condition, engendering further worry or depression, etc.

Patients learn about psoriasis mainly from doctors (Lanigan & Layton 1991), but, despite this, in one study, 35% of people with psoriasis in the community thought that their psoriasis was an allergy and 12% an infection (Nevitt & Hutchinson 1996). Many are critical of their general practitioners (Savin 1970; Jobling 1976) who may be seen as not interested, or merely as prescribers, routinely handing out ineffective and often unpleasant treatments. In contrast, after attending one hospital clinic, 70% of one group of patients became happier with their psoriasis (McHenry & Doherty 1992), although in Japan only one-quarter of hospital psoriasis patients were satisfied with their current treatment, and dermatologists were often seen as self-satisfied (Yasuda *et al.* 1990). Many patients—in one series more than 60% (Jobling 1976)—have also attended fringe practitioners.

3.6 Psoriasis and personality traits

Most agree that there is no specific 'psoriasis personality', but the debate continues. A recent report of four different personality clusters in psoriatic patients (Rubino *et al.* 1995) was criticised, as the control group had no patients with other disfiguring chronic skin conditions.

No clear-cut picture emerges from the literature, in which traits (the stable characteristics of an individual) are often muddled with states (temporary moods or conditions). Psoriatic people have variously been found to be less able to express anger than controls (Ginsburg *et al.* 1993), and to score highly for spontaneous aggression (Matussek *et al.* 1985). Patients whose psoriasis is stress responsive may be less angry about their skin condition than those with non-stress-responsive psoriasis (Gupta *et al.* 1989). Patients with equal amounts of psoriasis sometimes react quite differently, and their 'coping styles' are presumably based on differing character traits (Arnetz *et al.* 1991).

3.7 Psychological treatments for psoriasis

As stress seems to worsen psoriasis, many methods (group therapy, psychotherapy, treatment for depression, biofeedback training and hypnosis) have been used to reduce it. Modest improvements in the skin have sometimes been achieved (Zachariae *et al.* 1996), but so far the results have not led to the routine use of these methods in many centres.

3.8 Practical applications in the clinic

All doctors who treat patients with psoriasis should be aware of its psychosocial effects, so that they can deal with them sensitively and sympathetically. However, many of the studies quoted in this chapter are of populations, and their findings cannot easily be transferred directly to the management of individuals. In addition, most psychosocial approaches are tremendously time-consuming, and not suitable for use in busy clinics.

There are further problems. Dermatologists know about the adverse effects on psoriasis of smoking, and of drinking excessive amounts of alcohol, but this does not always mean that they can change their patients' habits. Similarly, misconceptions about psoriasis can be 'fixed' and resist prolonged explanations. Nevertheless, every patient with psoriasis should be given a full explanation of the condition, couched in simple language, and backed up by written information sheets.

An experienced dermatologist will also be on the look-out for depression and the risk of suicide, and counselling may be of value in selected cases. Patient support groups, such as the Psoriasis Association, continue to help large numbers of patients.

References

Al'abadie, M.S., Kent, G.G. & Gawkrodger, D.J. (1994) The relationship between stress and the onset and exacerbation of psoriasis and other skin conditions. *British Journal of Dermatology* **130**, 199–203.

Arnetz, B.B., Fjellner, B., Eneroth, P. & Kallner, A. (1991) Endocrine and dermatological concomitants of mental stress. *Acta Dermato-Venereologica Supplementum.* **156**, 9–12.

Beare, J.M., Burrows, D. & Merrett, J.D. (1978) The effects of mental and physical stress on the incidence of skin disorders. *British Journal of Dermatology* **98**, 553–558.

Finlay, A.Y. (1997) Quality of life measurement in dermatology: a practical guide. *British Journal of Dermatology* **136**, 305–314.

Finlay, A.Y. & Coles, E.C. (1995) The effect of severe psoriasis on the quality of life of 369 patients. *British Journal of Dermatology* **132**, 236–244.

Finlay, A.Y., Khan, G.K., Luscombe, D.K. & Salek, M.S. (1990) Validation of the Sickness Impact Profile and Psoriasis Disability Index in psoriasis. *British Journal of Dermatology* **123**, 751–756.

Fortune, D.G., Main, C.J., O'Sullivan, T.M. & Griffiths, C.E.M. (1997) Quality of life in patients with psoriasis: the contribution of clinical variables and psoriasis—specific stress. *British Journal of Dermatology* **137**, 755–760.

Ginsberg, I.H. & Link, B.G. (1989) Feelings of stigmatisation in patients with psoriasis. *Journal of the American Academy of Dermatology* **20**, 52–63.

Ginsberg, I.H. & Link, B.G. (1993) Psychosocial consequences of rejection and stigma feelings in psoriasis patients. *International Journal of Dermatology* **32**, 587–591.

Ginsburg, I.H., Prystowsky, J.H., Kornfield, D.S. & Wolland, H. (1993) Role of emotional factors in adults with atopic dermatitis. *International Journal of Dermatology* **32**, 656–660.

Gupta, M.A. & Gupta, A.K. (1995) Age and gender differences in the impact of psoriasis on the quality of life. *International Journal of Dermatology* **34**, 700–703.

Gupta, M.A. & Gupta, A.K. (1997) Psoriasis and sex: a study of moderately to severely affected patients. *International Journal of Dermatology* **36**, 259–262.

Gupta, M.A., Gupta, A.K., Kirby, S. *et al.* (1989) A psychocutaneous profile of psoriasis patients who are stress reactors. *General Hospital Psychiatry* **11**, 166–173.

Gupta, M.A., Gupta, A.K., Kirkby, S. *et al.*(1988) Pruritus in psoriasis. A prospective study of some psychiatric and dermatologic correlates. *Archives of Dermatology* **124**, 1052–1057.

Gupta, M.A., Gupta, A.K., Schork, N.J. & Ellis, C.N. (1994) Depression modulates pruritus perception: a study of pruritus in psoriasis, atopic dermatitis, and chronic idiopathic urticaria. *Psychosomatic Medicine* **56**, 36–40.

Gupta, M.A., Gupta, A.K. & Watteel, G.N. (1996) Early onset psoriasis (> 40 years age) is co-morbid with a greater psychopathology than late onset psoriasis: a study of 137 patients. *Acta Dermato-Venereologica* **76**, 464–466.

Gupta, M.A., Schork, N.J., Gupta, A.K. & Ellis, C.N. (1993) Suicidal ideation in psoriasis. *International Journal of Dermatology* **32**, 188–190.

Harvima, R.J., Viinamaki, H., Harvima, I.T. *et al.* (1996) Association of psychic stress with clinical severity and symptoms of psoriatic patients. *Acta Dermato-Venereologica* **76**, 467–471.

Harvima, I.T., Viinamaki, H., Naukkarinen, A. *et al.* (1993) Association of cutaneous mast-cells and sensory nerves with psychic stress in psoriasis. *Psychotherapy and Psychosomatics* **60**, 168–176.

Jobling, R.G. (1976) Psoriasis—a preliminary questionnaire study of sufferers' subjective experience. *Clinical and Experimental Dermatology* **1**, 233–236.

Kurwa, H.A. & Finlay, A.Y. (1995) Dermatology in-patient management greatly improves life quality. *British Journal of Dermatology* **133**, 575–578.

Lanigan, S.W. & Layton, A. (1991) Level of knowledge and information sources used by patients with psoriasis. *British Journal of Dermatology* **125**, 340–342.

Leuteritz, G. & Shimshoni, R. (1982) Psychotherapy in psoriasis—results at the Dead Sea. *Zeitschrift fur Hautkrankheiten* **57**, 1612–1615.

Lindegard, B. (1986) Diseases associated with psoriasis in a general population of 159,200 middle-aged, urban, native Swedes. *Dermatologica* **172**, 298–304.

Lomholt, G. (1963) *Psoriasis: Prevalence, Spontaneous Course and Genetics*. G.E.C.GAD. Copenhagen, p. 121.

Matussek, P., Agerer, D. & Seibt, G. (1985) Aggression in depressives and psoriatics. *Psychotherapy and Psychosomatics* **43**, 120–125.

Mazzetti, M., Mozzetta, A., Soavi, G.C. *et al.* (1994) Psoriasis, stress, and psychiatry: psychodynamic characteristics of stressors. *Acta Dermato-Venereologica* **186** (Suppl.), 62–64.

McHenry, P.M. & Doherty, V.R. (1992) Psoriasis: an audit of patients' views on the disease and its treatment. *British Journal of Dermatology* **127**, 13–17.

McKenna, K.E. & Stern, R.S. (1997) The impact of psoriasis on the quality of life of patients from the 16-center PUVA follow-up cohort. *Journal of the American Academy of Dermatology* **36**, 388–394.

Meulenberg, F. (1997) The hidden delight of psoriasis. *British Medical Journal* **315**, 1709–1711.

Mills, C.M., Srivastava, E.D., Harvey, I.M. *et al.* (1992) Smoking habits in psoriasis: a case control study. *British Journal of Dermatology* **127**, 18–21.

Misery, L. (1997) Skin, immunity and the nervous system. *British Journal of Dermatology* **137**, 843–850.

Morgan, M., McCreedy, R., Simpson, J. & Hay, R.J. (1997) Dermatology quality of life scales—a measure of the impact of skin diseases. *British Journal of Dermatology* **136**, 202–206.

Naldi, L., Parazzini, F. & Brevi, A. (1992) Family history, smoking habits, alcohol consumption and risk of psoriasis. *British Journal of Dermatology* **127**, 212–217.

Naldi, L., Parazzini, F., Peli, L., Chatenoud, L., Cainelli, T. and the Psoriasis Study Group of the Italian Group for Epidemiologic Research in Dermatology (1996) Dietary factors and the risk of psoriasis. Results of an Italian case-control study. *British Journal of Dermatology* **134**, 101–106.

Nevitt, G.J. & Hutchinson, P.E. (1996) Psoriasis in the community: prevalence, severity and patients' beliefs, and attitudes towards the disease. *British Journal of Dermatology* **135**, 533–537.

O'Neill, P. & Kelly, P. (1996) Postal questionnaire study of disability in the community associated with psoriasis. *British Medical Journal* **313**, 919–921.

Pincelli, C., Fantini, F., Magnoni, C. & Gianetti, A. (1994) Psoriasis and the nervous system. *Acta Dermato-Venereologica* **186** (Suppl.), 60–61.

Poikolainen, K., Reunula, T. & Karvonen, J. (1994) Smoking, alcohol and life events related to psoriasis among women. *British Journal of Dermatology* **130**, 473–477.

Poikolainen, K., Reunula, T., Karvonen, J., Lauharanta, J. & Karkkainen, P. (1990) Alcohol intake: a risk factor for psoriasis in young and middle aged men? *British Medical Journal* **300**, 780–783.

Ramsay, B. & O'Reagan, M. (1988) A survey of the social and psychological effects of psoriasis. *British Journal of Dermatology* **118**, 195–201.

Root, S., Kent, G. & Al-Abadie, M.S.K. (1994) The relationship between disease severity, disability and psychological distress in patients undergoing PUVA treatment for psoriasis. *Dermatology* **189**, 234–237.

Rubino, I.A., Sonnino, A., Pezzarossa, B., Ciani, N. & Bassi, R. (1995) Personality

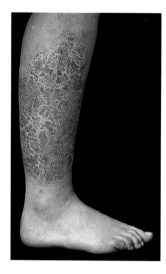

Plate 1.1 The macromorphological appearance of psoriatic lesions.

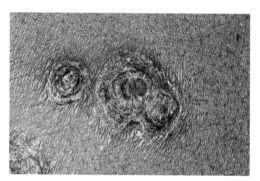

Plate 1.2 Rupoid psoriasis.

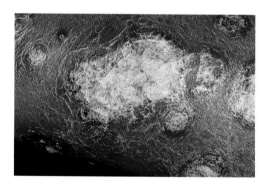

Plate 1.3 Inveterate psoriasis.

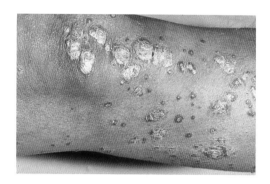

Plate 1.4 Small pin point papules, coalescing to a plaque.

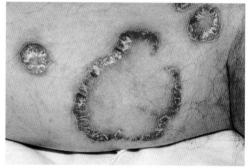

Plate 1.5 Annular psoriasis.

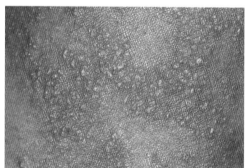

Plate 1.6 Guttate psoriasis.

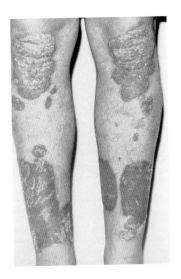

Plate 1.7 Chronic plaque psoriasis.

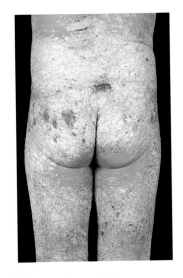

Plate 1.8 Geographic psoriasis.

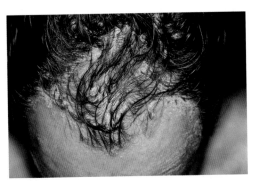

Plate 1.9 Psoriasis of the scalp.

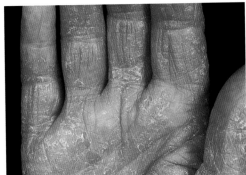

Plate 1.10 Chronic plaque psoriasis of palms.

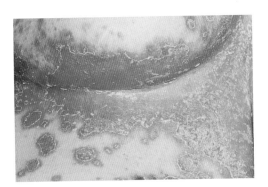

Plate 1.11 Submammary psoriasis.

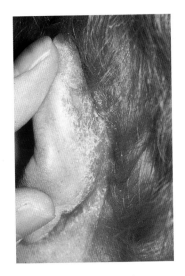

Plate 1.12 Retroauricular psoriasis.

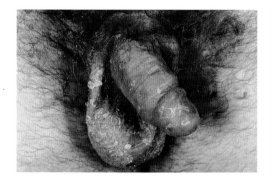

Plate 1.13 Penile psoriasis.

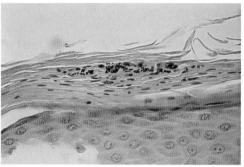

Plate 1.16 Microabscess of Munro.

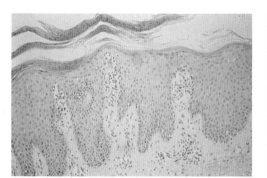

Plate 1.14 Parkeratotic foci with absence of the granular layer, epidermal acanthosis with elongation of rete ridges and thinning of the suprapapillary plate with a mixed inflammatory infiltrate.

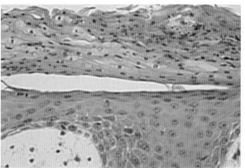

Plate 1.17 Papillary and suprapapillary arrangement.

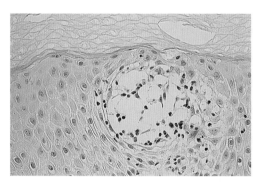

Plate 1.15 Micropustule of Kogoj.

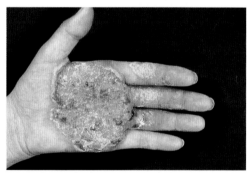

Plate 1.18 Pustulosis palmaris.

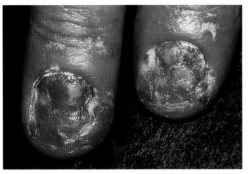

Plate 1.19 Acrodermatitis continua Hallopeau.

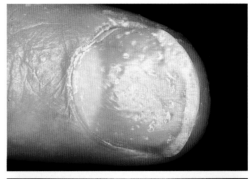

(a)

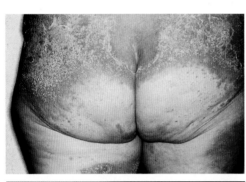

(a)

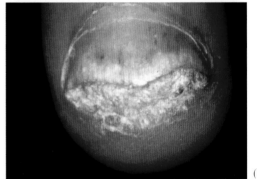

(b)

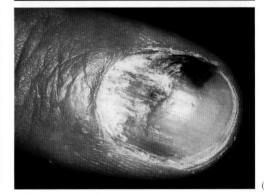

(b)

(c)

Plate 1.20 Generalized pustular psoriasis.
(a) Zumbusch pattern. (b) Annular pattern.

Plate 1.21 Nail abnormalities: (a) pits, (b) subungual keratosis and distal onycholysis, (c) ölfleck phenomenon.

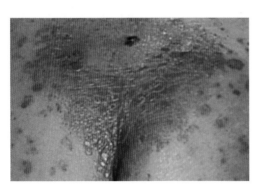

Plate 1.22 Lichenified psoriasis.

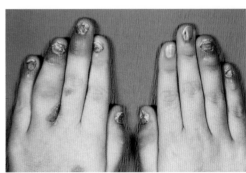

Plate 2.1 Psoriatic arthritis: hands, nail changes, rash, and arthritis. Reprinted from the Clinical Slide Collection on the Rheumatic Diseases, copyright 1991, 1995, 1997. Used by permission of the American College of Rheumatology.

disorders and psychiatric symptoms in psoriasis. *Psychological Reports* **77**, 547–553.

Savin, J.A. (1970) Patients' beliefs about psoriasis. *Transactions of the St. John's Hospital Dermatology Society* **56**, 135–142.

Savin, J.A., Adam, K., Oswald, I. & Paterson, W.D. (1990) Pruritus and nocturnal awakenings. *Journal of the American Academy of Dermatology* **23**, 767–768.

Schmid-Ott, G., Jaeger, B., Kuensbeck, H.W., Ott, R. & Lamprecht, F. (1996) Dimensions of stigmatisation in patients with psoriasis in a 'Questionnaire on Experience with Skin Complaints'. *Dermatology* **193**, 304–310.

Seville, R.H. (1977) Psoriasis and stress. *British Journal of Dermatology* **97**, 297–302.

Seville, R.H. (1978) Psoriasis and stress II. *British Journal of Dermatology* **98**, 151–153.

Shuster, S. (1979) Stress and psoriasis. *British Journal of Dermatology* **100**, 614–615.

van Dorssen, I.E., Boom, B.W. & Hengeveld, M.W. (1992) Experience of sexuality in patients with psoriasis and constitutional eczema. *Nederlands Tijdschrift Voor Geneeskunde* **136**, 2175–2178.

Yasuda, H., Koboyashi, H. & Ohkawara, A. (1990) A survey of the social and psychological effects of psoriasis. *Japanese Journal of Dermatology* **100**, 1167–1171.

Zachariae, R., Oster, H., Bjerring, P. & Kragballe, K. (1996) Effects of psychologic intervention on psoriasis: a preliminary report. *Journal of the American Academy of Dermatology* **34**, 1008–1015.

Zamboni, S., Zanetti, G., Grosso, G., Ambrosio, G.B., Gozzetti, S. & Peserico, A. (1989) Dietary behaviour in psoriatic patients. *Acta Dermato-Venereologica* **146** (Suppl.), 182–183.

Part 2
Etiology and Pathogenesis

In this part the epidemiology, genetics and pathophysiology will be high-lighted. Again the information is of practical relevance to dermatologists, residents and general practitioners.

In Chapter 4 the occurrence of psoriasis, the demographics, the characteristics of 'early onset' and 'late onset' and exogenous as well as endogenous triggering factors will be presented.

Chapter 5 provides an overview of the genetics of psoriasis. Information on progress with respect to the identification of responsible genes is given whilst practically relevant information on genetic markers for the course of psoriasis and genetic counselling is also reported.

In Chapter 6 the general pathogenetic aspects are considered.

Chapter 7 provides a review of immunopathogenesis. In particular the various antipsoriatic mechanisms are highlighted in order to provide an understanding of the modes of action of the various treatments.

Chapter 4: Epidemiology

J.J. Grob and G. Folchetti

4.1 Descriptive epidemiology: assessment of morbidity

4.1.1 Prevalence

All data about morbidity of psoriasis must be regarded with caution. Morbidity measures suppose that the disease is perfectly defined. Although the diagnosis of psoriasis is often considered as easy, the diagnostic criteria have never been assessed. In most epidemiological studies of psoriasis, diagnostic criteria are not described. Furthermore, the question of whether or not borderline conditions, such as severe seborrhoeic dermatitis, palmoplantar pustulosis or transient psoriasis guttata, are included in the study, is not always addressed.

Interview or postal survey (Rea *et al.* 1976; Braathen *et al.* 1989; Nevitt & Hutchinson 1996), and systematic examination (Lomholt 1963; Hellgren 1967; Johnson 1978) provide different measures of morbidity, since patients with mild forms of psoriasis are often unaware of their disease, or unaware of the name of the disorder. Postal surveys are also hindered by non-responders. As compared to population-based data (Lomholt 1963; Hellgren 1967), an excess of severe or persistent psoriasis probably biases hospital data obtained from in- and outpatients (Kavli *et al.* 1985).

Prevalence measurements must be carefully analysed: point prevalence is the rate of persons clinically affected by psoriasis at a given time (as assessed by systematic examination or interview), whereas cumulative prevalence is the number of people who have had in the past, or still have psoriasis (as assessed by interview). Based on the more-or-less persistent course of rather severe cases referred to hospital, cumulated prevalence and point prevalence are often considered as similar. However, in the community cases, mild psoriasis with long remissions are commonly observed.

Therefore, point prevalence of active psoriasis is certainly lower than cumulative prevalence. Additionally, prevalence of psoriasis usually means prevalence of the phenotype, which is lower than the prevalence of genotype. However, the quotient between the prevalence of the phenotype and the prevalence of genotype, which defines the penetrance of psoriasis, tends to increase with age. Therefore, the cumulated prevalence of the psoriasis phenotype in elderly people tends to be close to the prevalence of the genotype.

Due to the various limitations, all attempts to define the extent and severity of psoriasis in the population must be interpreted with caution. Direct comparison of data obtained by different methods, in differently biased samples, from different populations, are hardly comparable.

A large literature about psoriasis prevalence has been published over 30 years. Using data from systematic examination of the total population or from very large population-based samples, cumulative prevalence was measured at 2.8% in the Faroe islands (Lomholt 1964), 1.4% in Norway (Braathen *et al.* 1989) and UK (Nevitt & Hutchinson 1996) and 0.9% in the USA (Johnson 1978). These data must be considered as minimum prevalence, since it is likely that minor psoriasis can be overlooked. These results in Europe or North America cannot be extrapolated to the rest of the world, since psoriasis seems to be uncommon in other populations such as the Norwegian Laps (Kavli *et al.* 1985), people from Samoa Islands (Farber & Nall 1985) or from the South American Andes (Convit 1962), or more generally those of Mongoloid race (Shing 1984).

Prevalence of clinical subtypes

The prevalence of each clinical subtype of psoriasis is not easy to precisely estimate since the clinical aspect may change from non-pustular to pustular psoriasis or to erythroderma in the same patient.

Therefore the following must be interpreted as indicative only: prevalence of arthritis may range from 5 to 25% of psoriatics (Kononen *et al.* 1986; Farber *et al.* 1968), prevalence of nail disease has been reported at between 10 and 80%. One-quarter of erythroderma cases may be related to psoriasis (Boyd & Menter 1989).

4.1.2 Incidence

The incidence of psoriasis, i.e. the number of new psoriasis cases occurring in a given population in a defined time cannot be properly assessed, since individuals cannot be identified when they have their first detectable lesion. The only population-based study estimated incidence from the number of patients searching for medical advice per year concerning psoriasis, which is probably different from the true incidence (Bell *et al.* 1991). This study was carried out in Rochester and yielded a crude annual incidence of 58 per 100 000, which was corrected to 60 per 100 000 after adjustment to the US population.

4.1.3 Sex and socioeconomic distributions

In most surveys, psoriasis seems to affect males and females equally. A male preponderance has, however, been noted in some surveys (Hellgren 1967;

Bedi 1977). This may be due to reference biases. There is no evidence of different prevalence in various socioeconomic groups (Braathen *et al.* 1989)

4.1.4 Age of onset

There is no consensus about what defines onset. Birth is by definition the age of onset of the genotype. Onset of the phenotype is the first date when the first lesion appears, but the patient recall is subject to many inaccuracies.

The first time a patient seeks medical advice is more reliable, but is not strictly the disease onset. We can suspect that a minimal disease can precede by years the medical diagnosis. It has to be emphasized that the studies in the general population tend to over-represent the proportion of onset at young age. Of course, elderly people can declare an onset at a young age, whereas young people cannot declare an onset at old age.

Average age of onset varies considerably according to the study, but the definition of onset is usually not clearly defined: 12 years in Faroe Islands, 23 in Denmark, 28 in the USA and 36 in the Hong Kong Chinese population (Lomholt 1964; Farber & Nall 1974; Holgate 1974). Peak is usually described between 5 and 20 years, with perhaps a trend for a lower age at onset in females. A bimodal distribution of age of onset was suggested in different studies (Burch & Rowell 1965; Burch & Rowell 1981; Ross 1971; Gunawardena *et al.* 1978; Smith *et al.* 1993), with a peak at 15–20 years and a second peak at 55–60 years.

4.1.5 Periodicity and severity

Studies conducted in patients referred to hospital and in patients of psoriasis societies or associations are probably biased by an excess of severe forms. To our knowledge, no longitudinal study is available which could describe the course of the disease. Although many surveys addressed the question of the severity of the psoriasis, no study has assessed prospectively the median frequency of attacks, the mean duration of remissions and their correlation with environmental and genetic factors.

New tools, such as the quality-of-life instruments, which can present another assessment of psoriasis severity (McKenna & Stern 1996), have not yet been used in epidemiological studies. They could, however, bring useful information about the patient point of view in assessing severity.

4.1.6 Mortality

The mortality directly or indirectly linked to psoriasis is close to zero. In 1991, a comprehensive review of the literature over a century showed that only 72 lethal psoriasis cases were reported, these were due to visceral amyloidosis, fatal complications of methotrexate, cardiovascular failure or cachexia in erythrodermic patients, liver biopsies or PUVA-induced genital skin cancer

(Roth *et al.* 1991). However, the increasing demand for care and the use of potentially more aggressive systemic therapies for longer periods may lead to an increase in the mortality in the next decades.

4.1.7 Disease associations

When examining disease associations the possibility that the disease under study could influence the diagnosis of the associated disease or its referral must be taken into account. In Sweden, hospitalized psoriasis cases were compared to the urban catchment population of the hospital (Lindegard 1986). Psoriasis was associated with an excess of viral infections, alcoholism, hypertension, pneumonia, liver cirrhosis, urticaria and rheumatoid arthritis, in both sexes, with iritis and ankylosing spondylitis in males, and with lung cancer, diabetes, obesity, myocardial infarction and asthma in females. However, hospital data are suspected to be biased by an excess of associated disorders. Psoriasis was also shown to be more common in patients with Crohn's disease than in controls (Lee *et al.* 1990). Although severe psoriasis has been reported in human immunodeficiency virus (HIV)-infected patients, the estimated prevalence of psoriasis in HIV patients does not appear to be much higher than in the general population (Farber 1991). Review of the literature shows that autoimmune diseases including bullous pemphigoid have already been reported with psoriasis, but there is no epidemiological evidence that this is more than a chance occurrence.

4.2 Genetic epidemiology: analysis of inheritance and definition of disease subsets

4.2.1 Analyses of surveys

Two large population-based Scandinavian surveys (Lomholt 1963; Hellgren 1967) studied the relatives of psoriasis patients. Both found increased incidence of psoriasis in relatives compared to the general population providing evidence for a genetic transmission of psoriasis. These studies have been submitted to several reanalyses (Ananthakrishnan *et al.* 1973, 1974; Iselius & Williams 1984). First hypotheses suggested a multifactorial type of inheritance. The latest reanalysis suggested a single gene inheritance (Iselius & Williams 1984). More recently, Swanbeck *et al.* (1997a) using questionnaires sent to 22 000 members of the Swedish Psoriasis Association were able to estimate the proportion of psoriasis among parents and siblings. The lifetime risk of psoriasis, if no parent, one parent or both parents have psoriasis, was measured at 0.04, 0.28 and 0.65, respectively, in a questionnaire survey of 3717 families (Swanbeck *et al.* 1997b). Their data are compatible with a recessive mode of inheritance, with two or more involved genes. A genomic imprinting in psoriasis gene has been suspected since penetrance was different depending on whether father or mother was affected (Traupe *et al.* 1992). The reanalysis of the Faroe Islands epidemiological data (Lomholt 1963) confirmed the higher penetrance of psoriasis when the father was involved or the presumed carrier.

4.2.2 Twin studies

Using the Danish twin registry, Bandrup *et al.* (1982) found that 63% of monozygotic probands had a psoriatic twin, thus yielding a heritability of 91%. A similar study in Australia gave lower estimates at 80% (Duffy *et al.* 1993).

4.2.3 HLA correlation studies

HLA associations have been studied for many years. Association with Cw6 is noteworthy (Elder *et al.* 1994), with a several-fold higher risk of developing psoriasis in people with HLA Cw6.

4.2.4 Definition of disease subsets

On the basis of the epidemiological data showing bimodality in the age at onset, Henseler and Christophers (1985) showed that the patients from the early-onset subgroup were at higher risk of having affected parents than patients from the late-onset subgroup. Familial forms (siblings with psoriasis) tend to be more frequent in early-onset psoriasis (Melski & Stern 1981). A strong positive association of early-onset cases with HLA Cw6 was demonstrated (Brenner *et al.* 1978; Tiilikainen *et al.* 1980; Henseler & Christophers 1985). Furthermore, in families with multiple psoriasis cases, age of onset was significantly earlier in HLA Cw6-positive siblings than in Cw6-negative siblings. Finally, this has led to the concept of two forms of psoriasis based on the model of diabetes or rheumatoid arthritis: hereditary, HLA-associated, early-onset, and severe psoriasis vs. sporadic, HLA-unrelated, late-onset and mild psoriasis. This is, however, an oversimplification. More recently, using a very large sample of psoriatic patients, Swanbeck *et al.* (1995), studied the age of onset not only in probands but also in siblings. They were able to recognize three variants of psoriasis which could be caused by three different genes.

4.3 Investigative epidemiology: environmental risk factors

As most epidemiological studies about environmental factors and psoriasis are cross-sectional, the temporal relationship between psoriasis and environmental exposures is difficult to assess. It is impossible to state whether psoriasis is the consequence, the cause or shares common aetiological factors with these exposures. Cohort studies, and case–control studies, although complicated by many biases (Naldi *et al.* 1994), are better options. However, depending on the selection of psoriasis cases and control population, 'risk factors for psoriasis' may correspond to quite distinct problems: risk factors for having clinical manifestations of psoriasis, risk factors for an early onset of the disease, risk factors for a flare-up of the disease, or risk factors for having a severe form of the disease. Unfortunately, the type of risk studied is not always clearly described in the different studies.

4.3.1 Infections

The role of streptococcal infections has been suspected as a triggering factor for psoriasis for many decades, especially in children and guttate forms. A survey of children showed that half of those with medically documented upper respiratory tract infection had an accompanying exacerbation of the disease (Nyfors & Lemholt 1975).

The association of streptococcal infection with acute guttate psoriasis has been confirmed by a cross-sectional study in different types of psoriasis (Telfer *et al.* 1992). The role of HIV infection in the worsening of psoriasis is debated. The estimated prevalence does not appear to be much higher in HIV patients than in the general population (Duvic *et al.* 1987). An open study has suggested an association between hepatitis C and psoriasis (Yamamoto *et al.* 1995), but this has not been yet confirmed by any controlled study.

4.3.2 Alcohol consumption and smoking

Multiple studies addressed this question and are reviewed by Naldi & Peli (1997). There is some evidence that psoriasis is associated with a number of diseases strongly linked to alcohol consumption and smoking (Lindegard 1986; Recchia *et al.* 1989; Lindelof *et al.* 1990; Olsen *et al.* 1992). Several case–control studies provided discordant results (Poikolainen *et al.* 1990; Mills *et al.* 1992; Naldi *et al.* 1996; Poikolainen *et al.* 1994). To summarize, these results show that smoking and alcohol consumption are not major factors in the epidemiology of psoriasis. However, they do not discard the possibility that they could be weak triggering factors for psoriasis onset or flare-up: smoking especially in women, and alcohol consumption especially in men.

4.3.3 Diet

Diet has received less attention. Coffee consumption (Naldi *et al.* 1992) and vitamin A level (Safavi 1992) were not confirmed to be risk factors and fish oil (Soyland *et al.* 1993) failed to demonstrate a beneficial effect in controlled studies. Although there is some epidemiological evidence that other nutriments might play a role in psoriasis (Naldi *et al.* 1996), further research is needed to draw conclusions.

4.3.4 Stress

The widely accepted role of stress as a trigger factor in psoriasis has never been properly established. Review of the literature (Gupta & Gupta 1997) suggests that stress from major life events, and some personality traits such as difficulty in expressing emotion, may play a role in psoriasis. Several uncontrolled studies have found a stressful event in a large proportion of patients in the months before the clinical onset of psoriasis (Gupta & Gupta 1997). In a case–control study, patients reported stress in the month before the onset of psoriasis (Seville 1977). However, monozygotic twins discordant for psoriasis appeared to have the same stress history (Brandrup *et al.* 1982). The assessment of the role of stress in promoting psoriasis flare-up is further hampered by the fact that disfigurement by psoriasis results in significant stress.

4.3.5 Drugs

Many drugs including lithium, β-adrenergic-receptor-blocking agents, antimalarials, systemic corticosteroids and non-steroidal anti-inflammatory drugs have been suspected to trigger psoriasis (Abel *et al.* 1986). Many observations and series of cases have been reported but to the best of our knowledge no controlled epidemiological study has ever assessed the risk of drug-induced flare-up in psoriasis.

4.4 Prevention

On the basis of the information provided by these epidemiological investigations, some preventive measures (Farber & Nall 1984) may be proposed in patients with psoriasis, such as stress reduction techniques (Gaston *et al.* 1991), exclusion of at-risk drugs and smoking limitation.

4.5 Prospectives

Although psoriasis is generally considered as a benign disorder due to the absence of mortality, assessment of morbidity shows that psoriasis is a common disease, with a severe impact on quality of life. This accounts for an important economical burden related to the severity of the disease (Feldman *et al.* 1997). Psoriasis cost was estimated in the USA in 1993 as being between $1.6 billion and $3.2 billion (Sander *et al.* 1993). A better assessment of the impact of the disease using quality of life and socioeconomic tools is needed.

Epidemiological investigations have provided evidence of the familial transmission of psoriasis. They have permitted interesting insights in the pattern
of inheritance of the disease. New techniques of genetics combined with epidemiological tools may aid the localization of the psoriasis genes.

Based on the available data about environmental risk factors, prevention
is not yet expected to change the course of the disease in patients with the
psoriasis genotype. Further investigations should focus on the environmental factors responsible for a disease flare-up.

References

Abel, E., DiCicco, L., Orenberg, E., Fraki, J. & Farber, E. (1986) Drugs in exacerbation of
    psoriasis. *Journal of the American Academy of Dermatology* **15**, 1007–1022.
Ananthakrishnan, R., Eckes, L. & Walter, H. (1973) On the genetics of psoriasis: an
    analysis of Hellgren's data for a model of multifactorial inheritance. *Archiv fur
    Dermatologische Forschung* **247**, 53–58.
Ananthakrishnan, R., Eckes, L. & Walter, H. (1974) On the genetics of psoriasis: an
    analysis of Lomholt's data from Faroe Islands for a multifactorial model of inherit-
    ance. *Journal of Genetics* **61**, 142–146.
Bedi, T. (1977) Psoriasis in North India. *Dermatologica* **155**, 310–314.
Bell, L., Sedlack, R., Beard, C., Perry, H., Michet, C. & Kurland, L. (1991) Incidence of
    psoriasis in Rochester, Minn. 1980–83. *Archives of Dermatology* **127**, 1184–1187.
Boyd, A. & Menter, A. (1989) Erythrodermic psoriasis. *Journal of the American Academy of
    Dermatology* **21**, 985–991.
Braathen, L.R., Botten, G. & Bjerkedal, T. (1989) Prevalence of psoriasis in Norway. *Acta
    Dermato-Venereologica Supplementum* **142**, 5–8.
Brandrup, F., Holm, N., Grunnet, N., Henningsen, K. & Hansen, H. (1982) Psoriasis in
    monozygotic twins: variations in expression in individuals with identical genetic
    constitution. *Acta Dermato-Venereologica* **62**, 229–236.
Brenner, W., Gschnait, F. & Mayr, W. (1978) HLA B13, B17, B37 and Cw6 in psoriasis
    vulgaris: association with age of onset. *Archives of Dermatological Research* **262**, 337–
    339.
Burch, P.R.J. & Rowell, N.R. (1965) Psoriasis: aetiological aspects. *Acta Dermato-
    Venereologica* **45**, 366–380.
Burch, P.R.J. & Rowell, N.R. (1981) Mode of inheritance in psoriasis. *Archives of Dermatol-
    ogy* **117**, 251.
Convit, C. (1962) Investigation of the incidence of psoriasis among Latin American
    Indians. In: *Proceedings of the 12th International Congress of Dermatology,* International
    Congress Series No. 55, Amsterdam.
Duffy, D., Spelman, L. & Martin, N. (1993) Psoriasis in Australian twins. *Journal of the
    American Academy of Dermatology* **29**, 428–434.
Duvic, M., Johnson, T. & Rapini, R. (1987) Acquired immunodeficiency syndrome
    associated psoriasis and Reiter's syndrome. *Archives of Dermatology* **123**, 1622–1632.
Elder, J., Nair, R. & Voorhees, J. (1994) Epidemiology and the genetics of psoriasis.
    Journal of Investigative Dermatology **102**, 24–27.
Farber, E.M. (1991) Epidemiology: natural history and genetics. In: *Psoriasis* (eds
    Roenigk, H.H. & Mainbach, H.I.), 2nd edn, pp. 209–258. Marcel Dekker, New York.
Farber, E.M. & Nall, M. (1974) The natural history of psoriasis in 5600 patients. *Derma-
    tologica* **148**, 1–18.
Farber, E. & Nall, L. (1984) An appraisal of measures to prevent and control psoriasis.

Journal of the American Academy of Dermatology **10**, 511–517.

Farber, E.M. & Nall, M.L. (1985) Epidemiology of psoriasis. In: *Psoriasis* (eds Roenigk, H.H. & Mainbach, H.I.), p. 141. Marcel Dekker, New York.

Farber, E.M., Bright, R.D. & Nall, M.L. (1968) Psoriasis. A questionnaire survey of 2144 patients. *Archives of Dermatology* **98**, 248–259.

Feldman, S., Fleischer, A., Reboussin, D. *et al.* (1997) The economic impact of psoriasis increases with psoriasis severity. *Journal of the American Academy of Dermatology* **37**, 564–569.

Gaston, L., Crombez, J.C., Lassonde, M., Bernier Buzzanga, J. & Hodgins, S. (1991) Psychological stress and psoriasis: experimental and prospective correlational studies. *Acta Dermato-Venereologica Supplementum* **156**, 37–43.

Gunawardena, D.A., Gunawardena, K.A., Vasanthanathan, N.S. & Gunawardena, J.A. (1978) Psoriasis in Sri Lanka: a computer analysis of 1366 cases. *British Journal of Dermatology* **98**, 85–96.

Gupta, M. & Gupta, A. (1997) Psychological factors and psoriasis. In: *Epidemiology, Causes and Prevention of Skin Diseases* (eds Grob, J.J., Stern, R., Mackie, R. & Weinstock, W.). Blackwell Science, Oxford.

Hellgren, L. (1967) *Psoriasis: the prevalence in sex, age and occupational groups in total populations in Sweden. Morphology, inheritance and association with other skin and rheumatic diseases.* Almquist & Wiksell, Stockholm.

Henseler, T. & Christophers, E. (1985) Psoriasis of early and late onset: characterization of two types of psoriasis vulgaris. *Journal of the American Academy of Dermatology* **13**, 450–456.

Holgate, M.C. (1974) The age of onset of psoriasis and the relationship to parental psoriasis. *British Journal of Dermatology* **92**, 443.

Iselius, L. & Williams, W. (1984) The mode of inheritance of psoriasis: evidence for a major gene as well as a multifactorial component and its implication for genetic counselling. *Human Genetics* **68**, 73–76.

Johnson, M. (1978) Skin conditions and related need for medical care among persons 1–74 years. United States 1971–74. Vital and Health Statistics. Series 11. (Data from the) *National Health Survey* **212**, DHEW Publication: PHS 79–1660.

Kavli, G., Stenvold, S.E. & Vandbakk, O. (1985) Low prevalence of psoriasis in Norwegian lapps. *Acta Dermato-Venereologica* **65**, 262–263.

Kononen, M., Torppa, J. & Lassus, A. (1986) An epidemiological survey of psoriasis in the greater Helsinki area. *Acta Dermato-Venereologica Supplementum* **124**, 3–10.

Lee, F., Bellary, S. & Francis, C. (1990) Increased occurrence of psoriasis in patients with Crohn's disease and their relatives. *American Journal of Gastroenterology* **85**, 962–963.

Lindegard, B. (1986) Diseases associated with psoriasis in a general population of 159,200 middle aged, urban native Swedes. *Dermatologica* **172**, 298–304.

Lindelof, B., Eklund, O., Liden, S. & Stern, R. (1990) The prevalence of malignant tumors in patients with psoriasis. *Journal of the American Academy of Dermatology* **22**, 1056–1060.

Lomholt, G. (1964) Prevalence of skin diseases in a population: a census study from the Faroe Islands. *Danish Medicine Bulletin* **11**, 1–7.

McKenna, K. & Stern, R. (1996) The outcomes movement and new measures of the severity of psoriasis. *Journal of the American Academy of Dermatology* **34**, 534–538.

Melski, J. & Stern, R. (1981) The separation of susceptibility of psoriasis from age at onset. *Journal of Investigative Dermatology* **77**, 474–477.

Mills, C., Srivastava, E. & Harvey, M. (1992) Smoking habits in psoriasis: a case control study. *British Journal of Dermatology* **127**, 18–21.

Naldi, L. & Peli, L. (1997) Alcohol, smoking and psoriasis. In: *Epidemiology, Causes and Prevention of Skin Diseases* (eds Grob, J.J., Stern, R., Mackie, R. & Weinstock, W.).

Blackwell Science, Oxford.

Naldi, L., Parazzini, F., Pali, L., Chatenoud, L. & Cainelli, T. (1996) Dietary factors and the risk of psoriasis. Results of an Italian case-control study. *British Journal of Dermatology* **134**, 101–106.

Naldi, L., Tognoni, G. & Cainelli, T. (1994) Analytic epidemiology in psoriasis. *Journal of Investigative Dermatology* **102**, 19–23.

Nevitt, G.J. & Hutchinson, P.E. (1996) Psoriasis in the community: prevalence, severity and patients' beliefs and attitudes towards the disease. *British Journal of Dermatology* **135**, 533–537.

Nyfors, A. & Lemholt, K. (1975) Psoriasis in children. A short review and a survey of 245 cases. *British Journal of Dermatology* **92**, 437–442.

Olsen, J., Moller, H. & Frentz, G. (1992) Malignant tumors in patients with psoriasis. *Journal of the American Academy of Dermatology* **27**, 716–722.

Poikolainen, K., Reunala, T. & Karvonen, J. (1994) Smoking alcohol and life events related to psoriasis among women. *British Journal of Dermatology* **130**, 473–477.

Poikolainen, K., Reunala, T., Karvonene, J., Lauhranta, J. & Karkkainen, P. (1990) Alcohol intake: a risk factor for psoriasis in young and middle aged men? *British Medicine Journal* **300**, 780–783.

Rea, J.N., Newhouse, M.L. & Halil, T. (1976) Skin disease in Lambeth. *British Journal of Preventive and Social Medicine* **30**, 107–114.

Recchia, G., Urbani, F., Tasin, L., Cristofolini, P., Scappini, P. & Bianchi, R. (1989) Epidemiology of psoriasis: a case control study in the province of Trentino (preliminary reports). *Acta Dermato-Venereologica Supplementum* **146**, 180–181.

Ross, H.G. (1971) Untersuchungen uber das entstehungsalter der psoriasis vulgaris. *Methods of Information in Medicine* **10**, 108–115.

Roth, P., Grosshans, E. & Bergoend, H. (1991) psoriasis: évolution et complications mortelles. *Annales de Dermatologie et de Venereologie* **118**, 97–105.

Safavi, K. (1992) Serum vitamin A levels in psoriasis: results from the first national health and nutrition examination survey. *Archives of Dermatology* **128**, 1130–1131.

Sander, H.M., Morris, L.F., Phillips, C.M., Harrison, P.E. & Menter, A. (1993) The annual cost of psoriasis. *Journal of the American Academy of Dermatology* **28**, 422–425.

Seville, R. (1977) Psoriasis and stress. *British Journal of Dermatology* **97**, 297–302.

Shing, Y.Y. (1984) The prevalence of psoriasis in the Mongoloid race. *Journal of the American Academy of Dermatology* **10**, 965–968.

Smith, A., Kassab, J., Rowland Payne, C. & Beer, W. (1993) Bimodality in age of onset of psoriasis, in both patients and their relatives. *Dermatology* **186**, 181–186.

Soyland, E., Funk, J. & Rajka, G. (1993) Effect of dietary supplementation with very long chain n-3 fatty acids in patients with psoriasis. *New England Journal of Medicine* **328**, 1812–1816.

Swanbeck, G., Inerot, A., Martinsson, T. *et al.* (1995) Age at onset and different types of psoriasis. *British Journal of Dermatology* **133**, 768–773.

Swanbeck, G., Inerot, A., Martinsson, T. *et al.* (1997a) Genetic counselling in psoriasis: empirical data on psoriasis among first-degree relatives of 3095 psoriatic probands. *British Journal of Dermatology* **137**, 939–942.

Swanbeck, G., Inerot, A., Martinsson, T. *et al* (1997b) Chapter 13. *Epidemiology, Causes and Prevention of Skin Diseases* (eds Grob, J.J., Stern, R., Mackie, R. & Weinstock, W.). Blackwell Science, Oxford.

Telfer, N., Chalmers, R., Whale, K. & Colman, G. (1992) The role of streptococcal infection in the initiation of guttate psoriasis. *Archives of Dermatology* **128**, 39–42.

Tiilikainen, A., Lassus, A., Karvonene, J., Vartiainen, P. & Julin, M. (1980) Psoriasis and HLA Cw6. *British Journal of Dermatology* **102**, 1079–1184.

Traupe, H., Van Gurp, P., Happle, R., Bozeman, J. & van de Kerkhof, P. (1992) Psoriasis vulgaris, fetal growth, and genomic imprinting. *American Journal of Medicine Genetics* **42**, 649–654.

Yamamoto, T., Katayama, I. & Nishioka, K. (1995) Psoriasis and hepatitis C virus. *Acta Dermato-Venereologica* **75**, 482–483.

Chapter 5: The Complex Genetics

H. Traupe

5.1 Introduction

Psoriasis is a common chronic inflammatory and hyperproliferative skin disease affecting about 2–3% of Caucasian populations (Lomholt 1963). The development of clinically manifest psoriasis requires an interaction between a genetically determined predisposition for the disease and environmental stimuli. Clinical observation and recent immunological research has lead to new concepts explaining how well-known environmental stimuli such as the infection with β-haemolytic streptoccocci could trigger the disease, for example by the secretion of a super antigen stimulating T lymphocytes (Boehncke *et al.* 1997). However, why stimulation of T lymphocytes in some patients finally results in clinical psoriasis remains unclear and will require the identification of the other side of the coin, namely of the genes contributing to the psoriasis phenotype.

5.2 Population-based and family studies

In questionnaire studies or when taking direct histories of patients in clinical situations, about 30–50% of all patients with psoriasis indicate that they are aware of one or more affected first- or second-degree relative (Andreßen & Henseler 1982). A recent survey comprising 589 patients from the Münster Department of Dermatology showed that 41% have a positive family history for psoriasis (Traupe *et al.* 1998). In contrast, a census study performed by Lomholt (1963) on the Faroe islands involving the examination of 10 984 inhabitants reported an occurrence of 90% among first- and second-degree relatives.

This study is the most carefully controlled population-based study that clearly underlines the fact that psoriasis has a genetic basis. The discrepancy between the figure of 41% familial occurrence obtained in a Westfalian population sample in northern Germany and that of 90% on the Faroe islands has probably two reasons: The populations on the Faroe islands is highly interrelated (inbred) because most inhabitants are descendants of the Vikings and it is reasonable to assume a genetic founder effect for psoriasis in this population. Second, a questionnaire study may underestimate the true prevalence of psoriasis, especially in uncles and grandparents, as a very mild disease manifestation in distant relatives may be unknown to the family member completing the questionnaire. However, for first-degree relatives questionnaire studies give a pretty realistic picture (Swanbeck *et al.* 1994). Therefore it is reasonable to assume that about 50% of all psoriasis patients in Caucasian populations suffer from a familial type of psoriasis.

The reason for geneticists and clinicians worldwide concentrating their interests on these 50% is that we tacitly assume that the very same genes that can be found in familial psoriasis will also be of importance in sporadic or seemingly non-familial psoriasis.

It is of interest that the data obtained by Lomholt (1963) in his census study and by several questionnaire studies all show a variable genetic risk. In other words for siblings of an affected proband the genetic risk of developing psoriasis is not constant but depends on the individual family situation. In the Lomholt study this risk ranged from 12 to 14% when no parent was affected but rose to 34–39% when one parent had psoriasis (Lomholt 1963). Andreßen and Henseler (1982) found a risk of only 6.6% for a sibling of the index patient when no parent was affected, this risk rose to 40% when both the mother and father had the disease.

In clinical practice parents with psoriasis very often wish to know the risk of their child developing psoriasis. The answer should be based on the data taken from the Lomholt study from the Faroe islands as shown in Table 5.1. Recent data from a Swedish survey are also provided. These data (Swanbeck *et al.* 1997) were obtained from members of the Swedish Psoriasis Association and may not reflect the population of Sweden at large. However, in my personal experience with German patients the risk is considerably lower and should be halved for most situations.

Twin studies provide further strong data for a major genetic influence in psoriasis. In a carefully conducted study from Denmark Brandrup *et al.* (1982) using the Danish Twin Register found among 32 monozygotic twin pairs a pairwise concordance of 56% while earlier retrospective studies had even yielded concordance rates of up to 70% (Farber *et al.* 1974). Interestingly Brandrup and coworkers could not find major environmental factors or other

Table 5.1 Risk for a child to develop psoriasis.

Situation	Faroe Islands (%)	Sweden (%)	Germany (%)
(a) No parent or sibling affected	2.84	4	2
(b) Parents unaffected, one sibling affected	17	24	6.6
(c) One parent affected, so far no sibling affected	25	28	14
(d) One parent affected and one sibling affected	31	51	no data
(e) Both parents affected, so far no sibling affected	78	65	41
(f) Both parents affected and one sibling affected	no data	83	no data

Data are taken from Lomholt 1963 (Faroe Islands), Swanbeck *et al.* 1997 (Sweden), and Andreßen and Henseler 1982 (Germany). For situation (c) we found, in Münster, a risk of 13.6% if the parent is a father and a risk of 9.5% if the parent is a mother. Swanbeck and coworkers used a life-time risk approach.

exogeneous factors that influenced age of onset or course and severity of the disease. Rather, they emphasized that in concordant monozygotic twins morphology and age of onset were rather alike and thus also seemed to be under genetic control.

Interpreting these data one has to conclude that psoriasis is not a single gene disorder but that a limited number of genes (oligogenic gene concept) are involved (Elder *et al.* 1994; Traupe 1995).

5.3 Recessive or dominant genes?

The next question which arises is whether the genes involved in psoriasis are dominant or recessive.

Because it is possible to record a large number of pedigrees in which the disease runs in families from one generation to the other, most scientists assume that psoriasis is caused by autosomal dominant genes. The best example to date for this was reported by Abele *et al.* (1963) who studied a large kindred from North Carolina comprising 402 examined family members of which 44 were affected. In this family a penetrance of 60% was estimated based on the percentage of unaffected parents giving rise to affected children.

However, the situation may be more complex and recently Swanbeck *et al.* (1994) obtained questionnaire data from more than 5197 members of the Swedish Psoriasis Association. In this study group they found that only 36% of the probands had an affected parent, while 64% actually lacked such a parent. Interestingly they also found that among those lacking an affected parent the risk for further siblings to be affected approximated 25%. In Sweden psoriasis is very frequent and has a prevalence of about 5%. Therefore Swanbeck *et al.* (1994) argued that if one assumed a very high gene frequency of 25% for the psoriasis gene in the general population then the recessive gene hypothesis would fit the data very nicely. Under a recessive gene hypothesis and under the assumption of a very frequent mutant gene, the penetrance of this gene would approximate 92.5%.

The argument of Swanbeck and coworkers cannot be simply discarded because their line of reasoning would explain why the vast majority of our patients do not have an affected parent suffering from the disease. However, a gene frequency of 0.25 is very high and means that one-quarter of the population should have the predisposing gene. In other words the predisposing gene would not be a rare mutant but more like a common polymorphism that could be interpreted, for example, in terms of a gain of function mutation, for instance of a gene involved in cutaneous inflammation.

While this is of course possible a number of points argue against the recessive hypothesis. As already pointed out a gene frequency of 0.25 is extremely high and so far such common mutant genes have not been found in other multifactorial diseases such as diabetes mellitus. Moreover, it would be very difficult to explain the fact that psoriasis is often transmitted in some families through three or four generations and the phenomenon of a preferential paternal inheritance can hardly be explained by a recessive gene (see below).

It is very difficult to understand that even today we cannot firmly decide whether the major predisposing genes in psoriasis are inherited in an autosomal dominant or in a recessive mode, but the answer to this may well be that perhaps three of four genes are inherited as autosomal dominant traits and one acts in a recessive manner and that for an individual to develop manifest disease only two of the different predisposing genes may be required.

5.4 Preferential paternal inheritance

Substantial evidence for the involvement of at least one gene being inherited in an autosomal dominant mode comes from the observation of a preferential paternal inheritance of psoriasis in most studies. Traupe *et al.* (1992) found two independent lines of evidence suggesting a paternal effect on the inheritance of psoriasis. First the birth weight of children of psoriatic patients was influenced by the sex of the psoriatic parent, children of fathers with psoriasis being heavier than children of mothers with psoriasis ($p = 0.0004$). Second, a reanalysis of the pedigree material provided by Lomholt in his studies on the Faroe islands revealed that disease manifestation depends in part on the sex of the psoriatic parent. For this type of analysis only children above the age of 20 years were included because of the age dependency of psoriasis.

Traupe *et al.* (1992) found that offspring of fathers with psoriasis and male gene carriers were significantly ($p = 0.015$ and $p = 0.007$) more often affected than offspring of mothers with psoriasis and female gene carriers. A review of published series of pedigrees by Theeuwes and Morhenn (1995) confirms that most but not all studies show a small paternal effect. Surprisingly, the paternal effect on susceptibility to psoriasis does not seem to be associated with an earlier age of onset. In a German patient group from Münster comprising 589 patients paternal inheritance was present in 80 cases (13.6%) while maternal transmission was seen in 56 cases (9.5%, $p = 0.015$) but paternal inheritance did not result in an earlier age of onset (Traupe *et al.* 1998). It is also of interest that in an ongoing gene-mapping study selecting families from the Münster patient group the paternal effect was no longer present (Traupe *et al.* 1998). We attribute this to the selection procedure which required for example at least three available affected family members. Molecular genetic studies lend further support to the paternal effect on susceptibility to psoriasis: Burden *et al.* (1998) performed a sibling-pair study and could show that evidence for linkage to chromosome 6p was greatest when the allele was of paternal origin and was most significant in those families without psoriatic arthritis. In contrast there was no paternal effect seen for loci on chromosome 17q and chromosome 4q.

5.4.1 Possible mechanism for the paternal effect

While a paternal effect on the susceptibility to psoriasis is now firmly established, the mechanism by which this effect is achieved remains to be established. Traupe *et al.* (1992) originally suggested genomic imprinting. This concept is now often referred to as gametic imprinting because this latter term conceives the monoparental specificity of this type of imprinting behaviour and implies that modifications made in the gamete can be inherited by the zygote (Barlow 1994). Gametic imprinting implies the existence of at least two genes: a major gene that receives the imprint and a modifying gene that establishes this imprint (Hall 1990). Gametic imprinting is today considered as a reversible process whereby a gamete-specific modification in the parental generation can sometimes lead to functional differences between maternal and paternal genome in diploid cells of the offspring (Barlow 1994). At a molecular level methylation of so-called CpG islands has been found, for example, for the imprinted locus IGF2-MPR which encodes the insulin-like growth factor type 2 receptor and for IGF2 which encodes the insulin-like growth factor type 2 (reviewed by Barlow 1994). In the past it was often assumed that a paternal effect meant that the paternal gene copy had received a primary gametic imprint rendering it to be more active (Hall 1990). Molecular studies involving the insulin-like growth factor 2 and its receptor have shown the opposite. A paternally expressed gene usually accounts for a paternal effect because the maternal gene is repressed.

A second and alternative mechanism that can result in a paternal effect is the instability of a premutation in mitosis (Zheng *et al.* 1993). It has been well known for a long time that a number of diseases such as Huntington's chorea and the fragile X syndrome show a clear-cut paternal effect and that age of onset in these syndromes usually is much earlier when the genetic disposition is transmitted from the father. In both these disorders the underlying genes have been cloned and a new mutation mechanism has been discovered—an unstable premutation that is caused by a DNA repeat consisting of three base pairs. Such trinucleotide repeats can also be found in normal individuals, but they are increased in size in affected persons.

Once they are amplified above a critical size they interfere with normal gene expression and cause disease. Zheng *et al.* (1993) explained the paternal effect in Huntington's chorea and fragile X syndrome by the instability of the premutation in mitosis. They argue that in contrast to oogenesis, spermatogenesis is an ongoing process involving many more mitoses than oogenesis which would give the premutation a better chance to be amplified and to gain clinical relevance when being transmitted from the father. Both, Zheng *et al.* (1994) and Theeuwes and Morhenn (1995) have suggested interpreting the paternal effect in psoriasis by the 'allelic instability in mitosis' model. However, our recent observation that the paternal effect on the susceptibility to psoriasis is not associated with a decreased age of onset (see above) makes this mechanism less likely than classic gametic (genomic) imprinting (Traupe *et al.* 1998).

5.5 HLA associations and the age of onset

It has been known for a long time that the possession of certain HLA class I antigens such as A1, B13, B17, B37 and Cw6 is associated with an earlier age of onset in psoriasis (Russel *et al.* 1972; Brenner *et al.* 1978). Later it was found that the HLA class II antigens DR7 as well as other HLA D antigens such as DRB1*0701/2 is likewise associated with early onset psoriasis (Schmitt-Egenolf *et al.* 1993). About 90% of patients with early onset and 50% of patients with a late onset are Cw6 positive, compared with 7.4% in randomly assigned normal probands (Henseler & Christophers 1985). However, there is also an ethnic component in the HLA associations since in Japanese psoriasis patients the profile of HLA-associated antigens differs from that seen in Caucasian patients and only 26% of all psoriatic patients have Cw6; another 17% are positive for Cw7 (Ozawa *et al.* 1988).

A peculiar property of HLA antigens is that some of them preferentially associate with each other and are often transmitted in a fixed haplotype. For Japanese an extended risk haplotype conferring a high risk for psoriasis to the patients has been described. This haplotype comprises the antigens HLA A2, Cw11, Bw 46, C2C, BFS, C4A4, C4B2 and DRw8. Recently Schmitt-Egenolf was able to show that in German patients a similar extended haplotype exists which is preferentially associated with HLA antigens Cw6-B57-DRB1*0701-DQA1*0201-DQB1*0303 (Schmitt-Egenolf *et al.* 1996) and they were able to show that this haplotype is over-represented in familial early onset psoriasis but not in sporadic late onset psoriasis. This particular haplotype was found in about 35% of type I psoriasis patients but only in 2% of controls. Individuals having this haplotype therefore carry a 26-fold risk of developing early onset psoriasis than individuals who are negative for this haplotype.

From the above it becomes evident that a gene residing in the HLA region is involved in the genetics of psoriasis. Recently, several groups have been able to map such a gene to the HLA region on the short arm of chromosome 6 using—rather surprisingly—a model-free approach and the gene-hunter program (Nair *et al.* 1997; Trembath *et al.* 1997). Previously, several studies using dominant models had failed to show clear-cut linkage of the predisposing gene for psoriasis to the HLA region (reviewed in Traupe 1995). A sibling-pair study also confirms the chromosome 6 locus when analysing siblings with an affected father only (Burden *et al.* 1998).

While it is today more or less assumed that at least one predisposing gene resides in the HLA region, most likely this is not Cw6 itself. Rather, Cw6 seems to have a direct influence on the age of onset, that is, on the manifestation of psoriasis as was shown by Enerbäck *et al.* (1997) who demonstrated a significantly younger age at onset for the HLA Cw6-positive siblings in a series of siblings who both had psoriasis but were discordant for having Cw6.

5.5.1 Is type I psoriasis biologically distinct from type II psoriasis?

Different age of onset peaks in patients with psoriasis were detected by Henseler and Christophers (1985) and were interpreted by them in such a way that two different forms of psoriasis exist. According to their classification, type I psoriasis is characterized by associated HLA antigens such as Cw6 and DR7 and age of onset is before the age of 40 years with a peak at the age of 16 (female) or 22 (male) years. Patients with type II psoriasis according to Henseler and Christophers lack the HLA antigen DR7 and have an onset beyond 40 years with a peak at 60 years (female) or 57 years (male).

From these data Henseler and Christophers (1985) concluded that type I psoriasis and type II psoriasis should be biologically distinct. However, as discussed above these differences in age of onset may be influenced in part by HLA antigens such as Cw6 and by a number of other genetics systems. For example the α_1-antitrypsin gene and a polymorphism of the apolipoprotein E gene (Furumoto *et al.* 1997) have likewise been associated with an earlier age of onset in psoriasis. Other investigators (Swanbeck *et al.* 1995) have found evidence for three different maxima at puberty and 30 and 50 years of age. In gene-mapping studies age of onset has not proved so far to be clearly related to a specific predisposing gene. While a genetic contribution to the age of onset is now well established, the genes responsible, for example, for an early onset may not be the same as those that underlie the disease. It remains to be seen whether type I psoriasis is really biologically distinct from type II psoriasis.

5.6 Gene-mapping studies

From the above evidence it is clear that psoriasis has a strong genetic basis in about 40% of the patients, but that this basis is rather complex and that this genetic disposition cannot be easily interpreted along the lines of classical Mendelian inheritance. While new genetic concepts such as gametic (genomic) imprinting may explain the paternal effect other features such as the discordance among monozygotic twins remain rather puzzling. To gain more insights into the genetics of psoriasis a number of scientific groups worldwide have concentrated their efforts and perform genome-wide scans in large sets of psoriasis families with the aim of first mapping and finally cloning the predisposing genes for psoriasis. The current state of the field can be summarized as follows: there is clear-cut evidence now from several studies for a predisposing gene on the long arm of chromosome 17; however, this gene in most studies does not seem to account for a large proportion of the genetic disposition and can be found only in a small subset of the families (Tomfohrde *et al.* 1994; Nair *et al.* 1997; Trembath *et al.* 1997). The HLA region on the short arm of chromosome 6 certainly also contains a predisposing locus which as has been discussed above has been identified mainly in model-free so-called non-parametric analysis systems using the gene-hunter program (Trembath *et al.* 1997; Nair *et al.* 1997). According to the work of Trembath *et al.* (1997) this locus is found in about 35% of the British families. As already discussed the locus on 6p may be imprinted (maternally repressed), as a sibling-pair study shows a paternal effect (Burden *et al.* 1998). Recently Capon and coworkers found a third locus for psoriasis on the long arm of chromosome 1 close to the centromere (Capon *et al.* 1999). Surprisingly, our own group from Münster has been unable to identify this locus so far.

An Irish group (Matthews *et al.* 1996) has identified in Irish families a locus on the long arm of chromosome 4, but so far these results could not be replicated by other groups.

5.6.1 The need for replication

In this context it has to be stressed that replication is of course of paramount importance but that on the other hand ethnic differences may also exist. A gene that may be mutated and a driving force for psoriasis disposition in one population does not need necessarily to be as important in other populations. The group from Kiel has performed further studies on the 6p locus in the HLA region and has analysed a large number of trios with the so-called transmission disequilibrium test (TDT) (Jenisch *et al.* 1998). This test is especially suited to reveal whether a genetic marker is associated with the disease. The TDT was first introduced by Spielman *et al.* (1993) who studied the genetics of diabetes mellitus. In the TDT markers from the HLA region from a region of 330 kilobases which contained both HLA B and C genes showed significant *p* values for association with psoriasis, while flanking markers showed insignificant *p* values suggesting that the psoriasis gene in the HLA region should be located within this block of 330 kilobases between the HLA B and HLA C locus.

In addition to the gene which is probably located here other genetic components in the HLA region may also contribute to psoriasis. For example Höhler *et al.* (1997) using a case–control design recently reported the association between a promoter polymorphism at -238 in the tumour necrosis factor α (TNF-α) gene and early-onset psoriasis.

We ourselves wanted to replicate these findings and analysed 83 trios using the transmission disequilibrium test with regard to the promoter polymorphism at -238 in the TNF-α gene. Surprisingly, we could not confirm an association between this polymorphism by the TDT test (Jacob *et al.* 1998). This means that although it is possible that a polymorphism in this gene contributes to the manifestation of psoriasis, this polymorphism is not the major gene nor is it in linkage disequilibrium with the major gene causing the disease in the respective trios (Jacob *et al.* 1999).

5.7 Conclusions

Psoriasis has a complex genetic basis. Many aspects of the disease such as age of onset are under genetic control, but the genetic factors involved such as the HLA Cw6 gene are not necessarily those which provide the major predisposing genes in this disease. Rather they may act as enhancers for the genetic disposition. The same could be true for the promoter polymorphism in the TNF-α gene. By replicated studies, at present two chromosomal regions have been identified which contain a psoriasis-predisposing gene. These are a region on 17q, and a region on the short arm of chromosome 6 which has been narrowed down to a block of 330 kilobases between the genes for HLA B and C. There are a number of further candidate regions containing putative psoriasis genes and the locus heterogeneity of psoriasis may be greater than so far expected. Progress in the molecular genetics of psoriasis has been slow but steady and it is realistic to assume that within the next couple of years the two genes that have so far been mapped will also be cloned. Hopefully cloning will then also provide us with new insights into the function of these genes and give us a much better understanding why our patients finally develop the disease.

References

Abele, D.C., Dobson, R.L. & Graham, J.B. (1963) Heredity and psoriasis. *Archives of Dermatology* **88**, 38–47.

Andreßen, C. & Henseler, T. (1982) Erblichkeit der Psoriasis. *Hautarzt* **33**, 214–217.

Barlow, D.P. (1994) Imprinting: a gamete's point of view. *Trends in Genetics* **10**, 194–199.

Boehncke, W.H., Zollner, T.M., Dressel, D. & Kaufmann, R. (1997) Induction of psoriasiform inflammation by a bacterial superantigen in the SCID-hu xenogeneic transplantation model. *Journal of Cutaneous Pathology* **24**, 1–7.

Brandrup, F., Holm, N., Grunnet, N., Henningsen, K. & Hansen, H.E. (1982) Psoriasis in monozygotic twins: variations in expression in individuals with identical genetic constitution. *Acta Dermato-Venereologica* **62**, 229–236.

Brenner, W., Gschnait, F. & Mayr, W.R. (1978) HLA B13, B17, B37, and Cw6 in psoriasis vulgaris: association with the age of onset. *Archives of Dermatological Research* **262**, 337–339.

Burden, D., Javed, S., Bailey, M., Hodgins, M., Connor, M. & Tillman, D. (1998) Genetics of psoriasis: paternal inheritance and a locus on chromosome 6p. *Journal of Investigative Dermatology* **110**, 958–960.

Capon, F., Novelli, G., Semprini, S. *et al.* (1999) Scanning for psoriasis susceptibility genes in Italy: genome scan and evidence for a new locus on chromosome 1. *Journal of Investigative Dermatology* **112**, 32–35.

Elder, J.T., Nair, R.P., Guo, S.W., Henseler, T., Christophers, E. & Voorhees, J.J. (1994) The genetics of psoriasis. *Archives of Dermatology* **130**, 216–224.

Enerbäck, C., Martinsson, T., Inerot, A. *et al.* (1997) Significantly earlier age of onset for the HLA-Cw6-positive than for the Cw6-negative psoriatic sibling. *Journal of Investigative Dermatology* **108**, 695–696.

Farber, E.M., Nall, L. & Watson, W. (1974) Natural history of psoriasis in 61 twin pairs. *Archives of Dermatology* **109**, 207–211.

Furumoto, H., Nakamura, K., Imamura, T. *et al.* (1997) Association of apolipoprotein allele epsilon 2 with psoriasis vulgaris in the Japanese population. *Archives of Dermatological Research* **289**, 497–500.

Hall, J.G. (1990) Genomic imprinting: review and relevance to human diseases. *American Journal of Human Genetics* **46**, 857–873.

Henseler, T. & Christophers, E. (1985) Psoriasis of early and late onset: characterization of two types of psoriasis vulgaris. *Journal of the American Academy of Dermatology* **13**, 450–456.

Höhler, T., Kruger, A., Schneider, P.M. *et al.* (1997) A TNF-α promoter polymorphism is associated with juvenile onset psoriasis and psoriatic arthritis. *Journal of Investigative Dermatology* **109**, 562–565.

Jacob, N., Rüschendorf, F., Schmitt-Egenolf, M. *et al.* (1999) Promoter polymorphism at -238 of the tumor necrosis factor alpha gene is not associated with early onset psoriasis when tested by the transmission disequilibrium test. *Journal of Investigative Dermatology* **112**, 514–515.

Jenisch, S., Henseler, T., Nair, R.P. *et al.* (1998) Linkage analysis of human leukocyte antigen (HLA) markers in familial psoriasis: strong disequilibrium effects provide evidence for a major determinant in the HLA-B/-C region. *American Journal of Human Genetics* **63**, 191–199.

Lomholt, G. (1963) *Psoriasis. Prevalence, Spontaneous Course, and Genetics.* GEL Gad, Copenhagen.

Matthews, D., Fry, L., Powles, A., Weber, J. *et al.* (1996) Evidence that a locus for familial psoriasis maps to chromosome 4q. *Nature Genetics* **14**, 231–233.

Nair, R.P., Henseler, T., Jenisch, S. *et al.* (1997) Evidence for two psoriasis susceptibility loci (HLA and 17q) and two novel candidate regions (16q and 20p) by genome-wide scan. *Human Molecular Genetics* **6**, 1349–1356.

Ozawa, A., Ohkido, M., Inoko, H., Ando, A. & Tsuji, K. (1988) Specific restriction fragment length polymorphism of the HLA-C region and susceptibility to psoriasis vulgaris. *Journal of Investigative Dermatology* **90**, 402–405.

Russel, T.J., Schultes, L.M. & Kuban, D.J. (1972) Histocompatibility (HL-A) antigens associated with psoriasis. *New England Journal of Medicine* **287**, 738–740.

Schmitt-Egenolf, M., Boehncke, W.H., Ständer, M., Eiermann, T.H. & Sterry, W. (1993) Oligonucleotide typing reveals association of type I psoriasis with the HLA-DRB1* 0701/2-DQA1*0201-DQB1*0303 extended haplotype. *Journal of Investigative Dermatology* **100**, 749–752.

Schmitt-Egenolf, M., Eiermann, T.H., Boehncke, W.H., Ständer, M. & Sterry, W. (1996) Familial juvenile onset psoriasis is associated with the human leukocyte antigen (HLA) class I side of the extended haplotype Cw6–B57-DRB1*0701-DQA1*0201-DQB1*0303: a population- and family-based study. *Journal of Investigative Dermatology* **106**, 711–714.

Spielman, R.S., McGinnis, R.E. & Ewens, W.J. (1993) Transmission test for linkage disequilibrium: the insulin gene region and insulin-dependent diabetes mellitus (IDDM). *American Journal of Human Genetics* **52**, 506–516.

Swanbeck, G., Inerot, A., Martinsson, T. *et al.* (1997) Genetic counselling in psoriasis: empirical data on psoriasis among first-degree relatives of 3095 psoriatic probands.

British Journal of Dermatology **137**, 939–942.

Swanbeck, G., Inerot, A., Martinsson, T. & Wahlström, J.W. (1994) A population genetic study of psoriasis. *British Journal of Dermatology* **131**, 32–39.

Swanbeck, G., Inerot, A., Martinsson, T. *et al.* (1995) Age at onset and different types of psoriasis. *British Journal of Dermatology* **133**, 768–773.

Theeuwes, M. & Morhenn, V. (1995) Allelic instability in the mitosis model and the inheritance of psoriasis. *Journal of the American Academy of Dermatology* **32**, 44–52.

Tomfohrde, J., Silverman, A., Barnes, R. *et al.* (1994) Gene for familial psoriasis suscepti-bility mapped to the distal end of human chromosome 17q. *Science* **264**, 1141–1145.

Traupe, H. (1995) The puzzling genetics of psoriasis. *Clinics Dermatology* **13**, 99–103.

Traupe, H., van Gurp, J.M., Happle, R., Boezeman, J. & van de Kerkhof, P.C.M. (1992) Psoriasis vulgaris, fetal growth, and genomic imprinting. *American Journal of Medical Genetics* **42**, 649–654.

Traupe, H., Saar, K., Mehrens, C. *et al.* (1998) Further evidence for a paternal effect in susceptibility to psoriasis vulgaris and failure to confirm a locus on chromosome 20 in German families. *Archives of Dermatological Research* **290**, 56 (Abstract).

Trembath, R.C., Clough, R.L., Rosbotham, J.L. *et al.*(1997) Identification of a major susceptibility locus on chromosome 6p and evidence for further disease loci revealed by a two stage genome-wide search in psoriasis. *Human Molecular Genetics* **6**, 813–820.

Zheng, C.J., Byers, B. & Moolgavkar, S.H. (1993) Allelic instability in mitosis: a unified model for dominant disorders. *Proceedings of the National Academy of Sciences of the USA* **90**, 10178–10182.

Zheng, C.J., Thomson, G. & Peng, Y.N. (1994) Allelic instability in mitosis can explain 'genome imprinting' and other genetic phenomena in psoriasis. *American Journal of Medical Genetics* **51**, 163–164.

Chapter 6: Pathogenesis

P.C.M. van de Kerkhof

6.1 Introduction

It is widely accepted that a genetic defect underlies the pathogenesis of psoriasis. Most authors agree that the predisposition to psoriasis is due to a poly-
genic inheritance (Chapter 5). On the other hand triggering factors are
involved in the elicitation of psoriatic lesions in genetically predisposed subjects (Chapter 1).

   Both systemic factors and local factors are involved in the pathogenesis of
psoriasis (Chapter 1). Within the skin, several features are believed to have a
primary role in the pathogenesis of the disease. Systemic factors, cutaneous
inflammation, changes of the stroma, proliferation and differentiation of
keratinocytes, and signal transducing pathways are those which will be discussed in this chapter. In Chapter 7 the immune system will be described in
more detail. The immunopathogenesis of psoriasis provides the rationale for
recently developed immunomodulating treatments.

6.2 Systemic factors

Systemic factors are involved in the pathogenesis of psoriasis. Direct evidence for a causal relationship is provided by the following clinical observations.

1   The symptomless skin of psoriatic patients may respond to an injury with
the appearance of a psoriatic lesion (Koebner response). This is an all-or-
none phenomenon; if the elicitation occurs at one site, it occurs at all sites.
2   Several systemic factors may aggravate psoriasis:
   (a) psychological stress;
   (b) focal infections;
   (c) some drugs.
Several systemic abnormalities have been described. So far it is not clear as to
what extent these are causative for psoriasis or resulting from psoriasis.

6.2.1 Circulating blood polymorphonuclear leucocytes

Chemotactic responsiveness of polymorphonuclear leucocytes (PMN) has been
reported by various groups to be normal, increased or decreased. The most
likely explanation is the variation in clinical expression. Patients with chronic

stable plaque psoriasis had relatively low values and patients with actively spreading lesions had relatively high levels; The extent of the lesions was not correlated to PMN chemotaxis (Langner *et al.* 1983; Pease *et al.* 1987).

Using an *in vitro* assay to study PMN adherence to endothelium the following observations were reported by Sedgwick *et al.* (1980). Patients with minimal disease activity had normal adherence activity, patients with moderate and extensive disease had increased values for PMN adherence. Patients with inflammatory conditions other than psoriasis had increased PMN adherence values (Csato *et al.* 1983).

Recently, CD11b expression was measured on peripheral blood PMN (van Pelt *et al.* 1997). CD11b is part of the β2-integrin receptor MAC-1. CD11b proved to be decreased in psoriatic patients, irrespective of their clinical severity.

6.2.2 Psoriatic sera and modulation of polymorphonuclear leucocyte functions

Chemokinetic activity of psoriatic sera for PMN have been reported to be increased and decreased (Kawohl *et al.* 1980; Sedgwick *et al.* 1981).

In serum of psoriatic patients increased levels of skin-associated antileucoprotease (SKALP) have been demonstrated (Alkemade *et al.* 1995). SKALP is a proteinase inhibitor and might be of relevance to counteract elastase, released by the PMN. Elastase action is required for the movement of PMN into the epidermis.

6.2.3 Endocrine factors

Several hormones have been reported to have abnormal plasma levels in psoriasis. These hormones are: dehydroepiandrosterone (Holzman *et al.* 1976), aldosterone (van de Kerkhof 1982) and somatotropic hormone (Weber *et al.* 1981).

A causal role of these hormones in the pathogenesis has not yet been proven.

6.2.4 Other plasma and serum abnormalities

During the last decade a plethora of abnormalities have been reported (Table 6.1) which all are related to inflammation. None of these changes have been shown to have a causal significance.

6.3 Cutaneous inflammation and stroma

The inflammatory infiltrate of the psoriatic lesion varies with the manifestation of the disease. Recently the inflammatory infiltrate in psoriasis has been

Table 6.1 Other plasma and serum abnormalities in psoriasis.

Abnormality	Reference
Increased sedimentation rate	(Samitz and Pomerantz 1959)
Increased C-reactive protein	(Shuster 1958)
Increased α_2-macroglobulin	(Herschell 1971)
Increased IgA	(Kikindjanin and Milakov 1976)
Decreased IgM	(Kikindjanin and Milakov 1976)
Immunocomplexes	(Karsh 1978)
Inhibitor of E-rosette formation	(Glinski 1978)

reviewed extensively by Christophers and Mrowietz (1995). In this section, a few aspects are presented.

Important subpopulations are PMN, monocytes/macrophages and T lymphocytes.

Immunophenotypical studies have shown that infiltrate cells are in the activated state and express a variety of adhesion molecules and cytokines.

6.3.1 Polymorphonuclear leucocytes

PMN accumulation in the epidermis provides a specific aspect: the spongiforme pustulus of Kogoj and the microabscesses of Munro. PMN adhesion to psoriatic epidermis was found to be greatly enhanced compared to normal skin. Adhesion was most pronounced in areas were the expression of intercellular adhesion molecule 1 (ICAM-1) serves as an anchoring structure for PMN in the psoriatic epidermis. In the psoriatic plaque PMN are activated. This may be due to a large spectrum of activating factors including: complement-split product 5a (C5a), interleukin 8 (IL-8), GRO-α and arachidonic acid metabolites such as 12-hydroeicosatetraenoic acid and leucotriene B$_4$ (Barker *et al.* 1992; Schröder *et al.* 1992).

6.3.2 Monocytes and macrophages

Monocytes and tissue macrophages are consistently present in all manifestations of psoriasis. In about two-thirds of psoriatic lesions, lining macrophages may be found. They have been designated as such by their band-like appearance directly beneath the basal membrane (Wortmann *et al.* 1993; van de Oord & de Wolf-Peeter 1994). In more than one-third of patients, lining macrophages can be observed as a single cell layer immediately under the tips of the rete ridges.

Phenotypical characterization revealed that lining macrophages express monocyte markers such as CD11a, CD14 and CD36, but lack Langerhans cell markers CD1a and factor XIIIa, which are markers for dermal dendrocytes. Lining macrophages strongly express HLA DR which may indicate an activational state. Electron microscopy of lining macrophages revealed cellular protrusions through the basement membranes that were in contact with basal keratinocytes. Through this configuration, monocytes may directly influence keratinocyte growth by excretion of mediators such as IL-6 and IL-8 (Grossman *et al.* 1989; Krueger *et al.* 1990).

6.3.3 Dendritic cells and T lymphocytes

A more extensive review on the role of these cells in the (immuno)pathogenesis of psoriasis will be provided in Chapter 7.

6.3.4 Adhesion molecules

Leucocyte extravasation requires an interaction between adhesion molecules expressed by the endothelium and by the leucocytes. Three main classes of adhesion molecules are known (Smith & Barker 1995).

1 *Selectins* are a group of glycoproteins. Three selectins have been defined so far:

(a) E-selectin (endothelial leucocyte adherence molecule 1);

(b) P-selectin (granule membrane protein M_r);

(c) L-selectin (LEC-CAM-1).

P-selectin and E-selectin act as ligands for neutrophils, eosinophils, monocytes and memory T lymphocytes. L-selectin is expressed on all circulating leucocytes with the exception of a subpopulation of memory T lymphocytes.

2 *Integrins* are non-covalently linked α and β subunits. Various families are defined within the integrins according to the associated β subunit. Integrins are responsible for binding to the endothelium, leucocyte adhesion to tissue matrices and antigen presentation. The following integrins are relevant with respect to psoriasis:

(a) leucocyte function-associated antigen 1 (LFA-1, CD11a/CD18);

(b) MAC-1 (CD11b/CD18; CR3).

LFA-1 is found on all leucocytes. MAC-1 is confined to monocytes, eosinophils and PMN. Both molecules bind to members of the immunoglobulin supergene family.

3 *The immunoglobulin supergene family* are single-chain molecules with a variable number of immunoglobulin-like, extracellular domains and include ICAM-1, ICAM-2 and vascular cell adhesion molecule 1 (VCAM-1). Molecules of the immunoglobulin superfamily are predominantly expressed by endothelial cells.

In psoriasis, E-selectin expression is increased on psoriatic dermal endothelium, particularly at the tips of dermal papillae and correlates with sites of maximal neutrophil and lymphocyte intra- and perivascular accumulation (Groves *et al.* 1991).

ICAM-1 is significantly upregulated on psoriatic endothelial cells (Griffiths *et al.* 1989; Uyemura *et al.* 1993).

The relevance of ICAM-1 upregulation on psoriatic endothelium was provided by an experiment where T lymphocytes were overlaid onto frozen sections from psoriatic plaques; there was preferrential adherence of T lymphocytes to dermal endothelia within the papillary tips. Monoclonal antibodies to CD18 inhibited this adherence (Sackstein *et al.* 1988; Chin *et al.* 1990).

VCAM-1 is upregulated on endothelial cells in psoriatic lesional skin. Its expression is, however, relatively weak as compared with the expression of E-selectin and ICAM-1 (Groves *et al.* 1993).

6.3.5 The symptomless skin

Whereas cutaneous inflammation is markedly expressed in the lesional skin of psoriatic patients, the symptomless skin also expresses certain proinflammatory changes. Table 6.2 provides an overview of these abnormalities in the symptomless skin.

The stroma is already abnormal in the clinically uninvolved skin in several respects. Fibroblasts derived from the symptomless skin are hyperproliferative in culture and excrete increased quantities of glycosaminoglycans (Priestly 1991).

Increased expression of high endothelial venules has been reported and endoglin expression is decreased (Braverman & Sibley 1982; Heng *et al.* 1988). Decreased endoglin expression might result in increased concentrations of transforming growth factor β (TGF-β) (Rulo *et al.* 1995). TGF-β has an antiproliferative and anti-inflammatory effect. Indeed, the sharp demarcation of the psoriatic lesion implies that anti-inflammatory mechanisms exist in symptomless skin preventing the expansion of the psoriatic lesion.

Table 6.2 Stroma and T-lymphocyte trafficking on the symptomless skin.

		Reference
Stroma		
Fibroblast proliferation	I	(Priestly 1991)
Glycosaminoglycan	I	(Priestly 1991)
Vasodilatation	I	(Braverman and Sibley 1982)
High endothelial venules	I	(Heng *et al.* 1988)
Endoglin expression	D	(Rulo *et al.* 1995)
T-lymphocyte trafficking		
Number of CD4- and CD8-positive cells	I	(Baker *et al.* 1984; Placek *et al.* 1988)
Number of HLA-DR+/CD1a subclass antigen presenting cells	I	(Prens *et al.* 1991; Cooper *et al.* 1990)

I, Increased; D, decreased.

T-cell trafficking will be dealt with in Chapter 7. It is, however, important to realize that already in the symptomless psoriatic skin the number of CD4[+] and CD8[+] cells is increased (Baker *et al.* 1984; Placek *et al.* 1988), as well as the number of HLA-DR[+]/CD1a subclass of antigen-presenting cells (Cooper *et al.* 1990; Prens *et al.* 1991).

6.4 Proliferation and differentiation of keratinocytes

In the psoriatic plaque, but also in the symptomless skin of psoriatic patients the epidermis is abnormal. A major question is to what extent the epidermis is primarily involved in the pathogenesis or might respond to an abnormality in another compartment.

6.4.1 The psoriatic lesion

Numerous regulatory molecules in the epidermis of the psoriatic lesion have been suggested to be of pathogenetic significance, in particular molecules which are absent or only slightly expressed in normal epidermis but abundantly expressed in the psoriatic lesion have been claimed to be of major pathogenetic significance. Table 6.3 summarizes these characteristics. Suprabasal expression of keratins 6, 16 and 17 are associated with a disturbed integrity of the epidermis (de Jong *et al.* 1991). SKALP (Elafin) is expressed in psoriasis and other hyperproliferative conditions (Schalkwijk *et al.* 1990). SKALP binds to proteases, in particular elastase. Elastase is released by PMN and enables these infiltrate cells to penetrate into the skin by

Table 6.3 Molecules that are expressed in the psoriatic plaque but are absent or have a restricted expression in normal skin.

Molecule	Reference
Cytokeratin 6, 16 and 17	(de Mare *et al.* 1989; Weiss *et al.* 1984; de Jong *et al.* 1991a)
Skin-associated antileukoprotease	(Schalkwijk *et al.* 1990)
Psoriasis-associated fatty acid-binding protein	(Siegenthaler *et al.*, 1993)
Psoriasin	(Madsen *et al.* 1991)
Transforming growth factor α	(Elder *et al.* 1989; Turbitt *et al.* 1990)
Amphiregulin	(Cook *et al.* 1992)
Epidermal growth factor receptor	(Nanney *et al.* 1992)
Interleukin-1 ra	(Hamberger *et al.* 1992)
Interleukin-1 β	(Schmid *et al.* 1993)
Interleukin-6	(Nickoloff *et al.* 1991)
Interleukin-8	(Nickoloff *et al.* 1991)
GRO α/β/γ	(Tettelback *et al.* 1993)
Fibronectin	(Bernard *et al.* 1998)

degrading collagen type IV (Brigamen *et al.* 1984). In this respect it is of interest that antielastase activity was predominantly present in lesional skin of disorders with a mixed inflammatory infiltrate (Chang *et al.* 1990). The role of psoriasis-associated fatty acid binding protein and psoriasis remains to be established (Siegenthaler *et al.*, 1993).

TGF-α, calmodulin, epidermal growth factor receptor, IL-1α, IL-1β, IL-6 and -8. GRO-α, -β and -γ (Elder *et al.* 1989; Turbitt *et al.* 1990; Nickoloff *et al.* 1991; Cook *et al.* 1992; Hamberger *et al.* 1992; Nanney *et al.* 1992a; Schmid *et al.* 1993; Tettelbach *et al.* 1993) all are molecules which show an increased expression in the psoriatic epidermis and are associated primarily or secondarily with increased epidermal proliferation and cutaneous inflammation.

However, so far none of these changes has been shown to be specific for psoriasis and it remains to be established to what extent these changes are of significance for the pathogenesis of psoriasis.

In order to find out the role of epidermal proliferation it is important to characterize epidermal growth. It is particularly important to answer the question to what extent increased recruitment of cycling epidermal cells from the resting G_0 population and/or to what extent a decrease in cell cycle times are responsible for epidermal hyperproliferation in the psoriatic lesion.

Published data on the psoriatic plaque, the cell cycle time (T_c) and the duration of the S phase in the psoriatic plaque vary considerably (Table 6.4). Various methods have been used to measure the cell cycle times. The estimation of the fraction of labelled mitosis provided the most reproducible results and the most narrow range (Weinstein *et al.* 1985). Therefore 36–37 h can be regarded as a reliable estimation of the cell cycle time. Also the duration of the cell cycle times of normal skin has been measured by various groups (Table 6.5). However, all methods, including the fraction of labelled mitosis, revealed a wide variation (Weinstein *et al.* 1985). In this respect it is of relevance that the growth fraction in normal epidermis is 5–10% whereas the growth fraction of psoriatic lesion is at least 80% (van Rijzewijk *et al.* 1989).

Although the cell cycle time in the psoriatic lesion is well defined, the cell cycle time in normal skin shows a large variation. Therefore, some groups claim that the cell cycle time in psoriasis is shortened, some regard it to be

Table 6.4 Cell cycle parameters in the psoriatic lesion.

T_s	T_c	Reference
10	28	(van Erp *et al.* 1989)
8.5	36–37.5	(Weinstein *et al.* 1985)
7.7	54.5–62	(Duffill *et al.* 1977)
9.8	91	(Goodwin *et al.* 1974)
10.5	95	(Galasi *et al.* 1980)
14.4–19.9	114–202	(Pullmann *et al.* 1977)
11.2–14.0	173–279	(Steigleder *et al.* 1973)

T_s, Duration of S phase (h); T_c, cell cycle time (h).

T_s	T_c	Reference
9.7	27.8	(van Erp et al. 1988)
10	28	(van Erp et al. 1989)
10.2	39	(Boezeman et al. 1987)
11.5	59	(Chopra and Flaxman 1972)
9	98	(Gelfant 1982)
8	50–139	(Bauer 1986)
9	184	(Galasi et al. 1980)
10.2	213	(Heenen & Galand 1971)
7	224	(Gillenberg et al. 1980)
8.5–14	163–326	(Weinstein et al. 1985)
6.6–7.2	282–326	(Pullmann et al. 1977)

Table 6.5 Cell cycle parameters in normal skin.

T_s, Duration of S phase (h); T_c, cell cycle time (h).

normal and others state that the cell cycle time is lengthened compared with normal skin.

Recently a study was carried out to find out the duration of S phase and cell cycle time by *in vivo* labelling with iododeoxyuridine (van Erp *et al.*, 1996). Table 6.6 summarizes the epidermal cell kinetic parameters as computed from these studies. A T_c of $27.8 \pm 1.6\,h$ and a T_s of $9.7 \pm 0.6\,h$ could be demonstrated for normal skin. The same experimental approach to assess epidermal cell kinetic parameters for psoriatic lesion was not feasible as the primary medical ethical justification for carrying out these studies was to follow the results of chemotherapy in severe haematological malignancies. However, in view of the high density of mitoses in lesional psoriatic skin the value of 36–37.5 h for T_c and 9 h for T_s does not need further experimental re-evaluation. The large body of evidence indicates that the cell cycle time in psoriatic lesion is normal.

Immunohistochemical assessment of cycling epidermal cells is possible with the monoclonal antibody Ki-67 (van Erp *et al.* 1989; Schröder 1995). Nuclear staining with this antibody indicates that a cell has started progression through the cell cycle.

However, sensitivity of the staining methods introduces a lag period of approximately 12 h between the entrance into the cell cycle and detection of the epitope. Therefore, the number of cycling epidermal cells is slightly greater

	Normal	Psoriatic lesion
N_{diff}	60%	5%
N_{germ}	40%	5%
N_c/N_{germ}	≤ 0.1	0.3–1
T_s	10 h	10 h
T_c	30 h	30 h

Table 6.6 Cell kinetics of normal human epidermis (van Erp *et al.* 1996).

than the number of Ki-67-positive nuclei (Gerdes *et al.* 1984), using bromo-deoxyuridine (Brd-Urd) the number of cells in S phase can be counted (van Erp *et al.* 1989). In a double immunohistochemical staining procedure the number of cells in S phase and the number of cycling epidermal cells per millimetre length were assessed (van Erp *et al.* 1989). Table 6.7 summarizes the results.

The number of cycling cells is increased sevenfold in the psoriatic plaque. The number of cells in S phase is increased to the same extent, which implies that the ratio is equal for normal skin and psoriasis. In atopic dermatitis and following injury of the skin, similar values have been observed. Assuming cells progress through the cell cycle randomly, these findings again favour the view that the cell cycle in psoriasis is essentially normal. The grossly increased number of Ki-67-positive nuclei lends support to the concept of increased growth fraction as denominator of psoriatic hyperproliferation. From these observations it can be concluded that: (i) the recruitment of cycling epidermal cells is significantly increased in the psoriatic plaque without an abnormality in cell cycle times; (ii) the increased recruitment of cycling epidermal cells is not specific for the psoriatic lesion.

In order to answer the question of whether the increased recruitment of cycling cells in the psoriatic plaque might be the result of inflammatory phenomena a further description of the infiltrate present in the lesion as well as the investigations on the network of mediators of inflammation are of relevance.

The inflammatory infiltrate is composed of T lymphocytes, monocytes, macrophages, mast cells and PMN (Christophers & Mrowietz 1995). CD4+ and CD8+ cells invade the epidermis and macrophages are observed along the basement membrane with a high density close to the rete ridges. A large scale of mediators of inflammation has been identified in lesional skin of psoriatics (Schröder 1995). None of these aspects, however, has been shown to be specific to the psoriatic process. Two hypotheses for interaction between the inflammatory infiltrate and the recruitment of cycling epidermal cells are supported by experimental evidence.

1 In epidermal cells at the tips of the rete ridges, MCP-1 is expressed, which attracts monocytes. Macrophages can be seen accumulating at these sites just underneath the epidermis. Cellular protrusions of these cells through the basement membrane reaching the surface of keratinocytes have been

Table 6.7 Double immunohistochemical assessment of S phase cells (Brd-Urd+) and cycling cells expressing nuclear staining with the Ki-67 antibody (van Erp *et al.* 1989).

	Brd-Urd+	Ki-67+	mLI
Normal epidermis	8.6	24.7	0.35
Psoriatic plaque	76.1	196.9	0.39
Atopic dermatitis	48.8	135.3	0.37

mLI, modified labelling index.

demonstrated (Wortmann *et al.* 1993; van Oord and de Wolf-Peeter 1994). At the tips of the rete ridges the density of Ki-67-positive nuclei is maximal. From this observation one could conclude that the tips of the rete ridges play a role in attracting monocytes and T cells, and such cells might induce recruitment of cycling epidermal cells.

2   TGF-α activates the epidermal growth factor receptor, causing transcription of TGF-α. Activation of the TGF-α loop results in enhanced epidermal proliferation (Coffey *et al.* 1987). Recently, it was shown that TNF-α, interferon γ (IFN-γ) and IL-8 enhance the activation of this loop (Tuschil *et al.* 1992; Valgi-Nagy *et al.* 1992).

Infiltrate cells seem to have at least the potential to enhance epidermal proliferation and indeed the physical contact between infiltrate cells and epidermal keratinocytes seems to permit such interaction. However, to what extent does the inflammatory infiltrate determine abnormal epidermal proliferation and differentiation?

6.4.2 The symptomless psoriatic skin

Whereas the psoriatic lesion is burdened with a plethora of pathological changes, the symptomless skin of psoriatic patients seems to provide a more simple approach. Indeed the micromorphological picture of the symptomless skin by haematoxylin and eosin (H & E) staining is essentially normal. However, again many abnormalities have been shown in the epidermis of the symptomless skin at the cellular and molecular level. Table 6.8 summarizes these changes.

The interpretation of these results, however, is difficult. Some authors have sampled the symptomless skin adjacent to the psoriatic plaques. Some groups have included in their patients those who where admitted for inpatient treatment and had widespread and/or relapsing psoriasis. It is obvious

Table 6.8 Changes in the symptomless skin.

Epidermis		Reference
Thymidine units	I	(Marks 1978)
% SG$_2$M phase	I	(Bauer *et al.* 1981)
Ki-67+nuclei	N	(Gerritsen 1997)
Involucrin+cells	N	(Gerritsen 1997)
Filaggrin+cells	N	(Gerritsen 1997)
Protein kinase C activity	D	(Horn *et al.* 1987)
Ornithine decarboxylase activity	I	(Lowe *et al.* 1982)
Arachidonic acid release	I	(Ziboh *et al.* 1984)
Phospholipase A$_2$ activity	I	(Forster *et al.* 1983; Verhagen *et al.* 1984)
Calmodulin	N/I	(van de Kerkhof & van Erp 1983; Tucker *et al.* 1984)

N, normal; D, decreased; I, increased.

that in such biopsies 'preclinical lesion' might have been present. A further difficulty in interpreting the data is that changes in the symptomless skin theoretically might be the result of systemic dysregulation caused by factors stemming from psoriatic plaques or psoriatic arthritis.

In the symptomless skin thymidine labelling and percentage of cells in SG_2M phase (flow cytometry) have been reported to be significantly but slightly increased, comparing groups of patients and normal subjects (Bauer *et al.* 1981). However, the extent of body surface involved with lesions and the activity of the psoriatic process were not specified in these patients.

In the distant uninvolved skin of patients with limited stable plaque psoriasis (less than 5% of the body surface involved) we could not demonstrate an increase in the percentage of cells in SG_2M phase and an increase in the recruitment of cycling epidermal cells using the antibody Ki-67 (de Jong *et al.* 1991; Gerritsen 1997).

The question remains to be answered as to what extent the psoriatic epidermis, independent of the dermis and of systemic factors, will express abnormalities with respect to epidermal growth characteristics compared with normal epidermis.

6.4.3 The epidermis in isolation

Transplantation experiments of lesional symptomless psoriatic skin and normal skin to nude mice provide an experimental approach to assess changes of these donor skin specimens in the absence of systemic human factors (Krueger *et al.* 1981; Krueger *et al.* 1990). Six weeks after transplantation, synthesis of DNA by epidermal cells was unchanged for normal skin.

The symptomless skin of psoriatic patients displayed increased DNA synthesis in the epidermal cells, well above DNA synthesis level in the skin of normal subjects, reaching similar values as observed in the psoriatic lesional skin following transplantation. Although this implies that the uninvolved skin is persistently abnormal in isolation from the systemic factors, this approach still does not answer the question whether the epidermis is intrinsically abnormal. It is remotely possible that factors from the stroma or sessile infiltrate cells (macrophages) persist to trigger the epidermis to enhanced growth. The transplantation experiment does, however, suggest that systemic factors exist which suppress epidermal proliferation.

What about epidermal cells in culture? So far, studies on epidermal growth characteristics of total populations of psoriatic keratinocytes in culture failed to demonstrate an extrinsic abnormality (Table 6.9). Recently an extensive investigation was carried out by van Ruissen *et al.* (1996) on keratinocytes in secondary culture in defined medium without a feeder layer. At 30–40% confluence no significant abnormalities of growth characteristics were shown for psoriatic keratinocytes, using flow cytometrical analysis following iododeoxyuridine labelling. Growth characteristics were also assessed follow-

Table 6.9 Cell cycle parameters in cultured human skin.

Source	T_s	T_c	Reference
Normal skin	6.6	27.0	(van Ruissen *et al.* 1994)
Normal skin	8	12.6–47	(Dover & Potten 1983)
Normal skin	11.5	59	(Flaxman & Chopra 1972)
Psoriatic lesion	6.5		(Chopra & Flaxman 1974)

T_s, duration of S phase (h); T_c, cell cycle time (h).

ing growth arrest by TGF-β and subsequent restimulation of growth. Again, growth characteristics of normal and psoriatic keratinocytes proved to be similar. Therefore, considering total populations of keratinocytes, there are no apparent differences between psoriatic and normal cell lines with respect to epidermal growth characteristics.

Recently, it was reported by Bata-Csorgo *et al.* (1993) that in primary keratinocyte cultures soluble factors from CD4[+] T-lymphocyte clones derived from psoriatic plaques promote proliferation of the psoriatic CD29[+] keratin 10[-] subpopulation, whereas CD29[+] keratin 10[-] keratinocytes from normal subjects failed to have such a growth response following incubation with soluble factors from the same T-cell clones.

This experiment suggests that subpopulations of epidermal cells derived from psoriatic patients do respond abnormally to T-cell clones from psoriatic plaques.

6.5 The transition between symptomless and clinically involved skin

In order to answer the question as to what extent epidermal proliferation might be a primary pathogenetic event or the result of inflammatory changes, models have to be developed to study the transition between symptomless and lesional skin. Sequential studies following skin injury and studies in the margin zone of spreading psoriatic plaques are of relevance in this respect.

Heinrich Koebner (1878) described the artificial elicitation of the psoriatic plaque following trauma of the skin. This isomorphic response is an all-or-none phenomenon (Eyre & Krueger 1982). In 25% of psoriatic patients a fully developed lesion will appear at all injured sites (Eyre & Krueger 1982). Studies on various trauma lesions revealed that a selective dermal injury will not result in a psoriatic plaque (Farber *et al.* 1965); the epidermis has to be injured as well. Tape stripping is a relatively non-invasive trauma that has been reported to be sufficient to induce a psoriatic lesion. Therefore, comparative studies on the response to tape stripping in psoriatic patients and non-psoriatic volunteers might provide further information on the dynamics of the pathogenesis of psoriasis. In patients with unstable plaque psoriasis an increased accumulation of PMN was observed, whereas a decreased accumulation of PMN occurred in patients with stable plaque psoriasis following tape stripping of the symptomless skin (Chang *et al.* 1987).

An enhanced proliferative response of the epidermis has been observed by some authors in psoriatic patients compared with non-psoriatic subjects 48 h following tape stripping (Wiley & Weinstein 1979; Ricoh *et al.* 1985). Others failed to show this 48-h overresponse but observed an increased response of epidermal proliferation in the late phase (6–9 days) following tape stripping (van de Kerkhof *et al.* 1983). In the latter study an early overresponsiveness of the endothelial marker alkaline phosphatase was shown. The response pattern of the symptomless skin of psoriatic to standardized injury suggests that inflammatory changes in the endothelium and PMN accumulation are involved early, whereas increased recruitment of cycling cells occurs in the late phase (6–9 days).

The margin of the spreading psoriatic plaque (de Jong *et al.* 1991b) is an alternative model for studying the sequence of events during the transition from symptomless to clinically involved skin. Changes occurring in areas distant to the psoriatic lesion, i.e. in the symptomless skin, are likely to precede the changes that are observed in the more central areas of the margin zone. From the morphological studies carried out on the margin of the psoriatic plaque a three-staged model can be defined:

1   The most distant and early stage is the involvement of the stroma. This phase is characterized by an increased expression of the extracellular matrix molecule tenascin and an increased expression of alkaline phosphatase, which is a marker mainly of endothelial cell activation.

2   The second phase is the appearance of the inflammatory infiltrate together with the expression of keratin 16.

3   The third phase is the simultaneous appearance of increased recruitment of cycling epidermal cells, observed as Ki-67-positive cells, together with a decreased expression of involucrin. However, in view of the induction time of the Ki-67 epitope it is remotely possible that the recruitment process precedes the changes with respect to epidermal differentiation.

The dynamics of appearance of molecules that have been suggested to be of relevance in the pathogenesis of psoriasis can be studied in this model. In this respect it has been demonstrated that calmodulin and SKALP are overexpressed in the more central zones of the psoriatic margin.

Therefore, studies in the margin of the spreading psoratic plaque suggest an early commitment of the dermis in the pathogenesis of psoriasis as a permissive factor for both epidermal proliferation and cutaneous inflammation. In both models the suprabasal compartment (keratin 16 expression) anticipates further epidermal changes.

6.6 Signal transduction pathways in epidermal proliferation and cutaneous inflammation

A network of communication between keratinocytes, stroma and inflammatory cells exist. For a detailed account on signal transduction the reader is referred to a detailed review (van Ruissen *et al.* 1995). In this section various components of the signalling network, as presented in this review, are summarized.

6.6.1 The human epidermal keratinocytes

Cyclic adenosine monophosphate (cAMP) is a 'second messenger' which is formed from adenosine triphosphate (ATP) via the plasma membrane-bound enzyme adenylcyclase. Adenylcyclase is activated via the G_s protein by β catecholamines, histamine, prostaglandins, thyroid-stimulating hormone, adrenocorticotrophic hormone, luteinizing hormone, parathormone, vasopressin, glucagon and adenine nucleotides. The activity of adenylcyclase is inhibited via its G_i protein by α_2-adrenergic receptors. cAMP activates protein kinase A. cAMP inhibits epidermal proliferation, whereas high levels stimulate epidermal proliferation (Okada *et al.* 1982). In the psoriatic lesion intracellular cAMP levels are essentially normal, whereas the β-catecholamine-stimulated cAMP levels are decreased in lesional skin of psoriasis (Gommans *et al.* 1979). However, no significant changes have been observed in the symptomless skin.

6.6.2 Phospholipase C isoenzymes

Phospholipase C isoenzymes, in particular phospholipase Cγ, play a major role in signal transduction in the epidermis.

Activation of this enzyme results in hydrolysis of phosphatidyl-inositol 4,5-bisphosphate (PIP$_2$) to 1,2-diacylglycerol (DAG) and inositol triphosphate (IP$_3$) after stimulation. PIP$_2$ is formed through the sequential phosphorylation of phosphatidylinositol (PI) by PI kinase and phosphatidylinositol-4-monophosphokinase. The isoenzyme phospholipase Cγ_1 is of particular significance as it phosphonylates and hence activates tyrosine kinase-linked receptors (e.g. epidermal growth factor (EGF) receptor and platelet-derived growth factor (PDGF)).

As mentioned previously, stimulation of phospholipase Cγ (PLC-γ) results in the hydrolysis of PIP$_2$, yielding two second messengers: DAG, which directly activates protein kinase C (PKC) and IP$_3$, which induces the release of calcium into the cell. Activation of PKC and elevation of intracellular calcium levels induce epidermal proliferation and differentiation.

Histamine, bradykinin, platelet-activating factor (PAF) and thrombin have been identified as stimulators of PIP$_2$ turnover in the skin.

PLC-γ_1 has been demonstrated in basal and suprabasal layers of the epidermis. In addition, immunoreactive PLC-γ_1 co-localizes with immunoreactive EGF receptor in normal and hyperproliferative epidermis (Nanney *et al.* 1992).

Membrane-bound and cytosolic PLC are increased in psoriatic lesional skin (Inoue *et al.* 1977; Bartel *et al.* 1987; Bergers *et al.* 1990; Fisher *et al.* 1990; Nanney *et al.* 1992b). Further PIP_2 hydrolysis is markedly increased in lesional skin of psoriasis (Fisher *et al.* 1990). However, no abnormalities have been shown in the symptomless skin of psoriatic patients.

6.6.3 Signal transduction coupled to protein kinase C

PKC is a family of ubiquitous Ca^{2+}- and phospholipid-dependent, serine/threonine dependent protein kinases (Stabel & Parker 1991).

The PKC isoenzymes are involved in growth control, gene expression, terminal differentiation and neoplastic transformation. PKCs are activated by physiological mediators such as EGF, PDGF, TGF-α, histamine, bradykinin and pharmacological mediators such as phorbol esters. It is known that activation of PKC results in phosphorylation of serine residues of PLC-γ_1, PLC-β and EGF receptor. Addition of tumour promoting agent (TPA) to cultured keratinocytes induces transglutaminase production, cornified envelope formation, loricrin and filaggrin formation (Parkinson *et al.* 1984; Duglosz & Yuspa 1993). In keratinocyte cultures inhibitors of PKC inhibited proliferation (Hegeman *et al.* 1994).

Psoriatic involved skin and symptomless skin of psoriatics had significantly lower PKC activity as compared with skin of normal subjects, no significant difference in this respect was shown between lesional and symptomless skin of psoriatic patients (Horn *et al.* 1987).

In normal and psoriatic skin, messenger RNA (mRNA) levels of PKC-α, -β, -δ, -ϵ, -ζ, and -η were not significantly different (Fisher *et al.* 1993). However, the expression of PKC-α and PKC-β were reduced and PKC-ζ protein was increased in lesional skin as compared with normal skin (Fisher *et al.* 1993).

In general, PKC activity is decreased in psoriasis. It is attractive to speculate that such is due to downregulation resulting from a continuous activation of PKC.

6.6.4 Arachidonic acid metabolites

Phospholiphase A_2 enhances the release of arachidonic acid (AA) from membranes. AA is metabolized into lipoxygenase products (leukotrienes) and cyclooxygenase products (prostaglandins).

In psoriasis (reviewed by van de Kerkhof 1991), both in the lesional and symptomless skin, phospholipase A_2 activity is increased and AA formation is enhanced. In the psoriatic lesion, virtually all AA metabolites are increased. Activation of phospholipase A_2 in psoriasis might result from PKC activation.

6.6.5 Tyrosine kinase and signal transduction

Many growth-factor receptors show protein tyrosine kinase (PTK) activity. Following binding to a growth factor, the kinase domain of the receptor is activated. This results in a cascade of protein kinase activation, including the activation of serine/threonine kinases, mitogen-activated protein kinase, including the activation of PKC activating principles such as PLC-γ and ras guanosine triphosphatase (GTPase)-activating proteins (GAPs). Activation of PTK results therefore in a wide range of biological effects including epidermal proliferation and inflammation. Indeed, phosphorylation of lipocortin I and II and increased formation of AA metabolites is of relevance in this respect.

In psoriasis, the EGF receptor is increased two- to fourfold (Yates *et al.* 1991). Also insulin growth factor (IGF) is overexpressed in the lesional psoriatic epidermis. In line with these observations are the increased activities of PTK and protein phosphotyrosine phosphatases as well as the increase of TGF-α activity in lesional psoriatic epidermis (Gentleman *et al.* 1984; Elder *et al.* 1989). In the symptomless skin of psoriatic patients these parameters are not increased as compared with the symptomless skin.

Through the discovery of oncogenes, evidence has accumulated that proto-oncogenes are involved in epidermal growth control and also in the regulation of cutaneous inflammation.

In psoriatic lesional skin but also in normal skin, TGF-β_3, p53 and C-myc transcripts were clearly detectable (Schmid *et al.* 1993).

The expression of the proto-oncogenes C-fos and C-jun were significantly decreased in plaque type psoriasis but not in guttate psoriasis (Basset-Seguin *et al.* 1991). However, another group reported that C-fos expression was normal in psoriasis but p53, h-ras and C-myc proved to have a remarkable reactivity (Tadini *et al.* 1989). In lesional psoriatic epidermis the expression of ras[p21] was reported to be increased (Takahashi *et al.* 1990). So far, no abnormalities have been reported in this respect in the symptomless psoriatic skin.

6.6.6 Cytokines

Cytokines are a large family of extracellular protein mediators. These include:
1 ILs;
2 colony-stimulating factors (CSFs);
3 IFNs;
4 TNFs;
5 chemokines;
6 growth factors.

Cytokines have pleiotropic effects. The cytokine network is crucial in the control of epidermal proliferation, epidermal differentiation and inflammation as an integrated process.

6.6.7 Interleukins

After binding of an IL to its receptor, a cascade of events occurs with a major impact on epidermal behaviour and inflammation. Currently IL-1, IL-3, IL-6, IL-7, IL-8, IL-10 and IL-12 are expressed by keratinocytes.

IL-1 is secreted predominantly by macrophages but also by keratinocytes, fibroblasts, endothelial cells, Langerhans cells, B lymphocytes, some T lymphocytes and PMN (Billingham 1987). The IL-1 family of cytokines consist of three homologous molecules: two agonist (IL-1α and IL-1β) and the IL-1 receptor antagonist (IL-1ra) (Dinarello 1991; Dinarello & Thompson 1991). The actions of IL-1 include the induction of lymphocytotropic cytokines and the activation of vascular endothelial cells. In the psoriatic lesion IL-1ra has been reported to be increased according to some authors and decreased according to others (Hamberg *et al.* 1992; Kristensen *et al.* 1992). The IL-1ra/IL-1α protein ratio is significantly increased in psoriatic lesional skin vs. normal skin (Hamberg *et al.* 1992). In lesional psoriatic skin IL-1α mRNA was reported to be significantly reduced whereas IL-1β mRNA was significantly increased (Gearing *et al.* 1990; Schmid *et al.* 1993). IL-1 mRNAs have been shown already in the symptomless skin just adjacent to the psoriatic plaque. IL-1 release may be stimulated by TGF-α, IL-1α, TNF-α, CSF and IFN-γ (van Ruissen *et al.* 1995).

IL-3 is a member of haematopoeitic CSFs. It is synthesized by T lymphocytes, myeloid cell lines and keratinocytes. IL-3 has been shown to stimulate proliferation of keratinocytes.

IL-6 is produced by many different cell types including keratinocytes, fibroblasts, endothelial cells and monocytes. Like IL-1, IL-6 is released immediately after injury. IL-1, TNF-α, IFNs, PDGF, but also bacterial toxins may induce IL-6. IL-6 stimulates epidermal proliferation Yoshizaki *et al.* 1990). IL-6 mRNA and protein levels are increased in psoriatic lesional skin (Grossman *et al.* 1989; Ohta *et al.* 1991).

IL-7 is produced by murine and human keratinocytes (Heufler *et al.* 1993). Keratinocyte-derived IL-7 supports dendritic epidermal T-cell proliferation (Matsue *et al.* 1993). So far no levels of this cytokine have been reported in psoriatic skin.

IL-8 is produced by monocytes, T lymphocytes, endothelial cells, dermal fibroblasts, PMN keratinocytes. The production of this cytokine is stimulated by IL-1α, IL-1β, TNF-α and IFN-γ. IL-8 is chemotactic for PMN, T lymphocytes, basophils and lymphocytes. It also activates PMN by increasing the intracellular calcium concentration and inducing respiratory burst. IL-8 is chemotactic for normal human keratinocytes. IL-8 further promotes epidermal proliferation. Therefore it could be concluded that IL-8 plays an important role in the pathogenesis by mediating the influx of T cells and PMN and enhancing epidermal proliferation. IL-8 has been isolated in large quantities from psoriatic scales (Gearing *et al*. 1990). Lesional skin overexpresses IL-8 mRNA (Schmid *et al*. 1993).

IL-10 can be produced by T lymphocytes, B lymphocytes, macrophages/monocytes and activated keratinocytes. IL-10 profoundly alters the morphology of major histocompatibility complex (MHC) class II antigens. IL-10 has the ability to suppress the production of cytokines, including IL-2, IFN-γ and IL-1α and to upregulate IL-1ra. Therefore, it is possible that IL-10 might have a role in the treatment of psoriasis (Cork *et al*. 1993).

IL-12 induces the production of IFN-γ and is required in optimal Th1 cell development. Therefore, keratinocytes may influence Th-mediated immune responses by favouring Th1 stimulation (Enk *et al*. 1994).

6.6.8 Interferons

IFNs are a family of glycoproteins which have several effects on epidermal cell behaviour and inflammation. Of particular relevance is the fact that HLA expression on keratinocytes and keratinocyte differentiation are induced by IFN-γ, whereas normal human keratinocyte proliferation is inhibited. IFNs may play an important role in the pathogenesis of psoriasis. IFN-γ and IFN-α are present in the psoriatic lesion (Livden *et al*. 1989). The increased hyperproliferation in psoriasis may be due to functional inactivation of the growth-inhibitory pathway mediated by high-affinity IFN-γ receptors on lesional keratinocytes (Nickoloff *et al*. 1991).

6.6.9 Tumour necrosis factor α

TNF-α is produced by activated keratinocytes and dermal macrophages. TNF-α is capable of activating lymphocytes, neutrophils, eosinophils and macrophages. TNF-α induces the expression of HLA DR and the adhesion molecules ICAM-1, and ELAM, TNF-α markedly suppresses keratinocyte growth (Kristensen *et al*. 1992).

6.6.10 Growth factors

Growth factors are pivotal in keratinocyte growth.

TGF-α shows high homology to EGF and both bind to the same receptor. IGF-α is produced by keratinocytes and activated macrophages.

Elevated levels of TGF-α protein were seen in both basal and suprabasal layers of involved psoriatic skin (Turbitt *et al*. 1990). The level of TGF-α in psoriatic involved epidermis was about five times higher than that observed in normal skin (Higashiguma *et al*. 1991). TGF-α mRNA has been reported to be increased in the psoriatic lesion (Schmid *et al.* 1993).

TGF-β is synthesized by platelets and keratinocytes. TGF-β inhibits epidermal proliferation and has a remodelling effect on the extracellular matrix. It is possible that TGF-β has an antipsoriatic effect. Indeed active vitamin D_3 induces its transcription (Koli & Keski Oja 1993).

6.6.11 Other cytokines

An overexpanding group of chemokines has been and is being analysed. Some of these are overexpressed in psoriasis (for review see Schröder 1995).

GRO, a cytokine originally characterized as an autocrine growth factor for melanoma cells, is highly chemotactic for neutrophils and triggers the release of neutrophil elastase. Psoriatic lesional skin is characterized by increased amounts of GRO-α (Kim *et al.* 1992)

MCP-1/MCAF/human JE protein is produced by keratinocytes upon stimulation by IFN-γ or IFN-γ and TNF-α (Barker *et al.* 1991). In psoriatic lesional skin MCP-1 is abundantly expressed above the proliferating basal keratinocytes of the tips of the rete ridges and, to a lesser extent, in cells in the dermal papillae (Gillitzer *et al.* 1993).

6.7 Conclusions

The pathogenesis of psoriasis is a complex spectrum of abnormalities involving the immune system, the stroma, the epidermis and various aspects of cutaneous inflammation.

Systemic abnormalities have been reported, including abnormalities of circulating blood leucocytes, serum factors and abnormalities of the endocrine system. It has not been resolved to what extent these abnormalities might play a causal role or whether they might be a permissive factor or just secondary changes.

Relatively early in the pathogenesis of psoriasis, changes of the stroma and inflammation occur. The initial signals have not yet been resolved.

During transition of the symptomless skin into the lesional skin, increased epidermal proliferation and abnormal keratinization are observed subsequent to changes in stroma and to cutaneous inflammation. An increased recruitment of cycling epidermal cells with normal cell cycle times accounts for hyperproliferation of the epidermis in the psoriatic lesion.

Studies on symptomless skin, on skin following transplantation to nude mice and on keratinocytes in culture provide no evidence for an intrinsic growth defect. However, the increased susceptibility of the CD29[+] keratin 10[-] subpopulation to the growth-enhancing property of those T-cell clones derived from the psoriatic lesion lend support to the hypothesis of an abnormal responsiveness of the psoriatic keratinocyte to growth factors released by stroma or inflammatory infiltrate.

Intercell communication is abnormal in psoriasis. Not only mediators of inflammation but also signal transduction systems are abnormal in the psoriatic plaque, but also in the symptomless skin.

The search for the hierarchy within the order of events in psoriasis is of importance, not only for increasing our insight in the pathogenesis but also to define potential antipsoriatic principles.

References

Alkemade, J.A.C., de Jong, G.J., Arnold, W.P., van de Kerkhof, P.C.M. & Schalkwijk, J. (1995) Levels of skin derived antileukoproteinase (SKALP/Elafin) in serum correlate with disease activity during treatment of severe psoriasis with cyclosporin A. *Journal of Investigative Dermatology* **104**, 1–5.

Baker, B.S., Swain, A.F., Fry, L. *et al.* (1984) Epidermal T lymphocytes and HLA-DR expression in psoriasis. *British Journal of Dermatology* **110**, 555–564.

Barker, J.N., Groves, R.W., Allen, M.H. & MacDonald, D.M. (1992) Preferential adherence of T lymphocytes and neutrophils to psoriatic epidermis. *British Journal of Dermatology* **127**, 205–211.

Barker, J.N., Jones, M.L. & Swenson, C.L. (1991) Monocyte chemotaxis and activating factor production by keratinocytes in response to IFN-gamma. *Journal of Immunology* **146**, 1192–1197.

Bartel, R.L., Marcelo, C.L. & Voorhees, J.J. (1987) Partial characterization of phospholipase C activity in normal, psoriatic uninvolved and lesional epidermis. *Journal of Investigative Dermatology* **88**, 447–451.

Basset-Seguin, N., Escot, C. & Moles, J.P. (1991) c-fos and c-jun proto-oncogenes expression is decreased in psoriasis; an in situ quantitative analysis. *Journal of Investigative Dermatology* **97**, 672–678.

Bata-Csorgo, Z., Hammerberg, C., Voorhees, J.J. & Cooper, K.D. (1993) Flowcytometric identification of proliferative subpopulations within normal human epidermis and the localisation of the primary hyperproliferative population in psoriasis. *Journal of Experimental Medicine* **178**, 1271–1281.

Bauer, F.W. (1986) Cell kinetics. In: *Textbook of Psoriasis* (eds Mier, P.D. & van de Kerkhof, P.C.M.), pp. 100–112. Churchill Livingstone, Edinburgh.

Bauer, F.W., Crombach, N.H.C.M.N., Boezeman, J.B.M. & de Grood, R.M. (1981) Flowcytometry as a tool for the study of cell kinetics in skin 2. Cell kinetic data in psoriasis. *British Journal of Dermatology* **104**, 271–276.

Bergers, M., van de Kerkhof, P.C.M. & Happle, R. (1990) Membrane bound phospholipase C activity in normal and psoriatic epidermis. *Acta Dermato-Venereologica* **70**, 57–59.

Bernard, B.A., Asselineau, D., Schaffer Deshayes, I. & Darmin, M.Y. (1998) Abnormal sequence of expression of differentiation markers in psoriatic epidermis: Inversion of two steps in the differentiation programme. *Journal of Investigative Dermatology* **90**, 801–853.

Billingham, M.E. (1987) Cytokines as inflammatory mediators. *British Medicine Bulletin* **43**, 350–370.

Boezeman, J.B.M., Bauer, F.W. & de Grood, R.M. (1987) Flow cytometric analysis of the recruitment of G_0 cells in human epidermis *in vivo* following tape stripping. *Cell Tissue Kinetics* **20**, 90–107.

Braverman, I.M. & Sibley, J. (1982) Role of the microcirculation in the treatment and pathogenesis of psoriasis. *Journal of Investigative Dermatology* **78**, 12–17.

Brigamen, R.A., Schechter, N.M., Fraki, J. & Lazarus, G.S. (1984) Degradation of the epidermo-dermal junction by proteolytic enzymes from human skin and human polymorphonuclear leukocytes. *Journal of Experimental Medicine* **160**, 1027–1042.

Chang, A., de Jong, G.J., Mier, P.D. & van de Kerkhof, P.C.M. (1987) Enzymatic quantification of polymorphonuclear leukocytes in normal and psoriatic skin following standardized injury. *Clinical Experimental Dermatology* **13**, 62–66.

Chang, A., Schalkwijk, J., Happle, R. & van de Kerkhof, P.C.M. (1990) Elastase inhibiting activity in scaling disorders. *Acta Dermato-Venereologica* **70**, 147–151.

Chin, Y.H., Falanga, V. & Taylor, J.R. (1990) Adherence of human helper/memory T-cell subsets to psoriatic dermal endothelium. *Journal of Investigative Dermatology* **94**, 413–417.

Chopra, D.P. & Flaxman, B.A. (1972) Human epidermal cell cycle *in vitro. British Journal of Dermatology* **87**, 13–17.

Chopra, D.P. & Flaxman, B.A. (1974) Comparative proliferative kinetics of cells from normal human epidermis and benign epidermal hyperplasia (psoriasis) in vitro. *Cell Tissue Kinetics* **7**, 69–76.

Christophers, E. & Mrowietz, U. (1995) The inflammatory infiltrate in psoriasis. *Clinical Dermatology* **13**, 131–135.

Coffey, R.J., Derynck, R., Wilcon, J.N. *et al.* (1987) Production and autoinduction of transforming growth factor α in human keratinocytes. *Nature* **328**, 817–820.

Cook, P.W., Pittelkow, M.R., Keeble, W.W. *et al.* (1992) Amphiregulin messenger RNA is elevated in psoriatic epidermis and gastrointestinal carcinomas. *Cancer Research* **52**, 3224–3227.

Cooper, K.D., Baadsgaard, O., Ellis, C.N. *et al.* (1990) Mechanisms of cyclosporin inhibition of antigen presenting activity in uninvolved and lesional psoriatic epidermis. *Journal of Investigative Dermatology* **94**, 649–656.

Cork, M.J., Mee, J.B., Duff, G.W. & Priestley, G.C. (1993) Molecular aspects of dermatology. *Cytokines*, Vol. 7, pp. 129–146. John Wiley & Sons, New York.

Csato, M., Dobozy, A., Hunyadi, J. & Simon, N. (1983) Polymorphonuclear leukocyte function in psoriasis vulgaris. *Dermatologische Monatsschrift* **169**, 238–242.

de Jong, E.M.G.J., Vlijmen, I.M., Erp, P.E.J. *et al.* (1991a) Keratin 17: a useful marker in antipsoriatic therapies. *Archives of Dermatolological Research* **283**, 480–482.

de Jong, E.M.G.J., Schalkwijk, J. & van de Kerkhof, P.C.M. (1991b) Epidermal proliferation and differentiation, composition of the inflammatory infiltrate and the extracellular matrix in the margin of the spreading psoriatic lesion. *European Journal of Dermatology* **1**, 221–227.

de Mare, S., Erp, P.E.J. & van de Kerkhof, P.C.M. (1989) Epidermal hyperproliferation assessed by the monoclonal antibody K_s 8.12 on frozen sections. *Journal of Investigative Dermatology* **92**, 130–131.

Dinarello, C.A. (1991) Interleukin-1 and interleukin1 antagonism. *Blood* **77**, 1627–1652.

Dinarello, C.A. & Thompson, R.C. (1991) Blocking IL-1: Interleukin 1 receptor antagonist in vivo and in vitro. *Immunological Today* **12**, 404–410.

Dover, R. & Potten, C.S. (1983) Cell cycle kinetics of cultured human epidermal keratinocytes. *Journal of Investigative Dermatology* **80**, 423–429.

Duffill, M.B., Appleton, D.R., Dyson, P., Shuster, S. & Wright, N.A. (1977) The measurement of the cell cycle time in squamous epithelium using the metaphase arrest technique with vincristine. *British Journal of Dermatology* **96**, 493–502.

Duglosz, A.A. & Yuspa, S.H. (1993) Coordinate changes in gene expression which mark the spinous to granular cell transition in epidermis are regulated by protein kinase C. *Journal of Cell Biology* **120**, 217–225.

Elder, J.T., Fisher, G.J., Lindquist, P.B. *et al.* (1989) Overexpression of transforming growth factor alpha in psoriatic epidermis. *Science* **243**, 811–814.

Enk, A.H., Mueller, G. & Salogam, J. (1994) Human keratinocyte derived interleukin-12 affects LC induced primary T cell responses. *Journal of Investigative Dermatology* **103**, 429.

Eyre, R.W. & Krueger, G.P. (1982) Response to injury of skin involved and uninvolved with psoriasis, and its realtion to disease activity. Koebner reactions. *British Journal of Dermatology* **106**, 153–159.

Farber, E.M., Roth, R.J., Aschheim, E., Eddy, J. & Epinette, W.V.V. (1965) Role of trauma in isomorphic response in psoriasis. *Archives of Dermatology* **91**, 246–251.

Fisher, G.F., Talwar, H.S. & Baldassare, J.J. (1990) Increased phospholipase C-catalysed hydrolysis of phosphotidyl-inositol-4,5-bisphosphate and 1,2-sn-diaglycerol content in psoriatic involved compared to uninvolved and normal epidermis. *Journal of Investigative Dermatology* **95**, 428–435.

Fisher, G.J., Tavakkol, A. & Leach, K. (1993) Differential expression of protein kinase C isoenzymes in normal and psoriatic adult human skin: reduced expression of protein kinase C-beta II in psoriasis. *Journal of Investigative Dermatology* **101**, 553–559.

Flaxman, B.A. & Chopra, D.P. (1972) Cell cycle of normal and psoriatic epidermis in vitro. *Journal of Investigative Dermatology* **59**, 102–105.

Forster, S., Ilderton, E., Summerly, R. & Yardley, H.J. (1983) The level of phospholipase A_2 activity is raised in the uninvolved epidermis of psoriasis. *British Journal of Dermatology* **108**, 103–108.

Galasi, A., Pullmann, H. & Steigleder, G.K. (1980) Abnormal epidermal cell proliferation on the elbow in psoriatic and normal skin. *Archives of Dermatological Research* **267**, 105–107.

Gearing, A.J., Fincham, M.J. & Bird, C.R. (1990) Cytokines in skin lesions of psoriasis. *Cytokine* **2**, 68–75.

Gelfant, S. (1982) On the existence of non-cycling germinative cells in human epidermis in vivo and cell cycle aspects of psoriasis. *Cell Tissue Kinetics* **15**, 393–397.

Gentleman, S., Martensen, T.M. & Digiovanna, J.J. (1984) Protein tyrosine kinase and protein phosphotyrosine phosphatase in normal and psoriatic skin. *Biochemica et Biophysics Acta* **798**, 53–59.

Gerdes, J., Lemke, H., Baisch, H. *et al.* (1984) Cell cycle analysis of a cell proliferation associated human nuclear antigen defined by the monoclonal antibody Ki-67. *Journal of Immunology* **133**, 1710–1715.

Gerritsen, M.J.P., Elbers, M.E., de Jong, E.M. & van de Kerkhof, P.C.M. (1997) Recruitment of cycling epidermal cells and expression of fillaggrin, involucrin and teuoscin in the margin of the active psoriatic plaque, in the uninvolved skin of psoriatic patients and in normal healthy skin. *Journal of Dermatological Science* **14**, 179–188.

Gillenberg, A., Immel, C. & Orfanoc, C.E. (1980) Retinoid-Einfluss auf die Zellkinetic gesunder menschlicher Epidermis. *Archives of Dermatological Research* **269**, 331–335.

Gillitzer, R., Wolff, K., Tong, D. *et al.* (1993) MCP-1 mRNA expression in basal keratinocytes of psoriatic lesions. *Journal of Investigative Dermatology* **101**, 127–131.

Glinski, W. (1978) Defective function of T-lymphocytes in psoriasis. *Journal of Investigative Dermatology* **70**, 105–110.

Gommans, J.M., Bergers, M., van Erp, P.E.J. *et al.* (1979) Studies on the plasma membrane of normal and psoriatic keratinocytes 2. Cyclic AMP and its response to hormonal stimulator. *British Journal of Dermatology* **101**, 413–419.

Goodwin, P., Hamilton, S. & Fry, L. (1974) The cell cycle in psoriasis. *British Journal of Dermatology* **90**, 517–524.

Griffiths, C.E.M., Voorhees, J.J. & Nickoloff, B.J. (1989) Characterization of intercellular adhesion molecule-1 and HLA-DR expression in normal and inflamed skin: modulation by recombinant gamma interferon and tumour necrosis factor. *Journal of the American Academy of Dermatology* **20**, 617–629.

Grossman, R.M., Krueger, J. & Yourish, D. (1989) Interleukin-6 is expressed in high levels in psoriatic skin and stimulates proliferation of cultured human keratinocytes. *Proceedings of the National Academy of Sciences of the USA* **86**, 6367–6371.

Groves, R.W., Allen, M.H. & Barker, J.N.W.N. (1991) Endothelial leucocyte adhesion molecule-1 (ELAM-1) expression in cutaneous inflammation. *British Journal of Dermatology* **124**, 117–123.

Groves, R.W., Ross, E., Barker, J.N.W.N. & MacDonald, D.M. (1993) Vascular cell adhesion molecule-1 (VCAM-1): Expression in normal and diseased skin and regulation in-vivo by interferon-gamma. *Journal of the American Academy of Dermatology* **29**, 67–72.

Hamberger, C., Arend, W.P., Fisher, G.J. *et al.* (1992) Interleukin-1 receptor antagonist in normal and psoriatic epidermis. *Journal of Clinical Investigations* **90**, 571–583.

Heenen, M. & Galand, P. (1971) Cell population kinetics in human epidermis: In vitro autoradiographic study by double-labelling method. *Journal of Investigative Dermatology* **56**, 425–429.

Hegeman, L., Kempenaar, J. & Ponec, M. (1994) The involvement of protein kinase C in proliferation and differentiation of human keratinocytes – an investigation using inhibitors of protein kinase C. *Archives of Dermatological Research* **286**, 278–284.

Heng, M.C.Y., Allen, S.G. & Chase, D.G. (1988) High endothelial venules in involved and uninvolved psoriatic skin: Recognition by homing receptors on cytotoxic T lymphocytes. *British Journal of Dermatology* **118**, 315–326.

Herschell, C.L. (1971) Serum profiles in psoriasis and arthritis. *Archives of Dermatology* **85**, 14–17.

Heufler, C., Topar, G. & Grasseger, A. (1993) Interleukin-7 is produced by murine and human keratinocytes. *Journal of Experimental Medicine* **178**, 1109–1114.

Higashiguma, N., Matsumoto, K. & Hashimoto, K. (1991) Increased production of transforming growth factor-alpha in psoriatic epidermis. *Journal of Dermatology* **18**, 117–119.

Holzman, H., Franz, J., Morsches, B. & Bröckelschen, H.A. (1976) Dehydroepiandrosterone and psoriasis. In: *Psoriasis: Proceedings of the Second International Symposium* (eds Farber, E.M. & Cox, A.J), pp. 81–90. York Medical Books, New York.

Horn, F., Marks, F., Fisher, G., Marcelo, C.L. & Voorhees, J.J. (1987) Decreased protein kinase C activity in psoriatic versus normal epidermis. *Journal of Investigative Dermatology* **88**, 220–222.

Inoue, M., Kishimoto, A. & Takai, Y. (1977) Studies on a cyclic nucleotide independent protein kinase and its proenzyme in mammalian tissues. II Proenzyme and its activation by calcium-dependent protease from rat brain. *Journal of Biological Chemistry* **252**, 7610–7616.

Karsh, J. (1978) Immune complexes in psoriasis with and without arthritis. *Journal of Rheumatology* **5**, 314–319.

Kawohl, G., Szperalski, B., Schröder, J.M. & Christophers, E. (1980) Polymorphonuclear leukocyte chemotaxis in psoriasis: enhancement by self activated serum. *British Journal of Dermatology* **103**, 527–533.

Kikindjanin, V. & Milakov, J. (1976) Serum immunoglobulin and complement levels in patients with psoriasis vulgaris. *Allergy Immunology* **22**, 143–146.

Kim, H.J., Abdelkader, N. & Katz, M. (1992) 1,25-dihydroxy-vitamin-D_3 enhances antiproliferative effect and transcription of TGF-β1 on human keratinocytes in culture. *Journal of Cell Physiology* **151**, 579–587.

Koebner, H. (1878) Klinische experimentelle und therapeutische Mitteilungen über Psoriasis. *Berliner Klinische Wochenschrift* **21**, 631–632.

Koli, K. & Keski Oja, J. (1993) Vitamin D3 and calcipotriol enhance the secretion of transforming growth factor β in cultured murine keratinocytes. *Growth Factors* **8**, 153–156.

Kristensen, M., Deleuran, B. & Eedy, D.J. (1992) Distribution of interleukin 1 receptor antagonist protein (IRAP), interleukin 1 receptor, and interleukin 1 alpha in normal and psoriatic skin. Decreased expression of IRAP in psoriatic lesional epidermis. *British Journal of Dermatology* **127**, 305–311.

Krueger, G.G., Chalmers, D.H. & Shelby, J. (1981) Involved and uninvolved skin from psoriatic subjects: are they equally diseased? Assessment by skin transplantation to congenitally athymic (nude) mice. *Journal of Clinical Investigations* **68**, 1548–1557.

Krueger, G.G., Jorgensen, C., Miller, C. *et al.* (1990) Effects of IL-8 on epidermal proliferation (Abstract). *Journal of Investigative Dermatology* **94**, 545.

Langner, A., Chorzelski, T.P., Fraczykowska, M., Jablonska, S. & Szymanczyk, J. (1983) Is chemotactic activity in polymorphonuclear leukocytes increased in psoriasis? *Archives of Dermatological Research* **275**, 226–228.

Livden, J.K., Nilsen, R. & Bjerke, J.R. (1989) In situ localization of interferons in psoriatic lesions. *Archives of Dermatolological Research* **281**, 392–397.

Lowe, N.J., Breeding, J. & Ruissel, D.H. (1982) Cutaneous polyamine in psoriasis. *British Journal of Dermatology* **107**, 21–26.

Madsen, P., Rasmussen, H.H., Leffers, H. *et al.* (1991) Molecular cloning, occurrence and expression of a novel partially secreted protein 'psoriasin' that is highly upregulated in psoriatic skin. *Journal of Investigative Dermatology* **97**, 701–706.

Marks, R. (1978) Epidermal activity in the involved and uninvolved skin of patients with psoriasis. *British Journal of Dermatology* **98**, 399–403.

Matsue, H., Bergstresser, P.R. & Takashima, A. (1993) Keratinocyte derived IL-7 serves as a growth factor for dendritic epidermal T cells in mice. *Journal of Immunology* **151**, 6012–6019.

Nanney, L.B., Yates, R.A. & King, L.E. (1992a) Modulation of epidermal growth factor receptors in psoriatic lesions during treatment with topical EGF. *Journal of Investigative Dermatology* **98**, 296–301.

Nanney, L.B., Gates, R.E., Todderud, G. *et al.* (1992b) Altered distribution of phospholipase C-gamma 1 in benign hyperproliferative epidermal diseases. *Cell Growth and Differentiation* **3**, 233–239.

Nickoloff, B.J., Karabin, G.D. & Barker, J.N. (1991) Cellular localization of interleukin-8 and its inducer tumor necrosis factor-alpha in psoriasis. *American Journal of Pathology* **138**, 129–140.

Ohta, Y., Katayama, I. & Funato, T. (1991) In expression of messenger RNA of interleukin-1 and interleukin-6 in psoriasis: Interleukin-6 involved in formation of psoriatic lesions. *Archives of Dermatological Research* **283**, 351–356.

Okada, N., Kitano, Y. & Ichihara, K. (1982) Effects of cholera toxin on proliferation of cultured human keratinocytes in relation to intracellular cyclic AMP levels. *Journal of Investigative Dermatology* **79**, 42–47.

Parkinson, E.K., Pera, M.F. & Emmerson, A. (1984) Differential effects of complete and second-stage tumour promoters in normal but not transformed human and mouse keratinocytes. *Carcinogenesis* **5**, 1071–1077.

Pease, C.T., Fennel, M., Staughton, R.C.D. & Brewerton, D.A. (1987) Polymorphonuclear leukocyte function in psoriasis. *British Journal of Dermatology* **117**, 161–167.

Placek, W., Haftek, M. & Thivolet, J. (1988) Sequence of changes in psoriatic epidermis: Immunocompetent cell redistribution precedes altered expression of keratinocyte differentiation markers. *Acta Dermato-Venereologica* **68**, 369–372.

Prens, E.B., Benner, K., van Joost, Th. *et al.* (1991) The autologous mixed epidermal cell-T lymphocyte reaction is elevated in psoriasis: a crucial role for HLA-DR+/CD1a-antigen presenting cells. *Journal of Investigative Dermatology* **96**, 880–887.

Priestly, G.C. (1991) The fibroblast in psoriasis: Master or slave? *European Journal of Dermatology* **1**, 185–191.

Pullmann, H., Lennartz, K.J. & Steigleder, G.K. (1977) Disturbance of DNA synthesis in early psoriasis. *Archives of Dermatological Research* **258**, 11–18.

Ricoh, M.J., Halprin, K.M., Baker, L., Cayer, M. & Taylor, J.R. (1985) Stimulated mitotic counts in the non-lesional skin of patients with psoriasis and controls. *British Journal of Dermatology* **113**, 185–188.

Rijzewijk, J.J., van Erp, P.E.J. & Bauer, F.W. (1989) Two binding sites for Ki-67 related to quiescent and cycling cells in human epidermis. *Acta Dermato-Venereologica* **69**, 512–515.

Rulo, H.F.C., Westphal, J.R., van de Kerkhof, P.C.M. *et al.* (1995) Expression of endoglin in psoriatic involved and uninvolved skin. *Journal of Dermatological Science* **10**, 103–109.

Sackstein, R., Falanga, V., Streilein, J.W. & Chin, Y.H. (1988) Lymphocyte adhesion to psoriatic dermal endothelium is mediated by a tissue-specific receptor/ligand interaction. *Journal of Investigative Dermatology* **91**, 423–428.

Samitz, M.H. & Pomerantz, H. (1959) Electrophoretic patterns in psoriatic exfoliative erythroderma. *Archives of Dermatology* **79**, 641–643.

Schalkwijk, J., Chang, A., Janssen, P., de Jongh, G.J. & Mier, P.D. (1990) Skin derived antileukoproteases (SKALP's): Characterization of two new elastase inhibitors from psoriatic epidermis. *British Journal of Dermatology* **122**, 631–641.

Schmid, P., Cox, D. & McMaster, G.K. (1993) In situ hybridization analysis of cytokine, protooncogene and tumour suppressor gene expression in psoriasis. *Archives of Dermatolological Research* **285**, 334–340.

Schröder, J.M. (1995) Inflammatory mediators and chemoattractants. In: *Pathogenic Aspects of Psoriasis* (eds van de Kerkhof, P.C.M. & Bos, J.D.), pp. 137–150. *Clinics in Dermatology,* Elsevier Vol. 13.

Schröder, J.M., Gregory, H., Young, J. & Christophers, E. (1992) Neutrophil-activating proteins in psoriasis. *Journal of Investigative Dermatology* **98**, 241–247.

Sedgwick, J.B., Bergstresser, P.R. & Hurd, E.R. (1980) Increased granulocyte adherence in psoriasis and psoriatic arthritis. *Journal of Investigative Dermatology* **74**, 81–84.

Sedgwick, J.B., Bergstresser, P.R. & Hurd, E.R. (1981) Increased superoxyde generation by normal granulocytes incubated in sera from patients with psoriasis. *Journal of Investigative Dermatology* **76**, 158–163.

Shuster, D.S. (1958) Electrophoretic studies in psoriasis. *Archives of Dermatology* **77**, 713–714.

Siegenthaler, G., Hotz, R., Chatellard-Gruaz, D., Jaconi, S. & Saurat, J.H. (1993) Characterization and expression of a novel human fatty acid-binding protein: The epidermal type (E-FABP). *Biochemistry and Biophysics Research Communications* **190**, 482–487.

Smith, C.H. & Barker, J.N.W.N. (1995) Pathogenic aspects of psoriasis: Cell trafficking and role of adhesion molecules in psoriasis. In: *Pathogenic Aspects of Psoriasis.* (eds van de Kerkhof, P.C.M. & Bos, J.D.) *Clinics in Dermatology,* Vol. 13, pp. 151–160.

Stabel, S. & Parker, P.J. (1991) Protein kinase C. *Pharmacological Therapy* **51**, 71–95.

Steigleder, G.K., Schumann, H. & Lennartz, K.J. (1973) Autoradiographic in vitro-examination of psoriatic skin before, during and after dithranol treatment. *Archives of Dermatology* **246**, 231–235.

Tadini, G., Cerri, A. & Crosti, L. (1989) P53 and oncogene expression in psoriasis. *Acta Dermato-Venereologica Supplementum* **146**, 33–35.

Takahashi, H., Iizuka, H. & Katagiri, M. (1990) No evidence for the mutation of ras gene in psoriatic epidermis. *Archives of Dermatological Research* **282**, 8–11.

Tettelbach, W., Nanccy, L., Ellis, D. *et al.* (1993) Localisation of MGSA/GRO protein in cutaneous lesions. *Journal of Cutaneous Pathology* **20**, 259–266.

Tucker, W.F.G., MacNeil, S., Bleehan, S.S. & Tomlinson, S. (1984) Biologically active calmodulin levels are elevated in both involved and uninvolved epidermis in psoriasis. *Journal of Investigative Dermatology* **82**, 298–299.

Turbitt, M.L., Akhurst, R.J. & White, S.I. (1990) Localization of elevated transforming growth factor-αin psoriatic epidermis. *Journal of Investigative Dermatology* **95**, 229–232.

Tuschil, A., Lam, C.R., Hulsberger, A. & Linley, I. (1992) Interleukin-8 stimulates calcium transients and promotes epidermal cell proliferation. *Journal of Investigative Dermatology* **99**, 294–299.

Uyemura, K., Yamamura, M. & Fivenson, D.F. (1993) The cytokine network in lesional and lesion-free psoriatic skin is characterized by a T-helper type 1 cell-mediated response. *Journal of Investigative Dermatology* **101**, 701–705.

Valgi-Nagy, I., Jensen, P.J., Albelda, S.M. & Rodeck, U. (1992) Cytokine induced expression of transforming growth factor and the epidermal growth factor receptor in neonatal skin explants. *Journal of Investigative Dermatology* **99**, 350–357.

van de Kerkhof, P.C.M. (1982) Plasma aldosterone and cortisol levels in psoriasis and atopic dermatitis. *British Journal of Dermatology* **106**, 423–428.

van de Kerkhof, P.C.M. (1991) Common pathways for epidermal growth and inflammation and their relevance in the pathogenesis of psoriasis. *International Journal of Dermatology* **30**, 755–762.

van de Kerkhof, P.C.M. & van Erp, P.E.J. (1983) Calmodulin levels are grossly elevated in the psoriatic lesion. *British Journal of Dermatology* **108**, 217–218.

van de Kerkhof, P.C.M., Rennes, H., de Grood, R.M. *et al.* (1983) Responses of the clinically involved skin of psoriasis to standardized injury. *British Journal of Dermatology* **109**, 287–294.

van de Oord, J.J. & de Wolf-Peeter, C. (1994) Epithelium lining macrophages in psoriasis. *British Journal of Dermatology* **130**, 589–594.

van Erp, P.E.J., Boezeman, B.J.M. & Brons, P.T. (1988) Cell cycle kinetics in normal human epidermis by in vitro administration of iododeoxy uridine and application of the differentiation marker RKSE$_{-60}$. *Journal of Investigative Dermatology* **90**, 801–853.

van Erp, P.E.J., Boezeman, J.B. & Brons, P.P. (1996) Cell cycle kinetics in normal human skin by *in vivo* administration of iododeoxyuridine and application of a differentiation marker – implications for cell cycle kinetics in psoriatic skin. *Annals of Cell Pathology* **11 (1)**, 43–54.

van Erp, P.E.J., de Mare, S., Rijzewijk, J.J., van de Kerkhof, P.C.M. & Bauer, F.W. (1989) A sequential double immunozymic staining procedure to obtain cell kinetic information in normal and hyperproliferative epidermis. *Histochemistry Journal* **21**, 343–347.

van Pelt, J.P.A., de Jong, E.M.G.J., van Erp, P.E.J. & van de Kerkhof, P.C.M. (1997) Decreased CD11 b expression on circulating polymorphonuclear leukocytes in patients with extensive plaque psoriasis. *European Journal of Dermatology* **7**, 324–328.

van Ruissen, F., de Jongh, G.J., Erp, P.E.J., Boezeman, J.B.M. & Schalkwijk, J. (1996) Cell kinetic characterization of cultured human keratinocytes from normal and psoriatic individuals. *Journal of Cell Physiology* **168**, 684–94.

van Ruissen, F., Erp, P.E.J., de Jong, G.J., Boezeman, J.B.M., van de Kerkhof, P.C.M. & Schalkwijk, J. (1994) Cell kinetic characterisation of growth arrest in cultured human keratinocytes. *Journal of Cell Science* **107**, 2219–2228.

van Ruissen, F., van de Kerkhof, P.C.M. & Schalkwijk, J. (1995) Signal transduction pathways in epidermal proliferation and cutaneous inflammation. In: *Pathogenetic Aspects of Psoriasis.* (eds van de Kerkhof, P.C.M. & Bos, J.D.) *Clinics in Dermatology*, Vol. 13, pp. 161–190.

Verhagen, A., Bergers, M., van Erp, P.R.J. *et al.* (1984) Confirmation of raised phospholipase A$_s$ activity in the uninvolved skin of psoriasis. *British Journal of Dermatology* **110**, 731–732.

Weber, G., Nederkort, M., Schmidt, A. & Geiger, A. (1981) The correlation of growth hormone and clinical picture of psoriasis. *Archives of Dermatological Research* **270**, 129–140.

Weinstein, G.D., MacCullough, J.L. & Ross, P.A. (1985) Cell kinetic basis for pathophysi-ology of psoriasis. *Journal of Investigative Dermatology* **85**, 579–583.

Weiss, R.A., Eichner, R. & Sun, T.T. (1984) Monoclonal antibody analysis of keratin expression in epidermal diseases: a 48- and 56k dalton keratin as molecular markers for hyperproliferative keratinocytes. *Journal of Cell Biology* **98**, 1397–1406.

Wiley, H.E. & Weinstein, G.D. (1979) Abnormal proliferation of uninvolved psoriatic epidermis: Differential induction by saline, propanolol and tape stripping *in vivo*. *Journal of Investigative Dermatology* **73**, 545–547.

Wortmann, S., Boehnke, W.H., Mielke, V. *et al.* (1993) Ultrastructure of macrophages lining the epidermal dermal border in psoriatic skin (lining cells). *Archives of Dermatolological Research* **285**, 85.

Yates, R.A., Nanney, L.B. & Gates, R.E. (1991) Epidermal growth factor and related growth factors. *International Journal of Dermatology* **30**, 687–694.

Yoshizaki, K., Nishimoto, N. & Matsumoto, K. (1990) Interleukin-6 and expression of its receptor on epidermal keratinocytes. *Cytokine* **2**, 381–387.

Ziboh, V.A., Tamara, L., Casebolt, B.S., Marcelom, C.L. & Voorheesm, J.J. (1984) Biosynthesis of lipoxygenase products by enzyme preparations from normal and psoriatic skin. *Journal of Investigative Dermatology* **83**, 426–430.

Chapter 7: Immunopathogenesis

S. Kang and J.J. Voorhees

7.1 Introduction

Prominent histological features of psoriasis are marked epidermal hyperplasia with parakeratotic stratum corneum, and modest inflammatory cell infiltrates. Elegant studies on cell kinetics have revealed that, in hyperplastic epidermis, basal keratinocytes not only undergo more frequent cell divisions, but also transit through the epidermal layer much more quickly than they do in normal skin (Weinstein & Frost 1968). Given the striking structural and functional alterations in psoriatic epidermis, it is quite clear why the prevailing view of psoriasis pathogenesis prior to the 1980s focused on keratinocyte biology. The less obvious inflammatory cell infiltrate was believed to be a secondary reaction to the epidermal pathology.

This understanding of psoriasis as a disease of defective keratinocytes was challenged by observations made by two rheumatologists, Mueller and Herrmann in 1979 (Mueller & Herrmann 1979). Their report described four patients with psoriatic arthritis being treated with oral cyclosporin A (CSA) for joint inflammation who experienced an unexpected, dramatic improvement of their skin disease. The clinical efficacy of CSA documented in Mueller and Herrmann's open study was subsequently confirmed in a double-blind, placebo-controlled trial of CSA in psoriasis (Ellis *et al.* 1986). With the proven clinical efficacy of CSA and rapidly accumulating evidence that the primary action of CSA is to inhibit lymphokine release and proliferation of T cells came a major paradigm shift. The view of psoriasis as a disease of epidermal origin began to shift to a view of psoriasis as an epidermal response to immunological injury. Although the cause of psoriasis remains unknown, enhanced immune response is known to be the critical factor in disease expression. This chapter summarizes evidence from detailed clinical and laboratory studies that provides the basis for this major paradigm shift.

7.2 T cells in psoriatic lesions

The cellular infiltrate in psoriasis is composed primarily of T cells, both CD4[+] and CD8[+] cells (Bjerke *et al.* 1978; Baker *et al.* 1984). Interestingly, these cell types are somewhat compartmentalized: CD4[+] cells are located mainly in the dermis, while CD8[+] cells are found mostly in the epidermis (Menssen *et al.* 1995). Changes in the relative ratio of these cell types may be important for both the genesis and resolution of psoriatic plaques. In acute guttate psoriasis, for example, one of the earliest observable events in the forming lesions is an intraepidermal influx of activated (HLA DR[+]) CD4[+] T cells (Valdimarsson *et al.* 1986). In spontaneous resolving guttate lesions, on the other hand, an influx of CD8[+] (HLA DR[+]) T cells is observed, along with a decrease in CD4[+] cells. Physical injury to the psoriatic uninvolved skin can lead to induction of the disease. In this 'Koebner phenomenon', CD4[+] cells predominate over CD8[+] T cells in the epidermis (Baker *et al.* 1988a). Several studies of psoriasis using different treatment regimens indicate that clearance of CD4[+] cells correlates with clinical improvement (Baker *et al.* 1985; Ellis *et al.* 1986; Gupta *et al.* 1989). In a recent study, however, reduction of the CD8[+] subset was most strongly correlated with resolution of the disease (Gottlieb *et al.* 1995). It is still unclear which of the two T-cell subsets is more important in the expression of psoriasis. Regardless of the phenotype, T cells in psoriatic skin display signs of activation [i.e., HLA DR[+] (Valdimarsson *et al.* 1986), interleukin 2 (IL-2) receptor (CD25[+]) (De Boer *et al.* 1994)]. For this reason, it is likely that both CD4[+] and CD8[+] cells contribute.

The presence of both CD4[+] and CD8[+] T cells in lesional skin is in accordance with the strong association between psoriasis and major histocompatibility complex (MHC) classes I (HLA Cw6) and II (DR7) molecules (Ozawa *et al.* 1988; Gottlieb & Krueger 1990; Elder *et al.* 1994). (See Chapter 5 for a more thorough review of the literature on the genetics of psoriasis.) Such studies are of interest to clinicians because inherited differences in HLA proteins may account for susceptibility to psoriasis. Since CD4[+] T cells interact with antigen-presenting cells (APCs) that express MHC class II molecules, and since CD8[+] T cells associate with APCs that carry MHC class I molecules, the strong correlation between psoriasis and both class I and II MHC molecules is consistent and compatible with the presence of both subsets of T cells (CD4[+] and CD8[+]) in psoriatic lesions.

7.3 Antigen-presenting cells in psoriasis

APCs represent a group of cells critical for T-cell function. They express MHC class I and II molecules on their surfaces, through which presentation of antigen is made to T cells. In normal human epidermis, bone-marrow-derived CD1a[+] Langerhans cells (HLA DR[+]) are the resident APCs. The Langerhans cells are present in similar numbers in lesional and non-lesional skin of psoriasis and thus are unlikely to be pathogenic APCs in lesions. In psoriatic epidermis, there are increased numbers of CD1a[-] DR[+] dendritic cells that are distinct from CD1a[+] Langerhans cells (Baadsgaard *et al.* 1989). The CD1a[-] DR[+] cells are not specific to psoriasis, since they are seen in other inflammatory dermatoses as well (Baker *et al.* 1988b). The ability of psoriatic epidermal cells to induce autologous T-cell activation and proliferation is significantly dependent on a population of CD1a[-] DR[+] macrophage-like cells, since depletion of this subset from cell suspensions markedly reduces the capacity for activation and proliferation (Baadsgaard *et al.* 1989). HLA DR⁺ keratinocytes that are abnormally represented in lesional skin do not contribute to heightened APC activity. Dermal dendrocytes appear to be another important type of APC in psoriatic dermis. Dermal dendrocytes are factor XIIIa⁺ and are located in the high papillary dermis around blood vessels (Headington 1986; Nickoloff & Griffiths 1990).

Several pathways of antigen processing and presentation in APCs are known (York & Rock 1996), but they will not be discussed in this chapter. Interested readers are referred to recent reviews (Barnaba 1996; Banchereau & Steinman 1998). Suffice to say, each pathway terminates with the MHC protein displaying an antigenic peptide on the surface of the APCs. This peptide–protein complex is specifically recognized by a particular T-cell receptor (TCR). It follows that a key element linking T cells and APCs is the antigen. The identity of this antigen in psoriasis has yet to be determined, but it is likely to be a peptide derived from foreign (i.e. infectious) agents and/or self proteins. As mentioned above, the interacting T cells are restricted to either CD8⁺ or CD4⁺ T cells, depending on whether the antigen is presented in the context of class I or II MHC molecules.

Thus, within psoriatic lesions reside abnormally large numbers of T cells and APCs, the cellular constituents necessary to initiate T-cell-mediated immune responses. Dividing memory T cells, often in direct apposition to non-Langerhans APCs, have been observed in psoriatic skin injected *in vivo* with ³H-deoxyuridine, using visualization by autoradiography and immunolabelling (Morganroth *et al.* 1991). These findings provide *in vivo* evidence that infiltrating APCs provide the necessary signals to activate intralesional T cells directly.

The critical importance of these two bone-marrow-derived cell types in psoriasis pathogenesis has been appreciated at the clinical level by recipients of bone-marrow transplants. Following successful allogeneic transplantation of bone-marrow cells, both resolution of psoriasis (Eedy *et al.* 1990), and the converse finding of transmission of psoriasis (Gardembas-Pain *et al.* 1990), have been reported.

7.4 T cell and antigen-presenting cell interaction

Successful engagement of T cells and APCs leads to stimulation of T cells. This process involves at least two activation signals from APCs. The first signal is generated through the so-called ternary complex (MHC/antigen/TCR) which imparts specificity to T-cell activation. The stimulation of a TCR is necessary, but not sufficient, to induce complete activation of T cells that results in cell proliferation and secretion of cytokines. For complete T-cell activation to occur, a second 'costimulatory signal' is required. The costimulation depends on interactions between several proteins working as ligand–receptor pairs that serve to regulate the activation cascade of T cells. Of these, the most important and well characterized is the B7 : CD28/CTLA-4 costimulatory pathway. It consists of two ligands, B7–1 and B7–2, on APCs that bind to two receptors on T cells, CD28 and CTLA-4 (Guinan *et al.* 1994). The CD28 and CTLA-4 proteins are similar in structure, with shared amino acid sequences, but are different in expression and function. CD28 is expressed by both resting and activated T cells (Bluestone 1995), whereas CTLA-4 is expressed only on activated T cells (Guinan *et al.* 1994). B7–1 and B7–2 have a greater affinity for binding with CTLA-4 than with CD-28. Unlike CD-28, however, CTLA-4 transmits an inhibitory signal that serves to terminate the immune response.

Together, signal 1 and signal 2 initiate a signal transduction cascade within T cells that ultimately affects T-cell function. This intracellular signalling is an extremely complex phenomenon that involves interactions between a number of signalling molecules. We will discuss only one, the nuclear factor of activated T cells (NF-AT) signalling pathway.

7.5 Nuclear factor of activated T cells activation pathway and cyclosporin/FK-506

Investigations into the immunosuppressive mechanism of action of CSA and FK-506 led to the identification of a unique signal transduction pathway in T cells (Fig. 7.1). One of the very early membrane-associated events in T-cell activation is phosphoinositide turnover following contact between the APC and the TCR–CD3 complex (Mizushima *et al.* 1987; Sawada *et al.* 1987; Dumont *et al.* 1990). Subsequently, there is a rise in intracellular calcium levels and activation of the protein kinase C (PKC) family, neither of which are influenced by CSA or FK-506. However, both drugs inhibit the expression of early lymphokine genes (i.e. IL-2, IL-3, IL-4, tumour necrosis factor-α (TNF-α), granulocyte/macrophage colony-stimulating factor (GM-CSF), and interferon-γ (IFN-γ)) that are usually expressed within 4 h of T-cell activation (Tocci *et al.* 1989). When either drug is administered after the expression of these early lymphokine messenger RNAs (mRNAs), there is no effect upon T cells (Dumont *et al.* 1990). Pathways that do not involve an increase in intracellular calcium, such as T-cell activation via the CD28 pathway, are not sensitive to the effects of CSA or FK-506 (June *et al.* 1987; Kay & Benzie 1989; Lin *et al.* 1991), suggesting that the two drugs affect a calcium-dependent signal transduction event. It is now known that elevation of calcium is required to activate the Ca^{2+}/calmodulin-dependent protein phosphatase, calcineurin (Friedman & Weissman 1991; Liu *et al.* 1991). Activated calcineurin phosphatase removes phosphate groups from transcription factor NF-ATc, a constitutive cytosolic component of the complex. The dephosphorylation of NF-ATc serves as a nuclear localization signal that leads to translocation of the transcription factor to the nucleus. There it combines with a nuclear NF-AT component of the

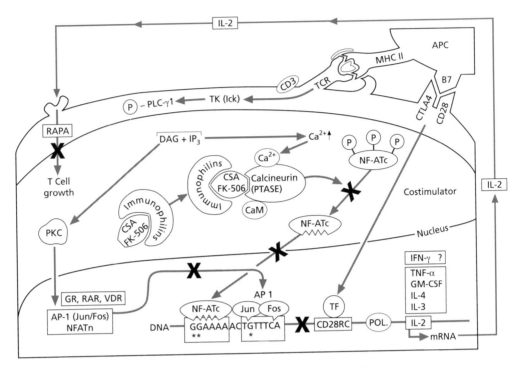

Fig. 7.1 T-cell activation signal transduction pathway: Regulation of cytokine gene transcription. See text for details. CSA, cyclosporin; RAPA, rapamycin; GR, RAR and VDR, glucocorticoid, retinoid, and vitamin D$_3$ receptors, respectively. X, the site of inhibition of antipsoriasis drugs. (From Voorhees 1996, with permission from The Japanese Dermatological Association.)

complex (NF-AT$_n$). The NF-AT$_c$/NF-AT$_n$ heterodimer binds to its regulatory site on several proinflammatory lymphokine gene promoters, such as IL-2, and induces their expression (Flanagan *et al.* 1991; McCaffrey *et al.* 1993).

Both CSA and FK-506 effectively inhibit IL-2 gene transcription in activated T cells. They bind to distinct intracellular receptors that possess similar properties. Cyclophilin A (CYP) and FKBP-12 are the major receptors for CSA and FK-506, respectively (Handschumacher *et al.* 1984; Siekierka *et al.* 1989). These receptors, referred to as immunophilins, are small cytosolic proteins that are both abundant and ubiquitous (Siekierka *et al.* 1990; Trandinh *et al.* 1992). One of the most interesting characteristics of CYP and FKBP-12 is their enzymatic activity whereby *cis*-to-*trans* isomerization of peptidyl-prolyl bonds is catalysed. The peptidyl-prolyl isomerase (PPIase) activity of CYP and FKBP-12 is lost when they are bound to their cognate ligands.

Initially, the inhibition of PPIase activity by CSA and FK-506 was believed to be related to their immunosuppressive effect. However, identification of CSA and FK-506 analogues that can potently inhibit their PPIase activity without an inhibitory effect on IL-2 transcription clearly indicated that PPIase inhibition is not sufficient to block T-cell activation. Rapamycin is one such analogue. It is chemically related to FK-506, and is equipotent in the ability to inhibit the PPIase activity of FKBP-12. However, rapamycin cannot block IL-2 transcription, and in fact, antagonizes the ability of FK-506 to do so (Fischer *et al.* 1989; Takahashi *et al.* 1989). The search for targets of CYP/CSA and FKBP/FK-506 led to the isolation of calcineurin phosphatase (Liu *et al.* 1991; Friedman & Weissman 1991). This calcium- and calmodulin-dependent serine–threonine phosphatase is inhibited by CSA and FK-506 bound to their respective immunophilins (Dumont *et al.* 1992). Indeed, a strong correlation exists between the immunosuppressive activity of CSA or FK-506 analogues and the ability of the receptor–analogue complex to bind calcineurin and inhibit its phosphatase activity (Dumont *et al.* 1992).

7.6 The human interleukin 2 gene promoter

The ultimate manifestation of T-cell activation is T-cell proliferation. IL-2 is a mitogen necessary for the amplification of T-cell-mediated immune responses. Understanding the regulation of this lymphokine gene is therefore important for knowing the key elements involved in T-cell activation, as well as for identifying novel therapeutic targets for immunosuppression. For these reasons, the human IL-2 promoter has been extensively studied. The region required for maximal expression of IL-2 mRNA extends about 300 base pairs upstream from the transcription initiation site (Ullman *et al.* 1990). Several enhancer sites have been identified through deletion and mutational analysis. They contain binding sites for transcription factors operational in other cell types such as NF-kB, AP-1 (Jun/Fos), and octamer/octamer-associated protein (Oct/OAP). In addition, two enhancer elements bind NF-AT and a CD28-responsive factor, which appear to be unique to T cells. Results from transfection assays indicate that calcineurin activates the IL-2 promoter via NF-AT (Frantz *et al.* 1994). Other transcription factors (AP-1 and CD28-TF) that also bind to enhancer elements of the IL-2 promoter are activated through different signalling elements, such as PKC, following successful engagement of T cells by APCs.

7.7 Inflammatory cytokines in psoriasis and their effect on keratinocytes

The same transcription factors that are activated in stimulated T cells to promote transcription of IL-2 govern the transcription of other proinflammatory cytokine genes to amplify immune responses. Activated T cells in general produce one of two types of cytokines, known as type 1 (T1) and type 2 (T2) cytokines.

T1 cytokines IL-2 and IFN-γ mediate cellular immunity. T2 cytokines IL-4, IL-5, and IL-10 mediate humoral immunity. Not only are T1 and T2 responses fairly discrete, they are self-reinforcing in that T1 cytokines tend to inhibit the production of T2 cytokines, and vice versa (Del Prete *et al.* 1994). Cells cloned from psoriatic lesions have been shown to produce IL-2 and IFN-γ (Uyemura *et al.* 1993; Schlaak *et al.* 1994). For this reason, psoriasis is considered to be a T1-dominant disease. The influence of IFN-γ on psoriatic keratinocytes is evident *in vivo* by their expression of MHC class II molecules and IFN-γ inducible protein 10 (IP-10) molecules, which are uniquely induced by the T-cell-specific lymphokine (Morhenn *et al.* 1982; Gottlieb *et al.* 1988; Baadsgaard *et al.* 1989). The critical importance of IL-2 and IFN-γ in disease expression is clear because each cytokine is capable of inducing the appearance of psoriasis when it is administered *in vivo* to patients with a propensity for psoriasis (Lee *et al.* 1988; Fierlbeck *et al.* 1990).

Not all keratinocytes in the epidermis are capable of proliferating. Two subsets of potentially proliferative keratinocytes are β1 integrin (CD29)$^+$ K1/K10$^-$ undifferentiated basal keratinocyte stem cells, and CD29$^+$ K1/K10$^+$ transient amplifying cells which reside suprabasally and are committed to differentiation (Bata-Csorgo *et al.* 1993). Involved psoriatic skin demonstrates a shift in the cell cycle of CD29$^+$ K1/K10$^-$ stem cells from the G_0 phase to an actively proliferating mode. The CD29$^+$ K1/K10$^-$ stem cells from uninvolved psoriatic skin, but not from normal skin, are stimulated to proliferate by cytokines and growth factors from T cells isolated from psoriatic plaques. If neutralizing antibodies to IFN-γ are added to the supernatants prior to addition to keratinocyte cultures, cell growth is inhibited. These data indicate that IFN-γ released from T cells of type T1 within lesions is a critical factor in disease pathogenesis.

7.8 Pharmacological evidence for psoriasis as an immunological disease

If the initiating signal that triggers psoriatic keratinocytes to hyperproliferate and manifest the clinical disease does indeed come from activated T cells, then agents that can interfere in the activation process should improve symptoms of psoriasis. Thus far in this chapter, CSA and FK-506 have been discussed in this context. In point of fact, almost all drugs that have successfully been used or are being experimentally used to treat psoriasis interfere in T-cell activation at some stage. The fact that effective pharmacological agents share a common mechanism of inducing immunosuppression provides strong complementary evidence that psoriasis is in fact an immune system-mediated disease. Selective examples of drugs that affect different steps in the T-cell activation signal transduction pathway are presented briefly. Figure 7.1 illustrates the sites of action of these pharmacological agents in the T-cell activation signalling pathways.

Starting at the T-cell surface, since the formation of intact ternary complex (signal 1) is necessary for immune mediation, impairment of any part of

the complex is expected to improve psoriasis. Indeed, intravenous administration of monoclonal antibodies targeted at CD3, a pan T-cell marker, and
CD4 have shown substantial efficacy (Weinshenker *et al.* 1989; Prinz *et al.*
1991). The requirement for costimulation (signal 2) in T-cell activation indicates that effective interference in this pathway would also be therapeuti-
cally beneficial. CTLA-4 immunoglobulin is a soluble chimeric protein
consisting of the extracellular domain of human CTLA-4 and the Fc portion
of human IgG1 (Linsley *et al.* 1991). By binding to B7 molecules on APCs,
CTLA-4 immunoglobulin can block the CD28-mediated costimulatory signal
required for T-cell activation.

In a recently completed phase I study, intravenous infusion of CTLA-4
immunoglobulin showed clinical promise for treatment of psoriasis (Abrams
et al. 1999), and warrants further investigation.

The ability of CSA and FK-506 to impair signal transduction within T
cells was discussed earlier. Rapamycin acts more distally in the signalling
pathway than do CSA and FK-506. Although it binds to FKBP, the rapamycin–
FKBP complex does not inhibit calcineurin phosphatase. Instead, it associ-
ates with target-of-rapamycin (TOR) and prevents it from activating p70
S6-kinase (p70^{S6K}) (Chung *et al.* 1992). Phosphorylation of S6 ribosomal protein by p70^{S6K} is essential for progression of the cell cycle through the G1
phase. By inhibiting S6-kinase, rapamycin blocks T-cell growth and proliferation, the ultimate consequence of T-cell activation. Because the requirement for phosphorylated S6 ribosomal protein in cell-cycle progression is
not unique to T cells, rapamycin would be expected to affect other proliferating cells, such as psoriatic keratinocytes. Indeed, oral administration of
rapamycin has been shown to block the cell cycle at the G_1 phase in
keratinocyte stem cells from psoriatic lesions (Javier *et al.* 1997).

Steroids, vitamin D and retinoids represent three distinct groups of pharmacological agents that are known to improve psoriasis. They possess multiple mechanisms of action, one of which involves blocking T-cell signalling at
the level of NF-AT/AP-1 and NF-kB transcription of lymphokine genes in T
cells (Alroy *et al.* 1995; Scheinman *et al.* 1995). Therefore, they too possess
immunosuppressive activity. In fully activated T cells in psoriatic skin, the
T1/T2 cytokine balance is shifted in favour of T1 expression (IL-2, IFN-γ).
Attempts to restore the balance by utilizing opposing T2 cytokines (IL-4, IL-5
or IL-10) offer an exciting therapeutic avenue. An open study with IL-10 has
demonstrated this pharmacological principle in psoriasis (Asadullah *et al.*
1998).

Even methotrexate, a well-characterized antimetabolite, is now known
to possess anti-inflammatory/immunosuppressive properties. At therapeutic
doses used to treat psoriasis (on average 10–20 mg per week) its ability to
inhibit dihydrofolate reductase appears to be a minimal feature. Rather, by
inhibiting an enzyme called 5-aminoimidazole carboxamidoribonucleotide
(AICAR) transformylase, methotrexate causes intracellular accumulation of

AICAR, which in turn promotes adenosine release by a mechanism that is not fully understood (Cronstein *et al.* 1993). The adenosine released at sites of inflammation binds to specific A_2 receptors on lymphocytes, resulting in inhibition of cytokine production and lymphocyte proliferation (Cronstein 1995). Sulphasalazine appears to act through a similar mechanism of adenosine accumulation to improve psoriasis and rheumatoid arthritis (Gandangi *et al.* 1996).

7.9 Conclusion

A serendipitous observation that CSA was effective in the treatment of psoriasis was the beginning of a major paradigm shift in viewing the pathogenesis of psoriasis. Since then, both clinical and basic investigations have generated a significant body of evidence that immunological mechanisms are critical in psoriasis pathophysiology. The advances in cellular and immunological characterization of psoriasis have been greatly facilitated by the immunopharmacological agents discussed in this chapter. Indeed, the weight of evidence supporting psoriasis as an immune-mediated disease would be substantially less if the complementary data from immunotherapeutics did not exist. Better understanding of the key steps involved in T-cell activation should enable identification of pharmacological targets that may lead to highly selective immunosuppressive therapy.

References

Abrams, J.R., Lebwohl, M.G., Guzzo, C.A. *et al.* (1999) CTLA4Ig-mediated blockade of T cell costimulation in patients with psoriasis vulgaris. *Journal of Clinical Investigation* **103**, 1243–1252.

Alroy, I., Towers, T.L. & Freedman, L.P. (1995) Transcriptional repression of the interleukin-2 gene by vitamin D_3: Direct inhibition of NFATp/AP-1 complex formation by a nuclear hormone receptor. *Molecular and Cell Biology* **15**, 5789–5799.

Asadullah, K., Sterry, W., Stephanek, K. *et al.* (1998) IL-10 is a key cytokine in psoriasis. Proof principle by IL-10 therapy: a new therapeutic approach. *Journal of Clinical Investigations* **101**, 783–794.

Baadsgaard, O., Gupta, A.K., Taylor, R.S., Ellis, C.N., Voorhees, J.J. & Cooper, K.D. (1989) Psoriatic epidermal cells demonstrate increased numbers and function of non-Langerhans antigen-presenting cells. *Journal of Investigative Dermatology* **92**, 190–195.

Baker, B.S., Powles, A.V., Lambert, S., Valdimarsson, H. & Fry, L. (1988a) A prospective study of the Koebner reaction and T lymphocytes in uninvolved psoriatic skin. *Acta Dermato-Venereologica* **68**, 430–434.

Baker, B.S., Lambert, S., Powles, A.V., Valdimarsson, H. & Fry, L. (1988b) Epidermal DR⁺T6⁻ dendritic cells in inflammatory skin diseases. *Acta Dermato-Venereologica* **68**, 209–217.

Baker, B.S., Swain, A.F., Fry, L. & Valdimarsson, H. (1984) Epidermal T lymphocytes and HLA-DR expression in psoriasis. *British Journal of Dermatology* **110**, 555–564.

Baker, B.S., Swain, A.F., Griffiths, C.E.M., Leonard, J.N., Fry, L. & Valdimarsson, H.

(1985) Epidermal T lymphocytes and dendritic cells in chronic plaque psoriasis: the effects of PUVA treatment. *Clinical Experimental Immunology* **61**, 526–534.

Banchereau, J. & Steinman, R.M. (1998) Dendritic cells and the control of immunity. *Nature* **392**, 245–251.

Barnaba, V. (1996) Viruses, hidden self-epitopes and autoimmunity. *Immunological Reviews* **152**, 47–66.

Bata-Csorgo, Z., Hammerberg, C., Voorhees, J.J. & Cooper, K.D. (1993) Flow cytometric indentification of proliferative subpopulations within normal human epidermis and the localization of the primary hyperproliferative population in psoriasis. *Journal of Experimental Medicine* **178**, 1271–1281.

Bjerke, J.R., Krough, H.K. & Matre, R. (1978) Characterization of mononuclear cell infiltrate in psoriatic lesions. *Journal of Investigative Dermatology* **71**, 340–343.

Bluestone, J.A. (1995) New perspectives of CD28–B7-mediated T cell costimulation. *Immunity* **2**, 555–559.

Chung, J.K., Kuo, C.J.R.C.G. & Blenis, J. (1992) Rapamycin-FKBP specially blocks growth-dependent activation of and signaling by the 70kd S6 protein kinase. *Cell* **69**, 1227–1236.

Cronstein, B.N. (1995) A novel approach to the development of anti-inflammatory agents: adenosine release at inflamed sites. *Journal of Investigative Medicine* **43**, 50–57.

Cronstein, B.N., Naime, D. & Ostad, E. (1993) The antiinflammatory mechanism of methotrexate: increased adenosine release at inflamed sites diminishes leukocyte accumulation in an in vivo model of inflammation. *Journal of Clinical Investigations* **92**, 2675–2682.

De Boer, O.J., van der Loos, C.M., Hamerlinck, F., Bos, J.D. & Das, P.K. (1994) Reappraisal of *in situ* immunophenotypic analysis of psoriasis skin: interaction of activated HLA-DR⁻ immunocompetent cells and endothelial cells is a major feature of psoriatic lesions. *Archives of Dermatological Research* **286**, 87–96.

Del Prete, G., Maggi, E. & Romagnani, S. (1994) Biology of disease. Human Th1 and Th2 cells: functional properties, mechanisms of regulation, and role in disease. *Laboratory and Investigations* **70**, 299–305.

Dumont, F., Staruch, M., Koprak, S., Melino, M. & Sigal, N. (1990) Distinct mechanisms of suppression of murine T cell activation by the related macrolides FK-506 and rapamycin. *Journal of Immunology* **144**, 251–258.

Dumont, F., Staruch, M., Koprak, S. *et al.* (1992) The immunosuppressive and toxic effects of FK-506 are mechanistically related: pharmacology of a novel antagonist of FK-506 and rapamycin. *Journal of Experimental Medicine* **176**, 751–760.

Eedy, D.J., Burrows, D., Bridges, J.M. & Jones, F.G.C. (1990) Clearance of severe psoriasis after allogeneic bone marrow transplantation. *British Medicine Journal* **300**, 908.

Elder, J.T., Nair, R.P., Guo. S. *et al.* (1994) The genetics of psoriasis. *Archives of Dermatology* **130**, 216–224.

Ellis, C.N., Gorsulowsky, D.C., Hamilton, T.A. *et al.* (1986) Cyclosporine A improves psoriasis in a double-blind study. *Journal of the American Medical Association* **256**, 3110–3116.

Fierlbeck, G., Rassner, G. & Muller, C. (1990) Psoriasis induced at the injection site of recombinant interferon gamma. Results of immunohistologic investigations. *Archives of Dermatology* **126**, 351–355.

Fischer, G., Wittmann, L., Lang, K., Kiefhaber, T. & Schmid, F. (1989) Cyclophilin and peptidyl-prolyl cis-trans isomerase are probably identical proteins. *Nature* **337**, 476–478.

Flanagan, W., Corthesy, B., Bram, R. & Crabtree, G. (1991) Nuclear association of a T-cell transcription factor blocked by FK-506 and cyclosporin A. *Nature* **352**, 803–807.

Frantz, B., Nordby, E., Bren, G. *et al.* (1994) Calcineurin acts in synergy with PMA to inactivate I kappa B/MAD3, an inhibitor of NF-kappa B. *EMBO Journal* **13**, 861–870.

Friedman, J. & Weissman, I. (1991) Two cytoplasmic candidates for immunophilin action are revealed by affinity for a new cyclophilin: one in the presence and one in the absence of CsA. *Cell* **66**, 799–806.

Gandangi, P., Longaker, M., Naime, D. *et al.* (1996) The anti-inflammatory mechanism of sulfasalazine is related to adenosine release at inflamed sites. *Journal of Immunology* **156**, 1937–41.

Gardembas-Pain, M., Irah, N., Foussard, C., Boassom, M., Andre, J.P.S. & Verret, J.L. (1990) Psoriasis after allogenic bone marrow transplantation. *Archives of Dermatology* **126**, 1523.

Gottlieb, S.L., Gilleaudeau, P., Johnson, R. *et al.* (1995) Response of psoriasis to a lymphocyte-selective toxin ($DAB_{389}IL-2$) suggests a primary immune, but not keratinocyte, pathogenic basis. *Nature Medicine* **1**, 442–447.

Gottlieb, A.B. & Krueger, J.G. (1990) HLA region genes and immune activation in the pathogenesis of psoriasis. *Archives of Dermatology* **126**, 1083–1086.

Gottlieb, A.B., Luster, A.D., Posnett, D.N. & Carter, D.M. (1988) Detection of a gamma interferon-induced protein IP-10 in psoriatic plaques. *Journal of Experimental Medicine* **168**, 941–948.

Guinan, E.C., Gribben, J.G., Boussiotis, V.A. *et al.* (1994) Pivotal role of the B7: CD28 pathway in transplantation tolerance and tumor immunity. *Blood* **84**, 3261–3282.

Gupta, A.K., Baadsgaard, O., Ellis, C.N., Voorhees, J.J. & Cooper, K.D. (1989) Lymphocytes and macrophages of the epidermis and dermis in lesional psoriatic skin, but not epidermal Langerhans cells, are depleted by treatment with cyclosporin A. *Archives of Dermatological Research* **281**, 219–226.

Handschumacher, R., Harding, M., Rice, J., Druggs, R. & Speicher, D. (1984) Cyclophilin: a specific cytosolic binding protein for cyclosporin A. *Science* **226**, 544–547.

Headington, J.T. (1986) The dermal dendrocyte. In: *Advances in Dermatology* (eds Callen, J.P., Dahl, M.V. & Golitz, L.D.), Vol. 1, pp. 159–171. Chicago: Year Book Medical.

Javier, A.F., Bata-Csorgo, Z., Ellis, C.N., Kang, S., Voorhees, J.J. & Cooper, K.D. (1997) Rapamycin (Sirolimus) inhibits proliferating cell nuclear antigen expression and blocks cell cycle in the G_1 phase in human keratinocyte stem cells. *Journal of Clinical Investigations* **99**, 2094–2099.

June, C., Ledbetter, J., Gillespie, M., Lindsten, T. & Thompson, C. (1987) T-cell proliferation involving the CD28 pathway is associated with cyclosporine-resistant interleukin 2 gene expression. *Molecular Cell Biology* **7**, 4472–4481.

Kay, J. & Benzie, C. (1989) T lymphocyte activation through the C28 pathway is insensitive to inhibition by the immunosuppressive drug FK-506. *Immunological Letters* **23**, 155–159.

Lee, R.E., Gaspari, A.A., Lotze, M.T., Chang. A.E. & Rosenberg, S.A. (1988) Interleukin 2 and psoriasis. *Archives of Dermatology* **124**, 1811–1815.

Lin, C., Boltz, R., Siekierka, J. & Sigal, N. (1991) FK-506 and cyclosporin A inhibit highly similar signal transduction pathways in human T lymphocytes. *Cell Immunity* **133**, 269–284.

Linsley, P.S., Brady, W., Urnes, M. *et al.* (1991) CTLA-4 is a second receptor for the B cell activation antigen B7. *Journal of Experimental Medicine* **174**, 561–569.

Liu, J., Farmer, J.D. Jr, Lane, W.S., Friedman, J., Weissman, I. & Schreiber, S.L. (1991) Calcineurin is a common target of cyclophilin-cyclosporin A and FKBP-FK-506 complexes. *Cell* **66**, 807–815.

McCaffrey, P., Perrino, B., Soderling, T. & Rao, A. (1993) NF-ATp, a T lymphocyte DNA-binding protein that is a target for calcineurin and immunosuppressive drugs. *Journal of Biological Chemistry* **268**, 3747–3752.

Menssen, A., Trommler, P., Vollmer, S. *et al.* (1995) Evidence for an antigen-specific cellular immune response in skin lesions of patients with psoriasis vulgaris. *Journal of Immunology* **155**, 4078–4083.

Mizushima, Y., Kosaka, H., Sakuma, S. *et al.* (1987) Cyclosporin A inhibits late steps of T lymphocyte activation after transmembrane signaling. *Journal of Biochemistry* **102**, 1193–1201.

Morganroth, G.S., Chan, L.S., Weinstein, G.D., Voorhees, J.J. & Cooper, K.D. (1991) Proliferating cells in psoriatic dermis are comprised primarily of T cells, endothelial cells, and factor XIIIa⁺ perivascular dendritic cells. *Journal of Investigative Dermatology* **96**, 333–340.

Morhenn, V.B., Abel, E.A. & Mahrle, G. (1982) Expression of HLA-DR antigen in skin from patients with psoriasis. *Journal of Investigative Dermatology* **78**, 165–168.

Mueller, W. & Herrmann, B. (1979) Cyclosporin A for psoriasis. *New England Journal of Medicine* **301**, 555.

Nickoloff, B.J. & Griffiths, C.E.M. (1990) Lymphocyte trafficking in psoriasis: a new perspective emphasizing the dermal dendrocyte with active dermal recruitment mediated via endothelial cells followed by intra-epidermal T-cell activation. *Journal of Investigative Dermatology* **95**, 35S–37S.

Ozawa, A., Lhikodo, M., Ihako, H. *et al.* (1988) Specific restriction fragment length polymorphisim on the HLA-C region and susceptibility to psoriasis vulgaris. *Journal of Investigative Dermatology* **90**, 402–405.

Prinz, J., Braun-Falco, O., Meurer, M. *et al.* (1991) Chimaeric CD4 monoclonal antibody in treatment of generalized pustular psoriasis. *Lancet* **338**, 320–321.

Sawada, S., Suzuki, G., Kawase, Y. & Takaku, G. (1987) Novel immunosuppressive agent, FK506. In vitro effects on the cloned T cell activation. *Journal of Immunology* **139**, 1797–1803.

Scheinman, R.I., Cogswell, P.C., Lofquist, A.K. & Baldwin, A.S. Jr (1995) Role of transcriptional activation of IκBα in mediation of immunosuppression by gluco-corticoids. *Science* **270**, 283–286.

Schlaak, J.F., Buslau, M., Jochum, W. *et al.* (1994) T cells involved in psoriasis vulgaris belong to the Th 1 subset. *Journal of Investigative Dermatology* **102**, 145–149.

Siekierka, J., Hung, S., Poe, M., Lin, C. & Sigal, N. (1989) A cytosolic binding protein for the immunosuppressant FK506 has peptidyl-prolyl isomerase activity but is distinct from cyclophilin. *Nature* **341**, 755–757.

Siekierka, J., Wiederrecht, G., Greulich, H. *et al.* (1990) The cytosolic-binding protein for the immunosuppressant FK-506 is both a ubiquitous and highly conserved peptidyl-prolyl cis-trans isomerase. *Journal of Biological Chemistry* **265**, 21011–21015.

Takahashi, N., Hayano, R. & Suzuki, M. (1989) Peptidyl-prolyl cis-trans isomerase is the cyclosporin A-binding protein cyclophilin. *Nature* **337**, 473–475.

Tocci, M., Matkovich, D., Collier, K. *et al.* (1989) The immunosuppressant FK506 selectively inhibits expression of early T cell activation genes. *Journal of Immunology* **143**, 718–726.

Trandinh, C., Pao, G. & Saier, M. (1992) Structural and evolutionary relationships among the immunophilins: two ubiquitous families of peptidyl-prolyl cis-trans isomerases. *FASEB Journal* **6**, 3410–3420.

Ullman, K., Northrop, J., Verweij, C. & Crabtree, G. (1990) Transmission of signals from the T lymphocyte antigen receptor to the genes responsible for cell proliferation and immune function: the missing link. *Annual Review of Immunology* **8**, 421–452.

Uyemura, K., Yamamura, M., Fivenson, D.F., Modlin, R.L. & Nickoloff, B.J. (1993) The cytokine network in lesional and lesion-free psoriatic skin is characterized by a T-helper type I cell-mediated response. *Journal of Investigative Dermatology* **101**, 701–705.

Valdimarsson, H., Baker, B.S., Jonsdottir, I. & Fry, L. (1986) Psoriasis: a disease of abnormal keratinocyte proliferation induced by T lymphocytes. *Immunology Today* **7**, 256–259.

Voorhees, J.J. (1996) Dohi Memorial Lecture. Psoriasis – an immunological disease. *Journal of Dermatology* **23**, 851–857.

Weinshenker, B.G., Bass, B.H., Ebers, G.C. & Rice, G.P.A. (1989) Remission of psoriatic lesions with muromonab-CD3 (Orthoclone OKT3) treatment. *Journal of the American Academy of Dermatology* **20**, 1132–1133.

Weinstein, G.D. & Frost, P. (1968) Abnormal cell proliferation in psoriasis. *Journal of Investigative Dermatology* **50**, 254–259.

York, I.A. & Rock, K.L. (1996) Antigen processing and presentation by the class I major histocompatibility complex. *Annual Review of Immunology* **14**, 369–396.

Part 3: Therapy

In the last decade important developments have revolutionized the treatment of psoriasis. Various existing treatments have been optimized by enhancing clinical efficacy and/or decreasing the occurrence of side-effects. Each author in this section provides an introduction into the mode of action. Indications/contraindications, general methodology, remission induction characteristics (percentage clearing, reduction psoriasis area and severity index (PASI), reduction of erythema induration and scaling), relapse characteristics, differential response in subforms of psoriasis and side-effects are described.

Chapters 8–10 provide information on topical treatment with vitamin D_3 analogues, corticosteroids and dithranol. Chapter 11 highlights phototherapy (UVB) and photo(chemo)therapy (PUVA).

Chapters 12–14 provide an account on systemic treatments with methotrexate, cyclosporin and acitretin. Treatment guidelines are of central importance in these chapters.

In Chapter 15 combinations and comparisons of treatments are detailed.

Chapter 8: Vitamin D$_3$ Analogues

K. Fogh and K. Kragballe

8.1 Introduction

Impared differentiation and increased proliferation of epidermal keratinocytes are key features in psoriatic lesions together with a local activation of T lymphocytes. The active form of vitamin D$_3$ (1,25-dihydroxyvitamin D$_3$, 1,25(OH)$_2$D$_3$) is known to play an important role in the regulation of intestinal calcium absorption, bone mineralization and prevention of rickets. In addition to these actions 1,25(OH)$_2$D$_3$ has several additional biological effects including stimulation of cellular differentiation, inhibition of proliferation (Smith *et al.* 1986; Kragballe & Wildfang 1990) and immune modulation (Bhalla *et al.* 1983; Müller & Bendtzen 1996). These biological actions make 1,25(OH)$_2$D$_3$ a potential candidate for treatment of psoriasis (Kragballe 1989; Kragballe & Iversen 1993; Green *et al.* 1994). Improvement of psoriasis by 1,25(OH)$_2$D$_3$ has been demonstrated in one patient with osteoporosis, who received oral 1-α-OH-D$_3$ 0.75 µg/day, and had a dramatic improvement of her severe psoriasis (Morimoto & Kumahara 1985). This observation, together with evidence that the bioactive form of 1,25(OH)$_2$D$_3$ inhibits keratinocyte proliferation and promotes keratinocyte differentiation (Hosomi *et al.* 1983), led to a new era in 1,25(OH)$_2$D$_3$ research.

1,25(OH)$_2$D$_3$ itself may not be suitable for treatment of psoriasis due to its hypercalcaemic effects. As a consequence, several non-calcaemic vitamin D$_3$ analogues with potent biological effects on the cellular level have been developed (Binderup & Kragballe 1992). One of these analogues, calcipotriol has been extensively investigated and is now available for topical treatment of psoriasis in most countries. The present review deals with molecular actions, clinical efficacy and safety of vitamin D$_3$ analogues in psoriasis.

8.2 Vitamin D receptors: molecular mechanisms

The genomic effects of 1,25(OH)$_2$D$_3$ and its analogues are thought to be mediated by their interaction with the vitamin D receptor (VDR) present in target cells. The VDR belongs to the superfamily of nuclear receptors also comprising the thyroid, steroid and retinoid receptors (Evans 1988). A single VDR is common to all cells and binds 1,25(OH)$_2$D$_3$ with high affinity. The subsequent effect on gene transcription occurs after binding of the activated VDR to specific DNA sequences (vitamin D response element (VDRE)) in the promotor region of target genes (Evans 1988). A number of VDREs have been identified (Kerner *et al.* 1989; Demay *et al.* 1990; Ozono *et al.* 1990; Darwish & DeLuca 1992; Demay *et al.* 1992; Chen *et al.* 1994; Quélo *et al.* 1994). Natural VDREs are generally composed of two direct repeat (DR) hexanucleotide half-sites separated by three bases, a so-called DR3 response element. In general, this spacing (i.e. number of bases between the hexanucleotides) determines the specificity of VDREs (Umesono *et al.* 1991). In addition, variations in the hexanucleotide orientation and the spacing may be important (Carlberg *et al.* 1993). The trans-acting activity of $1,25(OH)_2D_3$ in cells transfected with DR3 response elements requires heterodimerization of the VDR with the retinoid X receptor (RXR) (Sone *et al.* 1991; Carlberg *et al.* 1993; MacDonald *et al.* 1993; Carlberg *et al.* 1994; Schräder *et al.* 1994). This provides the molecular basis for a cross-talk between the retinoid and vitamin D pathways.

As determined by ligand binding and immunoblotting the VDR has been detected in most cell types in the skin, including cultured keratinocytes (Feldman *et al.* 1980), Langerhans cells (Dam *et al.* 1996), melanocytes (Ranson *et al.* 1988), fibroblasts (Eil & Marx 1981) and endothelial cells (Merke *et al.* 1989). Furthermore, monocytes and activated T cells participating in inflammatory skin reactions express the VDR (Bhalla *et al.* 1983; Müller & Bendtzen 1996).

It is believed that $1,25(OH)_2D_3$ also has various rapidly occurring 'non-genomic' actions. The importance of these actions are unclear. They include accumulation of cyclic guanosine monophosphate (GMP), stimulation of phospholipase C and increase in cytosolic free calcium. It is also unknown whether the rapid actions are mediated by the classical intracellular VDR (Barsony & Marx 1991) or a putative membrane receptor (Farach-Carson *et al.* 1991; Norman *et al.* 1992).

8.3 Biological actions of $1,25(OH)_2D_3$ and vitamin D_3 analogues

8.3.1 1,25-dihydroxyvitamin D_3

The effects of $1,25(OH)_2D_3$ on epidermal keratinocytes have been extensively investigated. In cultured differentiating keratinocytes $1,25(OH)_2D_3$ stimulates proliferation, whereas proliferating, undifferentiated keratinocytes are inhibited by $1,25(OH)_2D_3$ (Gniadecki 1996; Svendsen *et al.* 1999). A similar paradoxical response to $1,25(OH)_2D_3$ is observed *in vivo*.

Topical application of $1,25(OH)_2D_3$ and its analogues to normal mice skin increases keratinocyte proliferation and causes epidermal hyperplasia (Lützow-Holm *et al.* 1993; Gniadecki & Serup 1995). In contrast, petrolatum-induced epidermal hyperplasia in guinea pigs is inhibited by $1,24(OH)_2D_3$ (Demay *et al.* 1990). This inhibitory activity corresponds to the antiproliferative effect observed in psoriatic hyperplasia. The levels of VDR may determine the responsiveness to vitamin D$_3$. It is therefore of interest that 1,25(OH)$_2$D$_3$ upregulates the VDR levels in human epidermal keratinocytes *in vitro* (Sølvsten *et al.* 1997) as well as *in vivo* (Sølvsten *et al.* 1999).

1,25(OH)$_2$D$_3$ is recognized to have immunoregulatory properties *in vitro*. Defined actions of the hormone on human peripheral blood mononuclear cells include inhibition of mitogen/antigen-stimulated proliferation (Tsoukas *et al.* 1984). 1,25(OH)$_2$D$_3$ also modulates the ability of monocytes to provide signals important in T-lymphocyte activation. Thus, 1,25(OH)$_2$D$_3$ decreases monocyte HLA DR expression, monocyte antigen presentation, and monocyte promotion of T-cell proliferation (Rigby & Waugh 1992).

8.3.2 Calcipotriol

The *in vitro* effects of calcipotriol on keratinocytes and on the immunocompetent cells are similar to those of 1,25(OH)$_2$D$_3$ both quantitatively and qualitatively. Calcipotriol binds to the VDR with the same affinity as 1,25(OH)$_2$D$_3$ in a number of different cell types. Calcipotriol inhibits cell proliferation and induces cell differentiation at concentrations similar to those of 1,25(OH)$_2$D$_3$ in the human histiocytic lymphoma cell line U937 (Binderup & Bramm 1988) and in cultured human keratinocytes (Kragballe & Wildfang 1990; Binderup *et al.* 1994).

In addition, calcipotriol induces VDR-mediated gene transcription in transfected cultures of human keratinocytes (Henriksen *et al.* 1997). Furthermore, topical application of calcipotriol twice daily for 4 days suppresses the number of Langerhans cells, the antigen-presenting cells (APCs) of the epidermis, as well as their accessory cell function (Dam *et al.* 1996). Compared with 1,25(OH)$_2$D$_3$, calcipotriol has much lower calcaemic potency in mice, rats, dogs and guinea pigs. After oral and intraperitoneal administration it was found that calcipotriol was 100–200 times weaker than 1,25(OH)$_2$D$_3$ with respect to serum calcium and calcium excretion (Binderup & Bramm 1988). Calcipotriol is a 1,25(OH)$_2$D$_3$ analogue containing a double bond and a ring structure in the side chain. As a consequence of this modification of the side chain, it is rapidly transformed into inactive metabolites (Binderup & Kragballe 1992). Therefore, calcipotriol is about 200 times less potent than 1,25(OH)$_2$D$_3$ in producing hypercalcemia and hypercalciuria after oral and intraperitoneal administration in rats. In contrast, calcipotriol and 1,25(OH)$_2$D$_3$ are equipotent in their affinity for the VDR and in their *in vitro* effects (Binderup & Kragballe 1992).

8.3.3 Tacalcitol

Tacalcitol (1,24(OH)$_2$D$_3$) is another synthetic vitamin D analogue developed for topical use in psoriasis. 1,24(OH)$_2$D$_3$ is equipotent with 1,25(OH)$_2$D$_3$ in its affinity for the VDR (Matsumoto *et al.* 1990) and in its capacity to inhibit keratinocyte proliferation and to stimulate keratinocyte differentiation *in vitro* (Matsunaga *et al.* 1990).

Recently, it has been indicated that the antipsoriatic affects of tacalcitol may involve chemokine production by epidermal keratinocytes (i.e. RANTES and interleukin 8) (Fukuoka *et al.* 1998) Also, tacalcitol is as effective as $1,25(OH)_2D_3$ in increasing cytosolic calcium levels in cultured keratinocytes (Matsunaga *et al.* 1990). Compared with $1,25(OH)_2D_3$, tacalcitol induces a smaller increase of serum calcium levels after a single intravenous dose to rats (Matsunaga *et al.* 1990). However, the doses inducing hypercalcemia are similar for tacalcitol and $1,25(OH_2)D_3$. Although tacalcitol may be advantageous over $1,25(OH)_2D_3$ for clinical use, it is much less selective than calcipotriol in its effects on calcium metabolism.

8.4 Expression of the vitamin D receptor in psoriatic skin

Because the available anti-VDR antibodies crossreact with non-VDR proteins, it has been difficult to assess VDR levels in psoriatic skin. In an immunohistochemical study, lesional psoriatic epidermis showed increased staining with the monoclonal 9A7γ anti-VDR antibody compared with non-lesional epidermis and normal epidermis (Milde *et al.* 1991). Using the same antibody, Western analysis showed similar levels of VDR in lesional and in non-lesional psoriatic skin (Sølvsten *et al.* 1996). These results were confirmed using a polyclonal rabbit anti-VDR antibody. Furthermore, the VDR messenger RNA (mRNA) levels were similar in both acute and chronic psoriatic lesions and expressed at the same level as in normal uninvolved psoriatic skin (Sølvsten *et al.* 1996).

The levels of RXRα, the heterodimeric partner for VDR, are also normal in psoriatic skin (Jensen *et al.* 1998).

Furthermore, the binding of psoriatic skin extracts to a VDRE of the DR3 type suggests that the genomic signalling pathway is normal in this skin disease (Jensen *et al.* 1998).

8.5 Vitamin D metabolism in psoriasis

Vitamin D metabolism in psoriatic patients has long been a matter of dispute. Morimoto *et al.* (1990) observed no difference in the mean levels of circulating $1,25(OH)_2D_3$ between psoriatic and normal subjects, whereas Staberg *et al.* (1987) reported reduced $1,25(OH)_2D_3$ concentrations in psoriatics with disseminated disease. More recently Smith *et al.* (1988) and Guilhou *et al.* (1990) found normal serum $1,25(OH)_2D_3$ levels in patients with moderate to extensive psoriasis. An inverse relationship between the severity of psoriasis and the serum $1,25(OH)_2D_3$ level may probably explain these conflicting results (Morimoto *et al.* 1990).

Severe psoriasis has been observed in association with hypoparathyroidism (Risum 1973) and hypocalcemia (Stewart *et al.* 1984). In these patients psoriasis improved when serum calcium levels were restored. Although these case reports demonstrate that fluctuation in serum calcium can precipitate psoriasis, all parameters of calcium and bone metabolism are normal in larger groups of psoriatic patients (Smith *et al.* 1988; Mortensen *et al.* 1993). Taken together the available data do not support the idea that psoriasis is a manifestation of abnormal vitamin D or calcium metabolism.

A related question is whether psoriatic skin is less sensitive to 1,25(OH)$_2$D$_3$ than normal skin.

It has been reported that cultures of dermal fibroblasts and epidermal keratinocytes from psoriatics are relatively resistant to the antiproliferative effect of 1,25(OH)$_2$D$_3$, despite normal binding to the VDR (McLaughlin *et al.* 1985; Abe *et al.* 1989). However, one of these was unable to repeat the results (Smith *et al.* 1988). Because other investigators have failed to show a difference between psoriatic and normal fibroblasts, there is apparently no intrinsic insensitivity of psoriatic fibroblasts or keratinocytes to 1,25 (OH)$_2$D$_3$. It is also of interest that the cutaneous formation of vitamin D$_3$ after exposure to a single dose of UVB is normal in psoriasis (Matsouka *et al.* 1990).

8.6 Clinical effects of vitamin D$_3$ and vitamin D$_3$ analogues in psoriasis

8.6.1 1,25-dihydroxyvitamin D$_3$

1,25(OH)$_2$D$_3$ used topically shows mixed results due to different drug concentrations and vehicles (Morimoto *et al.* 1986; Henderson *et al.* 1989; van de Kerkhof *et al.* 1989; Langner *et al.* 1991; Langner *et al.* 1993; Wishart 1994; Bourke *et al.* 1995). In an early, open study improvement was reported in 16 out of 19 patients applying 1,25(OH)$_2$D$_3$ ointment 0.5 µg/g (Morimoto *et al.* 1986). However, in double-blind studies 1,25(OH)$_2$D$_3$ solution 2 µg/g produced no improvement compared with placebo (Henderson *et al.* 1989; van de Kerkhof *et al.* 1989). The concentration of 1,25(OH)$_2$D$_3$ was raised in the subsequent studies. Treatment with 1,25(OH)$_2$D$_3$ ointment 3 µg/g in amounts ranging from 35 g/week to 142 g/week appears to be safe (Henderson *et al.* 1989).

Treatment with 1,25(OH)$_3$D$_3$ 3 µg/g was, however, less effective than calcipotriol 50 µg/g in a comparative trial (Bourke *et al.* 1995). Recently, it has been shown that topical 1,25(OH)$_2$D$_3$ 3 µg/g was also safe and well-tolerated for the long-term treatment of psoriasis (Langner *et al.* 1996).

While 1,25(OH)$_2$D$_3$ appears to be safe to use topically, it seems that oral 1,25(OH)$_2$D$_3$ will be of limited value for treating psoriasis, because of its potent calcaemic effect. Although oral 1,25(OH)$_2$D$_3$ appears efficacious in psoriasis (Smith *et al.* 1988; Morimoto & Yoshikawa 1989; Perez *et al.* 1996), frequent monitoring of blood and urine calcium levels and yearly renal ultrasound is recommended. It should also be noted that psoriasis is not an approved indication for oral $1,25(OH)_2D_3$.

8.6.2 Calcipotriol

The antipsoriatic effect of calcipotriol ointment 50 µg/g has been documented in a number of clinical trials involving several thousands of patients (Tables 8.1 and 8.2). Calcipotriol ointment 50 µg/g is marketed for the treatment of plaque-type psoriasis vulgaris under the trade names Daivonex, Dovonex and Psorcutan. A calcipotriol cream (Kragballe *et al.* 1988; Staberg *et al.* 1989; Harrington *et al.* 1996) and solution (Green *et al.* 1994; Klaber *et al.* 1994) has also been found to be effective.

Comparative studies

Comparison with placebo. In a dose-finding, randomized, double-blind, right–left comparative study, calcipotriol ointment (25, 50 and 100 µg/g) and vehicle were compared in 50 patients with psoriasis vulgaris (Kragballe 1989). After treatment for 8 weeks calcipotriol 50 µg/g had a significantly greater antipsoriatic effect than vehicle. Calcipotriol 50 µg/g was more effective than calcipotriol 25 µg/g ointment, whereas no difference was found between calcipotriol 50 µg/g and 100 µg/g. From this study (Kragballe 1989) it was concluded that a calcipotriol concentration of 50 µg/g in an ointment is optimal for the treatment of psoriasis. Treatment with this calcipotriol concentration induces a significant improvement after just 1 week, and a marked improvement is observed in about two-thirds of the patients after 8 weeks. The efficacy and safety of calcipotriol ointment 50 µg/g was later confirmed in a multicentre, double-blind, placebo-controlled, right–left study including 66 psoriatic patients (Dubertret *et al.* 1992). Calcipotriol was used as a twice-daily treatment and the mean PASI (psoriasis area and severity index) score fell in 4 weeks from 14.2 to 6.3 with calcipotriol and from 14.1 to 9.2 with placebo (Dubertret *et al.* 1992). However, calcipotriol has also been investigated as a once-daily regimen in a double-blind, multicentre, placebo-controlled study including 245 psoriatics evaluated over an 8-week period (Pariser *et al.* 1996). It was found that calcipotriol was effective and well-tolerated and was found to be significantly better in terms of efficacy than its vehicle as early as the first week of treatment and the difference was maintained throughout the study (Pariser *et al.* 1996). Patient compliance is better with a once-daily regimen than a twice-daily regimen.

Other formulations of calcipotriol have been investigated. In a double-blind study (Kragballe *et al.* 1988) it was found that calcipotriol cream resulted in a statistically significant decrease in erythema, thickness and scaling of psoriatic lesions compared with cream base alone. Calcipotriol was investigated at

Table 8.1 Comparative studies with topical calcipotriol in psoriasis.

Calcipotriol	Comparison	Outcome	References
Ointment 50 μg/g	Vehicle, calcipotriol 25 μg/g and 100 μg/g	50 μg/g better than vehicle and 25 μg/g but equal to 100 μg/g	(Dubertret et al. 1992, Kragballe et al. 1998)
Ointment 50 μg/g	Betamethasone 17-valerate Betamethasone-dipropionate + salicylic acid Fluocinonide	Calcipotriol better than corticosteroid	(Kragballe 1990) (Scarpa 1996) (Bruce et al. 1994)
Cream 10–100 μg/g	Vehicle	Calcipotriol better than vehicle	(Stewart et al. 1984; Kragballe 1989; Harrington et al. 1996)
Cream 50 μg/g	Betamethasone 17-valerate	Calcipotriol equal to corticosteroid	(Molin et al. 1997)
Ointment 50 μg/g	Dithranol	Calcipotriol better than dithranol	(Berth-Jones et al. 1993; Van der Vleuten et al. 1995; Veien et al. 1997)
Ointment 50 μg/g	Tar	Calcipotriol better than tar	(Quélo et al. 1994; Tosti et al. 1998)

Table 8.2 Combination studies with calcipotriol.

Calcipotriol	Comparison	Outcome	References
Ointment 50 µg/g	Ointment 50 µg/g and steroid	Calcipotriol and steroid equal to or better than calcipotriol alone	(Kragballe *et al.* 1988; Scarpa 1994; Lebwohl *et al.* 1996; Lebwohl *et al.* 1998)
Ointment 50 µg/g	Ointment 50 µg/g and UVB	Calcipotriol and UVB better than calcipotriol alone	(Morimoto & Kumahara 1985: Kerscher *et al.* 1993; Kragballe & Iversen 1993)
Ointment 50 µg/g and UVB	UVB	Calcipotriol and UVB better than UVB alone	(Kokelj *et al.* 1995; Koo 1996; Ramsay 1998)
Ointment 50 µg/g and PUVA	PUVA	Reduction of PUVA dose in combination therapy	(Frappaz & Thivolet 1993)
Ointment 50 µg/g and CSA* (2 mg/kg/day)	Placebo and CSA	Calcipotriol/CSA better than placebo/CSA	(Grossman *et al.* 1994; Kokelj *et al.* 1998)
Ointment 50 µg/g and acitretin (10–20 mg/day)	Placebo and acitretin	Calcipotriol/acitretin better than placebo/acitretin	(Van de Kerkhof *et al.* 1989; Van de Kerkhof *et al.* 1998a)

*Cyclosporin

three different concentrations: 10 µg/g, 33 µg/g and 100 µg/g. After 6 weeks it was found that moderate or excellent improvement in two of nine patients treated with 10 µg/g, in five of nine patients treated with 33 µg/g and seven of nine patients treated with 100 µg/g of calcipotriol (Kragballe *et al.* 1988). In another study (Staberg *et al.* 1989), 10 inpatients with chronic plaque psoriasis, the antipsoriatic effect of calcipotriol was evaluated. In each patient two symmetrical located psoriatic plaques were selected for the study. Topical treatment with calcipotriol cream containing 1200 µg calcipotriol per gram of cream was compared with placebo cream in a double-blind, controlled, left–right, randomized trial during 6 weeks of therapy. Compared with baseline, the clinical (erythema, scaling and infiltration) improvement was significant after 1 week of therapy with calcipotriol cream, while lateral comparison showed calcipotriol cream significantly better than cream base after 4 weeks of therapy. Calcipotriol has also been investigated for psoriatic skin lesions in intertriginous areas, in an open and uncontrolled trial (Kienbaum *et al.* 1996). Twelve patients with psoriasis vulgaris who presented with psoriatic lesions in the axilla, and inguinal and anal folds, were treated with calcipotriol ointment (50 µg/g) twice daily for 6 weeks. In this study it was found that only two of 12 patients showed insufficient response to therapy whereas calcipotriol improved intertriginous psoriasis after 3–6 weeks of treatment. Treatment was generally well tolerated. Minimal burning was reported in one patient, slight lesional and/or perilesional irritation in five patients, and, in the remaining, no side-effects occurred. This open study indicates that topical calcipotriol is an effective and safe treatment for intertriginous psoriasis.

From these studies it is also concluded that calcipotriol cream is useful in the treatment of psoriasis, although it seems likely that calcipotriol cream is less effective as compared with ointment. However, calcipotriol cream may be preferred as it is less greasy.

Calcipotriol has also been investigated as a solution for scalp psoriasis. Efficacy and safety of calcipotriol solution in the treatment of scalp psoriasis was compared with placebo (vehicle solution), in a multicentre double-blind, randomized, parallel-group study of 49 adult patients (Green *et al.* 1994). Calcipotriol solution (50 µg/mL), or placebo, was applied twice daily over a 4-week period. At the end of the study period 60% of patients on calcipotriol showed clearance or marked improvement of their psoriasis compared with 17% on placebo. Overall assessment of treatment response showed that calcipotriol was superior to placebo and the solution was generally well tolerated (Green *et al.* 1994). The use of calcipotriol for scalp psoriasis was investigated in a multicentre, prospective, randomized, double-blind, parallel group study (Dubertret *et al.* 1992). Four hundred and seventy-four patients with scalp psoriasis were investigated in a twice-daily regimen. Treatment was compared with betamethasone 17-valerate solution (1 mg/mL) over a 4-weeks treatment period. The decrease in total sign score (sum of scores for erythema, thickness and scaliness) at the end of treatment was statistically significantly greater in the betamethasone group (61%) than the calcipotriol group (45%). Adverse events (lesional or perilesional irritation) were reported more frequently in the calcipotriol group (87 patients) than in the betamethasone group (31 patients). If the scales are very thick, the treatment of scalp psoriasis should be started with a descaling agent.

Recently, calcipotriol ointment was investigated for nail psoriasis in a double-blind randomized study (Tosti *et al.* 1998). Calcipotriol was compared with betamethasone/salicylic acid bath and it was found that calcipotriol is as effective as a combination of a topical corticosteroid with salicylic acid in the treatment of nail psoriasis.

From these studies it can be concluded that calcipotriol has marked antipsoriatic effects. Although not directly compared, it is the general impression that the ointment formulation is better than the cream and solution formulations. The cream formulation may be chosen for treatment of psoriasis located in the face and skin folds. In addition the cream formulation is less greasy than the ointment formulation. It is the impression that the effect of calcipotriol is more pronounced on lesional infiltration and scaling, whereas the effect is less pronounced on redness.

Comparison with topical corticosteroid. Efficacy of calcipotriol has been compared with a number of topical corticosteroids. Calcipotriol ointment 50 µg/g has been compared with betamethasone 17-valerate ointment 0.1% in a multicentre, randomized, double-blind, right–left comparison (Kragballe *et al.* 1991). Three hundred and forty-five patients with symmetrical, stable plaque-type psoriasis were randomized to treatment for 6 weeks. Both treatments produced a time-dependent improvement, and after 6 weeks the PASI was reduced by 68.8% with calcipotriol and 61.4% with betamethasone. Recently, calcipotriol cream 50 µg/g (210 patients) was compared with betamethasone 17-valerate cream, 1 mg/g (211 patients) in a multicentre, double-blind, parallel-group study (Molin *et al.* 1997).

It was found that both substances induced a significant reduction in PASI after 8 weeks of 47.8% and 45.4%, respectively. However, no difference was observed between the two groups. These results suggest that efficacy of calcipotriol ointment is superior to the cream formulation. Calcipotriol ointment was also shown to be more effective than the potent corticosteroids betamethasone dipropionate plus salicylic acid (Scarpa 1994) and fluocinonide (Bruce *et al.* 1994). In the latter study calcipotriol was compared with fluocinonide in a randomized, double-blind, parallel-group, active-controlled trial. Treatments were applied twice daily for 6 weeks. Mean scores for signs of scaling and plaque elevation in calcipotriol-treated subjects were significantly lower by week 2 than in the fluocinonide-treated subjects. These scores continued to be significantly lower than fluocinonide through week 6 and it was concluded that calcipotriol was superior to fluocinonide in the treatment of plaque psoriasis.

Taken together these comparative studies document that treatment with calcipotriol ointment and cream 50 µg/g is efficacious for psoriasis with a potency comparable to that of potent topical corticosteroids.

Comparison with dithranol and tar. Calcipotriol ointment 50 µg/g has been compared with dithranol (anthralin) used either as short-contact therapy in outpatients (Berth-Jones *et al.* 1992) or as conventional overnight inpatient therapy (van der Vleuten *et al.* 1995).

In a multicentre, open, randomized, parallel-group comparison patients were treated for 8 weeks with either calcipotriol 50 µg/g ointment applied twice daily or dithranol cream applied once daily for 30 min according to a short-contact regimen (Berth-Jones *et al.* 1992a).

Both the percentage reduction of PASI and the absolute reduction of PASI were significantly greater in the calcipotriol group (58.1%) than in the dithranol group (41.6%) at the end of treatment. Using of left–right comparative study design, 10 patients hospitalized with refractory psoriasis showed a better therapeutic response to calcipotriol ointment 50 µg/g than to dithranol after 2 weeks (van der Vleuten *et al.* 1995). Despite the low number of patients and the lack of follow-up of these patients, these results challenge one of the gold standards of antipsoriatic therapy.

Calcipotriol therapy has also been compared with tar treatment in a prospective, right–left, randomized, investigator-blinded, controlled study (Tham *et al.* 1994). Calcipotriol 50 µg/g was applied to one-half of the body and compared with a tar solution applied to the opposite side of the body. Twenty-seven patients were evaluated and it was found that a decrease in PASI score occurred on both sides at 2, 4 and 6 weeks. However, improvement was significantly better on the calcipotriol-treated side. High-dose calcipotriol (usage of an average of 377 g calcipotriol ointment for body lesions and 100 mL solution for scalp psoriasis per week) has also been compared with topical tar/dithranol in a 4-week multicentre, prospective, randomized, open, parallel-group study (van de Kerkhof 1998). It was found that PASI decreased significantly more in the calcipotriol group (58.4%) than the tar/dithranol group (35.6%).

Recently, calcipotriol ointment 50 µg/g was compared with a cream containing 5% coal tar/2% allantoin/0.5% hydrocortisone applied twice daily in a multicentre, randomized controlled study (Pinheiro 1997). One hundred and twenty-two patients participated in the study and it was found that calcipotriol was significantly better that 5% coal tar/2% allantoin/0.5% hydrocortisone.

Comparison with occlusion. The therapeutic response to calcipotriol ointment can be increased by occlusion under a polyethylene film (Bourke *et al.* 1993) or a hydrocolloid dressing (Nielsen 1993). Forty-eight patients with symmetrical chronic plaque psoriasis affecting the limbs were recruited for a single-blind, right–left, within-patient study to assess the effect of combining hydrocolloid occlusion with topical calcipotriol (Nielsen 1993). The combination of calcipotriol plus occlusion was significantly better than calcipotriol alone. The results indicate that occlusion improves the response to calcipotriol by enhancing its penetration. Indices of calcium metabolism remained unchanged throughout the study.

The beneficial effect of occlusion is probably due to better penetration and delivery of calcipotriol. Because of the risk of increased systemic absorption of calcipotriol, calcipotriol ointment should only be occluded in small areas. In particular very thick plaques benefit from occlusive therapy.

Combination therapies

Calcipotriol and corticosteroid. Calcipotriol monotherapy has been compared with combination therapy calcipotriol/corticosteroids (Lebwohl *et al.* 1996; Ruzicka & Lorenz 1998).

In the study by Ruzicka and Lorenz it was determined whether a combination of calcipotriol and betamethasone valerate after previous treatment with calcipotriol alone was more effective than the continuation of the monotherapy with calcipotriol. One hundred and sixty-nine psoriatic patients with the clinical diagnosis of chronic plaque-type psoriasis were treated twice daily for 2 weeks with calcipotriol, followed by a 4-week treatment with calcipotriol monotherapy in 87 patients or combined calcipotriol/ betamethasone valerate in 82 patients; all patients were followed for 8 weeks. The PASI was used to compare the two treatment groups. It was found that the combination therapy was more effective, as assessed by all evaluated variables; moreover, patients showing insufficient response to calcipotriol alone after 2 weeks showed a regression of psoriatic lesions using the combination regimen. These data indicate that in selected patients the use of a combination of calcipotriol and corticosteroid results in a greater antipsoriatic effect compared with calcipotriol as monotherapy.

Recently, calcipotriol cream was investigated with or without concurrent topical corticosteroid in a multicentre, double-blind, parallel-group study (Kragballe *et al.* 1998). It was found that calcipotriol applied twice daily was as effective as calcipotriol/clobetasone 17-butyrate, but slightly less effective than calcipotriol/betamethasone 17-butyrate. The incidence of skin irritation was less for patients using concurrent corticosteroids, whereas treatment with calcipotriol/vehicle did not reduce the incidence of skin irritation when compared with calcipotriol twice daily.

The combined therapy has been reviewed in detail by Lebwohl (Lebwohl 1997) and it can be concluded that regimens combining calcipotriol ointment with superpotent steroids such as halobetasol ointment can result in greater improvement and fewer side-effects.

Sequential therapy. In a double-blind, placebo-controlled, parallel-group study (Lebwohl *et al.* 1998) 44 patients with mild to moderate psoriasis were treated with calcipotriol ointment in the morning and halobetasol ointment in the evening for 2 weeks (phase 1). Thereafter, 40 patients who were at least moderately (50% or greater) improved were randomized to two treatment groups (phase 2). Twenty patients were randomized to receive halobetasol ointment twice daily on weekends and calcipotriol ointment twice daily on weekdays, and 20 patients were randomized to receive halobetasol ointment twice daily on weekends and placebo ointment twice daily on weekdays. It was found that 76% of patients applying halobetasol ointments on weekends and calcipotriol ointment on weekdays were able to maintain remission for 6 months compared with 40% of patients applying halobetasol ointment on weekends only with the vehicle on weekdays. These results indicate that the addition of calcipotriol ointment applied on weekdays to a weekend pulse therapy regimen of superpotent corticosteroids can increase the duration of remission of psoriasis. A third phase during which calcipotriol alone is used, may then follow for maintenance therapy.

Calcipotriol and UVB. There has been a considerable interest in combining topical calcipotriol with UVB phototherapy. In these trials the two treatments were started at the same time. Calcipotriol was then applied twice daily and UVB given 3 times weekly.

To avoid the risk of inactivation of calcipotriol by the UV light, patients applied calcipotriol ointment either at least 2 h before UVB exposure or after the UVB exposure. In the first studies the combination therapy was compared with calcipotriol monotherapy. After treatment for 8 weeks the combination therapy was more effective than calcipotriol alone (Kragballe 1990; Molin 1995). Broad-band UVB light sources were used in these studies, but the superiority of the combination therapy was also observed with narrow-band UVB light (Kerscher *et al.* 1993). In other trials the combination therapy was compared with UVB phototherapy alone. In a single-centre study including 19 patients the combination therapy had apparently a stronger antipsoriatic effect (Kokelj *et al.* 1995). However, in a larger multicentre study the advantage of the combination therapy was not statistically significant (Koo 1996).

Recently, UVB three times weekly was compared with calcipotriol cream plus UVB twice weekly in a multicentre, prospective, randomized, parallel-group, vehicle-controlled, single-blind study including 164 patients treated for 12 weeks (Ramsay 1998). It was found that the cumulative dose of UVB needed to induce 80% reduction in PASI score was less in the calcipotriol plus UVB group than in the group treated with UVB three times weekly.

Calcipotriol plus UVB results in a decreased number of UVB exposures. These results therefore seriously question the advocation of calcipotriol/UVB combination therapy.

One reason why UVB monotherapy was found to be almost as effective as the combination with calcipotriol may be that an aggressive UVB protocol was used (Koo 1996). This UVB treatment may by itself be so effective that an additional therapeutic effect of calcipotriol may be difficult to detect. However, in the case of suberythematogenic UVB doses the addition of calcipotriol does improve the therapeutic response to UVB, in particular during the first treatment weeks.

There are no follow-up data from UVB studies. It is therefore unknown whether the combination of UVB and calcipotriol improves the remission time compared with monotherapy.

It has consistently been found that the skin irritation induced by calcipotriol is not enhanced when UVB therapy is added. In general, calcipotriol and UVB should be started simultaneously. If calcipotriol is added to ongoing UVB therapy, patients should be aware of skin irritation (McKenna & Stern 1995). The risk of skin irritation can be reduced if the UVB dose is temporarily reduced when calcipotriol therapy is started.

Calcipotriol and PUVA. Calcipotriol improves the response to photochemotherapy with psoralen and UVA (PUVA). In a bilateral comparison of calcipotriol and ointment vehicle ($n = 13$), topical treatment was commenced on the first day of PUVA therapy (Speight & Farr 1994). Lesions treated with calcipotriol cleared earlier or were consistently judged to the better. In a larger, multicentre study calcipotriol or vehicle treatment was started 2 weeks prior to PUVA and then maintained during the therapy (Frappaz & Thivolet 1993).

Using this protocol, the combination of calcipotriol and PUVA reduced the cumulative UVA dose and the number of PUVA treatments required for clearance of psoriasis (Frappaz & Thivolet 1993). Because the combination of PUVA and calcipotriol can reduce UVA exposure and thereby the potential long-term hazards of PUVA (skin carcinomas), this combination therapy may be considered as a real progress in the management of psoriasis.

Calcipotriol and cyclosporin (CSA). Treatment with CSA (3–5 mg/kg/day) is very effective in patients with severe psoriasis. Because of the associated risk of nephrotoxicity, there has been an interest in combining low-dose (2 mg/kg/day) CSA with calcipotriol. In a double-blind, placebo-controlled, multicentre study including 69 patients calcipotriol/CSA was more effective than placebo/CSA (Grossman *et al.* 1994). It is unknown whether the superiority of the combination therapy is due to an additive effect or to a synergistic effect of calcipotriol on the CSA-induced suppression of interleukin 2 secretion (Gupta *et al.* 1989). Recently, calcipotriol has been shown useful in combination with high-dose of CSA (Kokelj *et al.* 1998). Twenty patients were enrolled in a right–left open study. All the patients admitted were treated with cyclosporin at an initial dose of 4.5 mg/kg/day; in case of clinical improvement this dosage was reduced by 0.5 mg/kg/day every 15 days. Calcipotriol ointment was applied only on the right lesion, twice a day, until the healing of the lesion or for 1 month. Patients were checked at baseline and every 15 days.

Eighteen patients completed the study and 17 of the 18 presented more evident improvement on the side treated with combined therapy, while only one patient showed a better result on the side treated with cyclosporin alone.

These results underline the usefulness of the association of calcipotriol and cyclosporin in order to decrease the total dosage of cyclosporin.

Calcipotriol and acitretin. Acitretin monotherapy may not induce sufficient improvement of plaque-type psoriasis. It has been shown that a combination of acitretin and topical calcipotriol results in a better treatment response after 12 weeks than acitretin alone (van de Kerkhof & Hutchinson 1996). This observation has recently been confirmed in a multicentre, randomized, double-blind, placebo-controlled study (van de Kerkhof *et al.* 1998). Patients were randomized to receive calcipotriol or placebo. All patients were treated with a starting dose of 20 mg acitretin per day and doses were adjusted at 2-weekly intervals with increments of 10 mg per day up to a maximum of 70 mg per day. The dose requirement for acitretin, clinical signs and adverse events were recorded. Seventy-six patients were randomized to treatment with calcipotriol 50 µg/g ointment twice daily and 59 patients to treatment with the vehicle only twice daily. Clearance or marked improvement was achieved by 67% of the patients in the calcipotriol group and by 41% of the patients in the placebo group ($P = 0.006$). Calcipotriol treatment proved to have a statistically significant additional effect to acitretin on the PASI, redness, thickness and scaliness as compared with placebo.

Clearance or marked improvement was achieved with a statistically significantly lower cumulative dose of acitretin by the patients in the calcipotriol group as compared with the placebo group. The number of patients reporting adverse events was pronounced and largely related to acitretin. No significant differences were observed between the two treatment groups with respect to adverse events (van de Kerkhof *et al.* 1998).

These results indicate that the addition of calcipotriol ointment to acitretin treatment contributes to the efficacy, reduces the cumulative dose of acitretin to reach marked improvement or clearance, and is well-tolerated and safe.

Long-term therapy

Because psoriasis is a chronic and relapsing disease, it becomes important to determine whether the beneficial effect of calcipotriol seen in the short-term studies can be maintained when patients are treated on a long-term basis.

This question has been assessed in two prospective, non-comparative, open studies. Included were patients who had a good clinical response to calcipotriol previously. In the first study, 15 patients from a single centre were treated with calcipotriol 50 µg/g ointment twice daily (maximally 100 g ointment per week) for at least 6 months (Kragballe & Fogh 1991). Assessment of efficacy at the end of therapy showed at least a moderate improvement in 80% of the treated patients.

These results have been confirmed and extended in multicentre study including 167 patients (Ramsay *et al.* 1994). In most patients the beneficial effect seen in short-term trials was maintained over the course of 1 year.

Although approximately 10% of the patients had to be withdrawn because of insufficient effect of calcipotriol, the dose required to maintain efficacy did not need to be increased with time. Thus, the mean quantity of ointment used fell from 35 g/week to 23 g/week during the last 6 months of therapy (Ramsay *et al.* 1994). Therefore, there was no suggestion of the development of a pharmacological tolerance to calcipotriol.

The major advantage of calcipotriol over corticosteroids may be that it does not induce skin atrophy during long-term treatment (Ramsay *et al.* 1994).

In a third study, the long-term safety and effectiveness of calcipotriol 0.005% ointment has been evaluated in the treatment of 397 patients with stable plaque psoriasis (Cullen 1996). In this multicentre, open-label clinical investigation, the psoriasis characteristics of scaling, erythema and plaque elevation, and overall disease severity, were evaluated periodically. At the end of the study, 235 subjects were considered assessable. Psoriatic plaques were cleared by week 8 in 25% of the subjects. The median time to initial clearing was between 16 and 17 weeks. This study showed that calcipotriol 0.005% ointment is safe and effective for long-term use in the treatment of plaque psoriasis (Cullen 1996).

Tolerability

Skin irritation is the only important local side-effect seen with calcipotriol therapy. It is registered in about 15% of the treated patients, but only 1–2% stop treatment for this reason. The skin irritation usually develops within the first few weeks of treatment, and no additional skin irritation is observed during long-term treatment.

The lesional or perilesional irritation consists of a burning or stinging sensation. It is, in general, transient and has no clinical consequence. In more severe cases, erythema and scaling are present. The face is particularly sensitive to calcipotriol (Kragballe 1989). Facial irritation may be seen not only after local application, but also after transfer of calcipotriol ointment applied elsewhere.

Facial irritation can be avoided, if the face is not treated, and if the patients are instructed to wash hands after applying the ointment (Kragballe *et al.* 1991; Cunliffe *et al.* 1992). In a patch-test study, calcipotriol was confirmed to be a weak irritant (Fullerton *et al.* 1996). Unfortunately, it is not possible to predict which patients become irritated by calcipotriol.

Safety

The potential effect on calcium and bone metabolism is the dose-limiting factor in the use of calcipotriol. In the clinical trials, patients were provided with 100 g or 120 g ointment per week. In neither short-term nor long-term trials did serum calcium change, except in one patient (Cunliffe *et al.* 1992). This patient applied approximately 400 g of calcipotriol ointment 50 µg/g during 10 days, i.e. about 3 times the amount permitted according to the protocol. There is another case of hypercalcemia during excessive use of calcipotriol ointment (Dwyer & Chapman 1991). This psoriatic patient had a 'moderate' degree of renal impairment. After applying approximately 200 g calcipotriol ointment to her extensive disease during the first week of treatment, she developed nausea, muscle weakness and abdominal pain, and the serum calcium rose from 2.44 mmol/L to 3.51 mmol/L. After stopping calcipotriol therapy, serum calcium normalized within 1 week.

No sequelae were reported. Changes in bone and calcium metabolism have been assessed in a randomized, double-blind, placebo-controlled, parallel-group comparison (Mortensen *et al.* 1993). Thirty-four psoriasis patients were randomized to receive treatment with either calcipotriol ointment 50 µg/g or placebo ointment for 3 weeks.

Calcipotriol-treated patients ($n = 17$) used on average 40.3 g ointment per week. During treatment there was no difference between the calcipotriol group and the placebo group in urinary calcium excretion or in the other biochemical indices assessed. The absence of an effect of calcipotriol treatment on bone and calcium metabolism has been confirmed in an open non-comparative study involving 12 psoriatics, who were treated for 4 weeks with an average of 100 g ointment per week (Gumowski-Sunek *et al.* 1991). Contradictory to these results, it was reported that the application of calcipotriol ointment 100 g/week for 4 weeks induced slight, but statistically significant changes in urinary calcium excretion (Berth-Jones *et al.* 1993) and serum parathyroid hormone (PTH) levels (Bourke *et al.* 1994). These results seem to indicate that the weekly calcipotriol dose should be kept below 100 g.

It has been a concern that long-term treatment with calcipotriol might have a cumulative effect on calcium and bone metabolism. Fortunately, the available data indicate that long-term calcipotriol treatment is as safe as short-term therapy. Thus, serum calcium levels and urinary calcium excretion did not increase in patients treated for 1 year with a mean of 30 g per week (Berth-Jones *et al.* 1993).

Patients with renal impairment may be at risk of developing hypercalcae-mia even when applying less than 100 g calcipotriol ointment per week. There-fore, at least two of the three reported cases of hypercalcaemia occurring after applying 70–80 g of calcipotriol ointment per week had some degree of renal impairment (Hardman & Heath 1993; Russell & Young 1994). These results may indicate that the small amounts of calcipotriol absorbed systemi-cally (less than 5%) may be sufficient to cause hypercalcemia in patients with a decreased renal capacity to regulate urinary calcium excretion.

Taken together the available evidence suggest that treatment with calcipotriol ointment 50 µg/g is safe when used in amounts up to 100 g per week. In patients requiring greater amounts of ointment, it is recommended to monitor serum PTH levels. A drop in serum PTH indicates a change in calcium homeostasis. In contrast, serum calcium is not sensitive enough to pick up minor changes of calcium metabolism.

Calcipotriol and the other vitamin D analogues are not teratogenic (data on file at the manufacturer Leo Pharmaceuticals, Denmark), but there is no clinical experience from treatment of pregnant patients. It is not known whether calcipotriol or its metabolites enter breast milk. If a patient becomes pregnant when treated with calcipotriol, treatment should be stopped, but elective abortion is not indicated.

Calcipotriol in the treatment of psoriasis in children

The use of topical calcipotriol in adults with psoriasis is safe and effective and should be regarded as the first line-topical drug for plaque-type psoriasis. Recently, the use of calcipotriol has been studied in children (Darley *et al.* 1996). Fifty-eight children were examined in an open study with application of calcipotriol 50 µg/g twice daily for up to 8 weeks. PASI scores were signifi-cantly reduced (from a mean of 6.1 to 2.7). Local skin irritation was reported in seven patients. No significant change in serum ionized calcium was ob-served (Darley *et al.* 1996).

The use of calcipotriol in 77 children was investigated in a multicentre, prospective, 8-week, double-blind, parallel-group study (Oranje *et al.* 1997). Response to treatment was assessed by means of the PASI score. The children were 2–14 years of age and had stable psoriasis, involving less than 30% of the body surface. Sixty-eight children completed the study. Both treatment groups (calcipotriol and placebo) showed significant improvement in PASI from baseline to the end of treatment, and the difference was not statistically significant. No serious side-effects, in particular including those relating to calcium and bone metabolism, were recorded. Calcipotriol ointment was sig-nificantly more effective statistically than its vehicle in terms of the investi-gator's overall assessment and reduction in redness and scaliness but not in terms of PASI score (Oranje *et al.* 1997).

These two studies show that calcipotriol is efficacious and safe for use in childhood psoriasis. However, use of calcipotriol in children needs further studies with respect to tolerability and long-term use.

8.6.3 Tacalcitol

In 1986 tacalcitol ointment $2\,\mu g/g$ and $4\,\mu g/g$ was reported to improve psoriasis in an open label study (Kato *et al.* 1986). In a subsequent controlled study, in which patients applied tacalcitol ointment twice daily to a single lesion for 4 weeks, a concentration of $2\,\mu g/g$ was superior to $1\,\mu g/g$ and as effective as $4\,\mu g/g$ (Nishimura *et al.* 1993).

In another dose-finding study, tacalcitol ointment was applied once daily to 2-cm² areas of lesional psoriasis for 4 weeks (Baadsgaard *et al.* 1995). Using this study design, $4\,\mu g/g$ was more effective than $2\,\mu g/g$ and similar to $8\,\mu g/g$ and $16\,\mu g/g$.

The differences in application frequency may explain the finding that optimal tacalcitol concentration was different in these two studies. When different body regions were treated with tacalcitol ointment $2\,\mu g/g$, the treatment was more effective on the face than on other skin areas (Nishimura *et al.* 1993). Tacalcitol $4\,\mu g/g$ was found to be as effective as 0.1% betamethasone ointment in a double-blind study in 63 patients (Scarpa 1996). Later, the effect of tacalcitol was further documented in a multicentre, placebo-controlled, double-blind study (van de Kerkhof *et al.* 1996) whereby 122 patients were evaluated and it was demonstrated that the once-daily application of $4\,\mu g/g$ tacalcitol ointment is an efficacious therapy for psoriasis vulgaris in Caucasian patients, and that its tolerance is good, wherever the lesion is located, including the face (van de Kerkhof *et al.* 1996). Tacalcitol has been compared with calcipotriol as a once-daily topical treatment of psoriasis with tacalcitol ointment ($4\,\mu g/g$) compared with twice-daily treatment with calcipotriol ointment ($50\,\mu g/g$) in a double-blind, randomized study over a treatment period of 8 weeks (Veien *et al.* 1997). It was found that although less effective than calcipotriol ointment used twice daily, tacalcitol ointment is an effective and useful once-daily treatment of chronic plaque psoriasis (Veien *et al.* 1997).

There is a limited knowledge about the efficacy of tacalcitol compared with topical antipsoriatic agents. Apparently treatment with tacalcitol ointment $2\,\mu g/g$ twice daily is as effective as hydrocortisone-butyrate, but slightly less effective than betamethasone 17-valerate (Nishimura *et al.* 1993). In a dose-finding study (Baadsgaard *et al.* 1995) calcipotriol ointment $50\,\mu g/g$ was included for comparison, but the results were not reported.

Used at a low concentration ($2\,\mu g/g$), tacalcitol ointment is well tolerated and skin irritation is uncommon (TV-02 Ointment Research Group 1991; Nishimura *et al.* 1993). Regarding safety, hypercalcaemia was not observed in two studies of a total of 210 patients (TV-02 Ointment Research Group

1991; Nishimura *et al.* 1993). There is, however, no information on the amount of tacalcitol ointment used by these patients. In a smaller study of 12 patients, an average cumulative dose of 340 µg (approximately 42 g of tacalcitol ointment 2 µg/g per week) did not increase serum calcium levels (Nishimura *et al.* 1994). There is no information available on the more sensitive markers of calcium metabolism (24-h calcium excretion and serum PTH) during tacalcitol therapy.

Conclusions

Topical calcipotriol is an efficacious and safe drug for topical treatment of chronic plaque psoriasis and should be regarded as the first-line topical drug for this condition. The effects are well documented in several clinical trials. However, few reports indicate that calcipotriol can be used in other clinical presentations of the disease such as generalized pustular psoriasis (Berth-Jones *et al.* 1992b) and erythrodermic psoriasis (Dwyer & Chapman 1991; Russell & Young 1994).

Calcipotriol can be used on all locations of the body and is available as an ointment, a cream and a scalp solution. The ointment formulation has been found to be the most efficacious of the three formulations.

The effect of calcipotriol begins within the first week of treatment and a marked improvement occurs in most patients after 8 weeks. It is recommended that calcipotriol usage is limited to a maximum of 100 g ointment/cream per week.

In general, the average remission time after stopping calcipotriol therapy is rather short. This means that patients may require repeated treatment courses. From the long-term studies there was no evidence of pharmacological tolerance. In contrast to corticosteroids, no evidence of skin atrophy was observed. Furthermore, it is important to note that calcipotriol treatment can be stopped without resulting in an exacerbation of psoriasis.

The data show that tacalcitol is also an efficacious and safe topical drug for psoriasis.

References

Abe, J., Kondo, S., Nishii, Y. & Kuroki, T. (1989) Resistance to 1,25-dihydroxyvitamin D$_3$ of cultured psoriatic epidermal keratinocytes from involved and uninvolved skin. *Journal of Clinical Endocrinology and Metabolism* **68**, 851–854.

Baadsgaard, O., Traulsen, J., Roed-Petersen, J. & Jakobsen, H.B. (1995) Optimal concentration of tacalcitol in once-daily treatment of psoriasis. *Journal of Dermatological Treatment* **6**, 145–150.

Barsony, J. & Marx, S.J. (1991) Rapid accumulatin of cGMP near activated vitamin D receptors. *Proceedings of the National Academy of Sciences of the USA* **88**, 1436–1440.

Berth-Jones, J., Bourke, J.F., Iqbal, S.J. & Hutchinson, P.E. (1993) Urine calcium excretion during treatment of psoriasis with topical calcipotriol. *British Journal of*

Dermatology **129**, 411–414.

Berth-Jones, J., Chu, A.C., Dodd, W.A.H. *et al.* (1992a) A multicentre parallel-group comparison of calcipotriol ointment and short-contact dithranol therapy in chronic plaque psoriasis. *British Journal of Dermatology* **127**, 266–271.

Berth-Jones, J., Bourke, J., Bailey, K., Graham-Brown, R.A. & Hutchinson, P.E. (1992b) Generalised pustular psoriasis: response to topical calcipotriol. *British Medical Journal* **305**, 868–869.

Bhalla, A.K., Amento, E.P. & Clemens, T.L. (1983) Specific high-affinity receptors for 1,25-dihydroxy-vitamin D$_3$ in human peripheral blood mononuclear cells: Presence in monocytes and induction in T-lymphocytes following activation. *Journal of Clinical Endocrinology and Metabolism* **57**, 1308–1310.

Binderup, L. & Bramm, E. (1988) Effects of a novel vitamin D analogue MC903 on cell proliferation and differentiation in vitro and on calcium metabolism in vivo. *Biochemistry and Pharmacology* **37**, 889–895.

Binderup, L., Carlberg, C., Kissmeyer, A. *et al.* (1994) In: *Vitamin D* (eds Norman, A.W., Bouillon, R. & Thomasset, M.), pp. 55–63. Walter de Gruyter, New York.

Binderup, L. & Kragballe, K. (1992) Origin of the use of calcipotriol in psoriasis treatment. *Review of Contemporary Pharmacotherapy* **23**, 401–409.

Bourke, J.F., Berth-Jones, J. & Hutchinson, P.E. (1993) Occlusion enhances the efficacy of topical calcipotriol in the treatment of psoriasis vulgaris. *Clinical Experimental Dermatology* **18**, 504–506.

Bourke, J.F., Berth-Jones, J., Mumford, R., Iqbal, S.J. & Hutchinson, P.E. (1994) High dose topical calcipotriol consistently reduces serum, parathyroid hormone levels. *Clinical Endocrinology* **41**, 295–297.

Bourke, J.F., Featherstone, S., Iqbal, S.J. & Hutchinson, P.E. (1995) A double-blind comparison of topical calcitriol (3µg/g) and calcipotriol (50µg/g) in the treatment of chronic plaque psoriasis vulgaris. *British Journal of Dermatology* **133**, 17 (Abstract).

Bruce, S., Epinette, W.W., Funicella, T. *et al.* (1994). Comparative study of calcipotriol (MC 903) ointment and fluocinonide ointment in the treatment of psoriasis. *Journal of the American Academy of Dermatology* **31**, 755–759.

Carlberg, C., Bendik, I., Wyss, A. *et al.* (1993) Two signalling pathways for vitamin D. *Nature* **361**, 657–660.

Carlberg, C., Mathiasen, I.S., Saurat, J.-H. & Binderup, L. (1994) The 1,25-dihydroxy-vitamin D$_3$ (VD) analogues MC903, EB1089 and KH1060 activate the VD receptor: Homodimers show higher ligand sensitivity than heterodimers with retinoid X receptors. *Journal of Steroid Biochemistry and Biology* **51**, 137–142.

Chen, M.L., Heinrich, G., Ohyama, Y. *et al.* (1994) Expression of 25-hydroxyvitamin D$_3$–24-hydroxylase mRNA in cultured human keratinocytes. *Proceedings of the Society of Experimental Biological Medicine* **207**, 57–61.

Cullen, S.I. (1996) Long-term effectiveness and safety of topical calcipotriene for psoriasis. *Southern Medicine Journal* **89**, 1053–1056.

Cunliffe, W.J., Claudy, A., Fairiss, G. *et al.* (1992) A multicentre comparative study of calcipotriol and betamethasone 17-valerate in patients with psoriasis vulgaris. *Journal of the American Academy of Dermatology* **26**, 736–743.

Dam, T.N., Møller, B., Hindkjær, J. & Kragballe, K. (1996) The vitamin D analog calcipotriol suppresses the number and antigen-presenting function of Langerhans cells in normal human skin. *Journal of Investigative Dermatology Symposium Proceedings* **1**, 72–77.

Darley, C.R., Cunliffe, W.J., Green, C.M. *et al.* (1996) Safety and efficacy of calcipotriol (Dovonex^R) in treating children with psoriasis vulgaris. *British Journal of Dermatology* **135**, 390–393.

Darwish, H. & DeLuca, H.F. (1992) Identification of a 1,25-dihydroxyvitamin D$_3$-

response element in the 5'-flanking region of the rat calbindin D-9k gene. *Proceedings of the National Academy of Sciences of the USA* **89**, 603–607.

Demay, M.B., Gerardi, J.M., DeLuca, H. & Kronenberg, H.M. (1990) DNA sequences in the rat osteocalcin gene that bind the 1,25-dihydroxyvitamin D₃ receptor and confer responsiveness to 1,25-dihydroxyvitamin D₃. *Proceedings of the National Academy of Sciences of the USA* **87**, 369–373.

Demay, M.B., Kiernan, M.S., DeLuca, H. & Kronenberg, H.M. (1992) Sequences in the human parathyroid hormone gene that bind the 1,25-dihydroxyvitamin D₃ receptor and mediate transcriptional repression in response to 1,25-dihydroxyvitamin D₃. *Proceedings of the National Academy of Sciences of the USA* **89**, 8097–8101.

Dubertret, L., Wallach, D., Souteyrand, P. *et al.* (1992) Efficacy and safety of calcipotriol (MC903) ointment in psoriasis vulgaris. *Journal of the American Academy of Dermatology* **27**, 983–988.

Dwyer, C. & Chapman, R.S. (1991) Calcipotriol and hypercalcaemia. *Lancet* **338**, 764–765.

Eil, C. & Marx, S. (1981) Nuclear uptake of 1,25-dihydroxycholecalciferol in dispersed fibroblasts cultured from normal human skin. *Proceedings of the National Academy of Sciences of the USA* **78**, 2562–2566.

Evans, R.M. (1988) The steroid and thyroid hormone receptor superfamily. *Science* **240**, 889–895.

Farach-Carson, M.C., Sergeev, I. & Norman, A.W. (1991) Nongenomic actions of 1,25-dihydroxyvitamin D₃ in rat osteosarcoma cells: structure-function studies using ligand analogs. *Endocrinology* **129**, 1876–1884.

Feldman, D., Chen, T., Hirst, M. *et al.* (1980) Demonstration of 1,25-dihydroxyvitamin D₃ receptor in human skin biopsies. *Journal of Clinical Endocrinological Metabiology* **51**, 1463–1465.

Frappaz, A. & Thivolet, J. (1993) Calcipotriol in combination with PUVA: a randomized double-blind placebo study in severe psoriasis. *European Journal of Dermatology* **3**, 351–354.

Fukuoka, M., Ogino, Y., Sato, H. *et al.* (1998) RANTES expression in psoriatic skin, and regulation of RANTES and IL-8 production in cultured epidermal keratinocytes by active vitamin D3 (tacalcitol). *British Journal of Dermatology* **138**, 63–70.

Fullerton, A., Avnstorp, C., Agner, T. *et al.* (1996) Patch test study with calcipotriol ointment in different patient groups, including psoriatic patients with and without adverse dermatitis. *Acta Dermato-Venereologica* **76**, 194–202.

Gniadecki, R. (1996) Stimulation versus inhibition of keratinocyte growth by 1,25-dihydroxyvitamin D₃: Dependence on cell culture conditions. *Journal of Investigative Dermatology* **106**, 510–516.

Gniadecki, R. & Serup, J. (1995) Stimulation of epidermal proliferation in mice with 1μ,25-dihydroxyvitamin D₃ and receptor-active 20-epi analogues of 1α,25-dihydroxyvitamin D₃. *Biochemistry and Pharmacology* **49**, 621–624.

Green, C., Ganpule, M., Harris, D. *et al.* (1994) Comparative effects of calcipotriol (MC903) solution and placebo (vehicle of MC903) in the treatment of psoriasis of the scalp. *British Journal of Dermatology* **130**, 483–487.

Grossman, R.M., Thivolet, J., Claudy, A. *et al.* (1994) A novel therapeutic approach to psoriasis with combination calcipotriol ointment and very low-dose cyclosporine: Results of a multicenter placebo-controlled study. *Journal of the American Academy of Dermatology* **31**, 68–74.

Guilhou, J.J., Colette, C., Monpoint, S. *et al.* (1990) Vitamin D metabolism in psoriasis before and after phototherapy. *Acta Dermato-Venereologica* **70**, 351–354.

Gumowski-Sunek, D., Rizzoli, R. & Saurat, J.H. (1991) Effects of topical calcipotriol on calcium metabolism in psoriatic patients: Comparison with oral calcitriol. *Dermato-*

logica **183**, 275–279.

Gupta, S., Fass, D. & Shimizu, M. (1989) Potentiation of immunosuppressive effects of cyclosporine A by 1-alpha, 25-dihydroxyvitamin D₃. *Cell Immunology* **121**, 290–297.

Hardman, K.H. & Heath, D.A. (1993) Hypercalcaemia associated with calcipotriol (Dovonex) treatment. *British Medical Journal* **306**, 896 (letter).

Harrington, C.I., Goldin, D., Lovell, C.R. *et al.* (1996) Comparative effects of two different calcipotriol (MC903) cream formulations versus placebo in psoriasis vulgaris. A randomized, double-blind, placebo-controlled, parallel group multi-centre study. *Journal of European Academy of Dermatology and Venereology* **6**, 152–158.

Henderson, C.A., Papworth-Smith, J., Cunliffe, W.J. *et al.* (1989) A double-blind placebo-controlled trial of topical 1,25-dihydroxycalciferol in psoriasis. *British Journal of Dermatology* **121**, 493–496.

Henriksen, L.Ø., Kragballe, K., Jensen, T.G. & Fogh, K. (1997) Transcriptional activation by 1,25-dihydroxyvitamin D₃ and synthetic vitamin D₃ analogues in transfected cultures of human keratinocytes. *Skin Pharmacology* **10**, 12–20.

Hosomi, J., Hosoi, J., Abe, E., Suda, T. & Kuroki, T. (1983) Regulation of terminal differentiation of mouse cultured epidermal cells by 1,25-dihydroxyvitamin D₃. *Endocrinology* **113**, 1950–57.

Jensen, T.J., Sølvsten, H. & Kragballe, K. (1998) The Vitamin D₃ and retinoid X receptors in psoriatic skin: the receptor levels correlate with receptor binding to DNA. *British Journal of Dermatology* **138**, 225–228.

Kato, T., Rokogu, M., Teuri, T. & Tagami, H. (1986) Successful treatment of psoriasis with topical application of the active vitamin D₃ analogue, 1,24-dihydroxy cholecalciferol. *British Journal of Dermatology* **115**, 431–433.

Kerner, S.A., Scott, R.A. & Pike, J.W. (1989) Sequence elements in the human osteo-calcin gene confer basal activation and inducible response to hormonal vitamin D₃. *Proceedings of the National Academy of Sciences of the USA* **86**, 4455–4459.

Kerscher, M., Volkenandt, M. & Plewig, G. (1993) Combination phototherapy of psoriasis with calcipotriol and narrowband UVB. *Lancet* **343**, 923 (letter).

Kienbaum, S., Lehmann, P. & Ruzicka, T. (1996) Topical calcipotriol in the treatment of tertriginous psoriasis. *British Journal of Dermatology* **135**, 647–650.

Klaber, M.R., Hutchinson, P.E., Pedvis, L. *et al.* (1994) Comparative effets of calcipotriol solution (50 µg/ml) and betamethasone 17-valerate solution (1 mg/ml) in the treatment of scalp psoriasis. *British Journal of Dermatology* **131**, 678–683.

Kokelj, F., Lavaroni, G. & Guadagnini, A. (1995) UVB versus UVB plus calcipotriol (MC 903) therapy for psoriasis vulgaris. *Acta Dermato-Venereologica* **75**, 386–387.

Kokelj, F., Torsello, P. & Plozzer, C. (1998) Calcipotriol improves the efficacy of cyclo-sporine in the treatment of psoriasis vulgaris. *Journal of European Academy of Dermatology and Venereology* **10**, 143–146.

Koo, J. (1996) Phototherapy in combination with vitamin D therapy. *Proceedings of Clinical Dermatology 2000*, 28–31 May, Vancouver, p. 88 (Abstract).

Kragballe, K. (1989) Treatment of psoriasis by the topical application of the novel cholecalciferol analogue calcipotriol (MC903). *Archives of Dermatology* **125**, 1647–1652.

Kragballe, K. (1990) Combination of topical calcipotriol (MC 903) and UVB radiation for psoriasis vulgaris. *Dermatologica* **181**, 211–214.

Kragballe, K. & Fogh, K. (1991) Long-term efficacy and tolerability of topical calcipotriol in psoriasis. *Acta Dermato-Venereologica* **71**, 475–478.

Kragballe, K. & Iversen, L. (1993) Calcipotriol (MC903) a new topical antipsoriatic. *Dermatological Clinics* **11**, 137–141.

Kragballe, K. & Wildfang, I.L. (1990) Calcipotriol (MC903), a novel vitamin D₃ analogue stimulates terminal differentiation and inhibits proliferation of cultured human keratinocytes. *Archives of Dermatological Research* **282**, 164–167.

Kragballe, K., Barnes, L. & Hamberg, K.J. (1998) Calcipotriol cream with or without concurrent topical corticosteroid in psoriasis: tolerability and efficacy. *British Journal of Dermatology* **139**, 649–654.

Kragballe, K., Beck, H.I. & Søgaard, H. (1988) Improvement of psoriasis by a topical vitamin D_3 analogue (MC903) in a double-blind study. *British Journal of Dermatology* **199**, 223–230.

Kragballe, K., Gjertsen, B.T., De Hoop, D. *et al.* (1991) Double blind, right-left comparison of calcipotriol and betamethasone valerate in treatment of psoriasis vulgaris. *Lancet* **337**, 193–196.

Langner, A., Ashton, P., van de Kerkhof, P.C.M. & Verjans, H. (1996) A long-term multicentre assessment of the safety and tolerability of calcitriol ointment in the treatment of chronic plaque psoriasis. *British Journal of Dermatology* **135**, 385–389.

Langner, A., Verjans, H., Stapar, V., Mol, M. & Fraczy-Kowska, A. (1993) Topical calcitriol in the treatment of chronic plaque psoriasis: a double-blind study. *British Journal of Dermatology* **128**, 566–571.

Langner, A., Verjans, H., Stapor, V., Mol, M. & Elzerman, J. (1991) Treatment of chronic plaque psoriasis by 1-alpha,25-dihydroxyvitamin D_3 ointment. In: *Vitamin D: Gene Regulation Structure-Function Analysis and Clinical Application* (eds Norman, A.W., Bouillon, R. & Thomasset, N.), pp. 430–431. Walter de Gruyter, Berlin.

Lebwohl, M. (1997) Topical application of calcipotriene and corticosteroids: combination regimens. *Journal of the American Academy of Dermatology* **37**, S55–S58.

Lebwohl, M., Siskin, S.B. & Epinette, W. (1996) A multicenter trial of calcipotriol ointment and halobetasol ointment compared with either agent alone for the treatment of psoriasis. *Journal of the American Academy of Dermatology* **35**, 268–269.

Lebwohl, M., Yoles, A., Lombardi, K. & Lou, W. (1998) Calcipotriene ointment and halobetasol ointment in the long-term treatment of psoriasis: effects on the duration of improvement. *Journal of the American Academy of Dermatology* **39**, 447–450.

Lützow-Holm, C., De Angelis, P., Grosvik, H. & Clausen, O.P. (1993) 1,25-dihydroxyvitamin D_3 and the vitamin D_3 analogue KH 1060 induce hyperproliferation in normal mouse epidermis. *Experimental Dermatology* **2**, 113–120.

MacDonald, P.N., Dowd, D.R., Nakajima, S. *et al.* (1993). Retinoid X receptors stimulate and 9-*cis* retinoic acid inhibits 1,25-dihydroxyvitamin D_3-activated expression of the rat osteocalcin gene. *Molecular Cell Biology* **13**, 5907–5917.

Matsouka, L.Y., Wortsman, J., Haddad, J. & Hollis, B. (1990) Cutaneous formation of vitamin D_3 in psoriasis. *Archives of Dermatology* **126**, 1107–1108.

Matsumoto, K., Hashimoto, K., Kiyoki, M., Yamamoto, M. & Yoshikawa, K. (1990) Effect of 1,24-dihydroxyvitamin D_3 on the growth of human keratinocytes. *Journal of Dermatology* **17**, 97–103.

Matsunaga, T., Yamamoto, M., Mimura, H. *et al.* (1990) 1,24 R-dihydroxyvitamin D_3, a novel active form of vitamin D_3 with high activity for inducing epidermal differentiation but decreased hypercalcemia activity. *Journal of Dermatology* **17**, 135–142.

McKenna, K.E. & Stern, R.S. (1995) Photosensitivity associated with combined UV-B and calcipotriene therapy. *Archives of Dermatology* **131**, 1305–1307.

McLaughlin, J.A., Gange, W. & Taylor, D. (1985) Cultured psoriatic fibroblasts from involved and uninvolved sites have partial, but not absolute resistance to the proliferation-inhibition activity of 1,25 dihydroxyvitamin D_3. *Proceedings of the National Academy of Sciences of the USA* **82**, 5409–5412.

Merke, J., Milde, P., Lewicka, S. *et al.* (1989) Identification and regulation of 1,25-dihydroxyvitamin D_3 receptor activity and biosynthesis of 1,25-dihydroxyvitamin D_3. *Journal of Clinical Investigation* **83**, 1903–1915.

Milde, P., Hauser, U., Simon, T. *et al.* (1991) Expression of 1,25-dihydroxyvitamin D_3

receptors in normal and psoriatic skin. *Journal of Investigative Dermatology* **97**, 230–236.

Molin, L. (1995) Calcipotriol combined with phototherapy (UVB and PUVA) in the treatment of psoriais. *Journal of European Academy of Dermatology* **5** (Suppl.), 184 (Abstract).

Molin, L., Cutler, T.P., Helander, I., Nyfors, B. & Downes, N. (1997) Comparative efficacy of calcipotriol (MC903) cream and betamethasone 17-valerate cream in the treatment of chronic plaque psoriasis. A randomised, double-blind, parallel group multicentre study. *British Journal of Dermatology* **136**, 89–93.

Morimoto, S. & Kumahara, Y. (1985) A patient with psoriasis cured by 1-alpha-hydroxy-vitamin D$_3$. *Medical Journal of Osaka University* **35**, 51.

Morimoto, S. & Yoshikawa, K. (1989) Psoriasis and vitamin D$_3$. A review of our experience. *Archives of Dermatology* **125**, 231–234.

Morimoto, S., Yoshikawa, K., Fukuo, K. *et al.* (1990) Inverse relationship between severity of psoriasis and serum 1,25-dihydroxyvitamin D level. *Journal of Dermatological Science* **1**, 277–282.

Morimoto, S., Yoshikawa, K., Kozuka, T. *et al.* (1986) An open study of vitamin D$_3$ treatment in psoriasis vulgaris. *British Journal of Dermatology* **115**, 421–429.

Mortensen, L., Kragballe, K., Wegman, E. *et al.* (1993) Treatment of psoriasis vulgaris with topical calcipotriol has no short-term effect on calcium and bone metabolism. *Acta Dermato-Venereologica* **73**, 300–304.

Müller, K. & Bendtzen, K. (1996) 1,25-Dihydroxyvitamin D$_3$ as a natural regulator of human immune functions. *Journal of Investigative Dermatology Symposium Proceedings* **1**, 68–71.

Nielsen, P.G. (1993) Calcipotriol or clobetasol propionate occluded with a hydrocolloid dressing for treatment of nummular psoriasis. *Acta Dermato-Venereologica* **73**, 394.

Nishimura, M., Hori, Y., Nishiyama, S. & Nakimizo, Y. (1993) Topical 1,24-dihydroxy-vitamin D$_3$ for the treatment of psoriasis. A review of the literature. *European Journal of Dermatology* **3**, 255–261.

Nishimura, M., Makino, Y. & Matugi, H. (1994) Tacalcitol ointment for psoriasis. *Acta Dermato-Venereologica* **186** (Suppl.), 166–168.

Norman, A.W., Nemere, I., Zhou, L.X. *et al.* (1992) 1,25 (OH)$_2$-vitamin D$_3$, a steroid hormone that produces biologic effects via both genomic and nongenomic pathways. *Journal of Steroid Biochemistry and Molecular Biology* **41**, 231–240.

Oranje, A.P., Marcoux, D., Svensson, A. *et al.* (1997) Topical calcipotriol in childhood psoriasis. *Journal of the American Academy of Dermatology* **36**, 203–208.

Ozono, K., Liao, J., Kerner, S.A., Scott, R.A. & Pike, J.W. (1990) The vitamin D-responsive element in the human osteocalcin gene. *Journal of Biological Chemistry* **265**, 21881–21888.

Pariser, M.D., Pariser, R.J., Breneman, D. *et al.* (1996) Calcipotriene ointment applied once a day for psoriasis: a double-blind multicenter placebo-controlled study. *Archives of Dermatology* **132**, 1527 (letter).

Perez, A., Raab, R., Chen, T.C., Turner, A. & Holick, M.F. (1996) Safety and efficacy of oral calcitriol (1,25-dihydroxy vitamin D$_3$) for the treatment of psoriasis. *British Journal of Dermatology* **134**, 1070–1078.

Pinheiro, N. (1997) Comparative effects of calcipotriol ointment (50 micrograms/g) and 5% coal tar/2% allantoin/0.5% hydrocortisone cream in treating plaque psoriasis. *British Journal of Clinical Practice* **51**, 16–19.

Quélo, I., Kahlen, J., Rascle, A., Jurdic, P. & Carlberg, C. (1994) Identification and characterization of a vitamin D$_3$ response element of chicken carbonic anhdrase-II. *DNA and Cell Biology* **13**, 1181–1187.

Ramsay, C. (1998) Calcipotriol cream and UVB phototherapy in psoriasis. *Journal of Investigative Dermatology* **110**, 686 (Abstract).

Ramsay, C.A., Berth-Jones, J., Brundin, G. *et al.* (1994). Long-term use of topical calcipotriol in chronic plaque-type psoriasis. *Dermatology* **189**, 260–264.

Ranson, M., Posen, S. & Manson, R. (1988) Human melanocytes as a target tissue for hormones. In vitro studies with 1,25-dihydroxyvitamin D_3, alpha-melanocyte stimulating hormone, and beta-estradiol. *Journal of Investigative Dermatology* **91**, 593–598.

Rigby, W.F.C. & Waugh, M.G. (1992) Decreased accessory cell function and costimulatory activity by 1,25-dihydroxyvitamin D_3 treated monocytes. *Arthritis and Rheumatism* **35**, 110–119.

Risum, G. (1973) Psoriasis exacerbated by hypoparathyroidism with hypocalcemia. *British Journal of Dermatology* **89**, 309–312.

Russell, S. & Young, M.J. (1994) Hypercalcaemia during treatment of psoriasis with calcipotriol. *British Journal of Dermatology* **130**, 795–796.

Ruzicka, T. & Lorenz, B. (1998) Comparison of calcipotriol monotherapy and a combination of calcipotriol and betamethasone valerate after 2 weeks' treatment with calcipotriol in the topical therapy of psoriasis vulgaris: a multicentre, double-blind, randomised study. *British Journal of Dermatology* **138**, 254–258.

Scarpa, C. (1994) Calcipotriol: clinical trial versus betamethasone dipropionate + salicylic acid. *Acta Dermato-Venereologica Supplementum* **186**, 47.

Scarpa, C. (1996) Tacalcitol ointment is an efficacious and well tolerated treatment for psoriasis. *Journal of European Academy of Dermatology and Venereology* **6**, 142–146.

Schräder, M., Müller, K.M., Becker-André, M. & Carlberg, C. (1994) Response element selectivity for heterodimerization of vitamin D receptors with retinoic acid and retinoid X receptors. *Journal of Molecular Endocrinology* **12**, 327–339.

Smith, E.L., Pincus, S.H., Donovan, L. & Holick, M.F. (1988) A novel approach for the evaluation and treatment of psoriasis. *Journal of the American Academy of Dermatology* **10**, 360–364.

Smith, E.L., Walworth, N.C. & Holick, M.F. (1986) Effect of 1,25-dihydroxyvitamin D_3 on the morphologic and biochemical differentiation of cultured human epidermal keratinocytes grown in serum-free conditions. *Journal of Investigative Dermatology* **86**, 706–716.

Sølvsten, H., Fogh, K., Svendsen, M. *et al.* (1996) Normal levels of the vitamin D receptor and its message in psoriatic skin. *Journal of Investigative Dermatology Symposium Proceedings* **1**, 28–32.

Sølvsten, H., Jensen, T.J., Sørensen, S. & Kragballe, K. (1999) Application of calcipotriol to normal human skin increases the level of the vitamin D receptor (VDR) and the binding of the VDR-retinoid X receptor heterodimer to a vitamin D response element, submitted.

Sølvsten, H., Svendsen, M.L., Fogh, K. & Kragballe, K. (1997) Upregulation of vitamin D receptor levels by 1,25 dihydroxyvitamin D_3 in cultured human keratinocytes. *Archives of Dermatological Research* **289**, 367–372.

Sone, T., Ozono, K. & Pike, J.W. (1991) A 55-kilodalton accessory factor facilitates vitamin D receptor DNA binding. *Molecular Endocrinology* **5**, 1578–1586.

Speight, E.L. & Farr, P.M. (1994) Calcipotriol improves the response of psoriasis to PUVA. *British Journal of Dermatology* **130**, 79–82.

Staberg, B., Oxholm, A., Klemp, P. & Christiansen, C. (1987) Abnormal vitamin D metabolism in patients with psoriasis. *Acta Dermato-Venereologica* **67**, 65–68.

Staberg, B., Roed-Petersen, J. & Menne, T. (1989) Efficacy of topical treatment in psoriasis with MC 903, a new vitamin D analogue. *Acta Dermato-Venereologica* **69**, 147–150.

Stewart, A.F., Battaglini-Sabetta, J. & Millstone, L. (1984) Hypocalcemia-induced pustular psoriasis of von Zumbusch. *Annals of Internal Medicine* **100**, 677–680.

Svendsen, M.L., Geysen, J., Binderup, L. & Kragballe, K. (1999) Proliferation and differentiation of cultured human kerationocytes is modulated by 1,25 (OH)$_2$D$_3$ and synthetic vitamin D$_3$ analogs in a cell-density-, calcium- and serum-dependent manner. *Pharmacological Toxicology* **80**, 49–56.

Tham, S.N., Lun, K.C. & Cheong, W.K. (1994) A comparative study of calcipotriol ointment and tar in chronic plaque psoriasis. *British Journal of Dermatology* **131**, 673–677.

Tosti, A., Piraccini, B.M., Cameli, N. *et al.* (1998) Calcipotriol ointment in nail psoriasis: a controlled double-blind comparison with betamethasone dipropionate and salicylic acid. *British Journal of Dermatology* **139**, 655–659.

Tsoukas, D.D., Provedini, D.M. & Manolagas, S.C. (1984) 1,25-dihydroxy vitamin D$_3$: a novel immunoregulatory hormone. *Science* **14**, 38–40.

TV-02 Ointment Research Group (1991) A Placebo controlled double-blind, right-left comparison study on the efficacy of TV-02 ointment for the treatment of psoriasis. *Nishinihon Journal of Dermatology* **53**, 1252–1256.

Umesono, K., Murakami, K.K., Thompson, C.C. & Evans, R.M. (1991) Direct repeats as selective response elements for the thyroid hormone, retinoic acid, and vitamin D$_3$ receptors. *Cell* **65**, 1255–1266.

van de Kerkhof, P.C.M. (1998) Topical use of high dose calcipotriol in psoriasis does not affect bone turnover or calcium metabolic profile. *56th Annual Meeting of the American Academy of Dermatology* (Abstract).

van de Kerkhof, P.C.M. & Hutchinson, P.E. (1996) Topical use of calcipotriol improves outcome in acitretin treated patients with severe psoriasis vulgaris. *British Journal of Dermatology* **135** (Suppl.), 30 (Abstract).

van de Kerkhof, P.C.M., van Bokhoven, M., Zultak, M. & Czarnetzki, M.B. (1989) A double-blind study of topical 1,25-dihydroxyvitamin D$_3$ in psoriasis. *British Journal of Dermatology* **120**, 661–664.

van de Kerkhof, P.C., Cambazard, F., Hutchinson, P.E., *et al.* (1998) The effect of addition of calcipotriol ointment (50 micrograms/g) to acitretin therapy in psoriasis. *British Journal of Dermatology* **138**, 84–89.

van de Kerkhof, P.C., Werfel, T., Haustein, U.F. *et al.* (1996) Tacalcitol ointment in the treatment of psoriasis vulgaris: a multicentre, placebo-controlled, double-blind study on efficacy and safety. *British Journal of Dermatology* **135**, 758–765.

van der Vleuten, C.J.M., de Jong, E.M.G.J., Ruto, E.H.F.C. *et al.* (1995) In-patient treatment with calcipotriol versus dithranol in refractory psoriasis. *European Journal of Dermatology* **5**, 676–679.

Veien, N.K., Bjerke, J.R., Rossmann-Ringdahl, I. & Jakobsen, H.B. (1997) Once daily treatment of psoriasis with tacalcitol compared with twice daily treatment with calcipotriol. A double-blind trial. *British Journal of Dermatology* **137**, 581–586.

Wishart, J.M. (1994) Calcitriol (1,25-dihydroxy-Vitamin D$_3$) ointment in psoriasis: a safety, tolerance and efficacy multicentre study. *Dermatology* **188**, 135–139.

Chapter 9: Corticosteroids

J. Hughes and M.H.A. Rustin

9.1 Introduction

Topical corticosteroids are important in the management of psoriasis. In the appropriate concentration they are generally effective and cosmetically acceptable. They are the treatment of choice in anatomical sites such as the flexures or genitals where other therapies, for example dithranol, tar or vitamin D analogues, may act as a primary irritant. Overuse may cause local side-effects and, rarely, serious systemic problems.

9.2 Background and pharmacology of synthetic corticosteroid analogues

The essential steroid ring structure is illustrated in Fig. 9.1. Modification of the steric configuration produces great changes in the biological activity of the steroid (Elks 1976). Sulzberger and Witten (1952) reported the first moderately successful use of topical corticosteroids (Compound F or hydrocortisone acetate) in inflammatory skin disease subsequent to the development of cortisone for the treatment of rheumatoid arthritis in 1949.

During the following decades it was found that the most successful modifications in improving the anti-inflammatory properties of corticosteroid analogues involved increasing lipophilicity by masking one or both of the 16- or

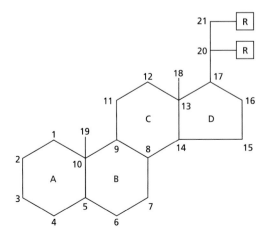

Fig. 9.1 The basic corticosteroid ring structure.

17-hydrophilic hydroxyl groups or introducing long carbon side chains, such as the acetonides, valerates or propionates.

9.3 Classification of corticosteroids

The vasoconstrictor assay is the most reliable bioassay to determine the relative potency of new or established topical corticosteroids (Mackenzie & Stoughton 1964).

This assay involves applying topical corticosteroids to the normal skin surface of healthy volunteers and observing the ability to induce blanching at the application site. The degree of vasoconstriction produced following application of a steroid in varying dilution for a standard length of time increases with the concentration of the steroid. Although this assay tests only one of numerous functions of topical corticosteroids, Barry (1983) and Cornell (1992) confirmed that the results correlate well with clinical effectiveness. There are exceptions to this rule, such as hydrocortisone valerate cream 0.2%, which has a higher blanching score than its actual efficacy in clinical use. The vasoconstrictor assay also helps to answer specific questions with regard to the clinical use of topical corticosteroids, for example how much the vehicle of a steroid affects its potency. Again, this test must be interpreted with caution as Cornell (1992) found that changing the vehicle of the potent steroid clobetasol propionate made a significant difference to percutaneous absorption without altering the results of the vasoconstrictor assay.

The chemical equivalence (brand name and generic products containing the same amount of steroid moiety) and biological equivalence (similar blanching scores in the vasoconstrictor assay) of a topical corticosteroid do not always imply therapeutic equivalence. Safety and efficacy data are required from randomized, double-blind clinical trials using topical corticosteroids in patients with chronic plaque psoriasis to assess therapeutic equivalence.

Kathchman et al. (1995) postulated that advances in the assessment of corticosteroids may lie in the transgenic mouse model as a biological assay of topical glucocorticosteroid potency. The transgenic mouse line expresses a human elastin promoter/CAT (chloramphenicol acetyltransferase) reporter gene construct that responds in a dose-dependent manner to steroid injections. This response is probably mediated by the three putative glucocorticoid responsive elements (GRE) in the promoter region.

Assaying CAT activity in these animals directly reflects the activity of the human elastin promoter, allowing preliminary testing of the strength of topical corticosteroids.

9.4 Corticosteroid mechanism of action

Topical corticosteroids have anti-inflammatory, immunosuppressive and antimitogenic action. They act via glucocorticoid receptors, first discovered in the late 1960s but the exact mechanism of all the multiple effects is still the subject of intensive research. Steroids are known to bind to receptors within the cells forming a complex that is rapidly transported to the nucleus of the cell, a process known as translocation. The steroid–receptor complex then binds to a region on the DNA of the cell known as the glucocorticoid responsive element (GRE) which can stimulate or inhibit transcription of the genes adjacent to the GRE, thus regulating the inflammatory process (Oakley & Cidlowski 1993). The glucocorticoid receptor is a 300-kDa structure that consists of two 90-kDa heat-shock proteins, a 59-kDa protein and a DNA-binding domain. Once steroid–receptor binding has occurred, the two heat-shock proteins and the p59 protein are lost, exposing the DNA-binding domain which allows transcription to occur.

Corticosteroids inhibit cytokine gene transcription (including the interleukins IL-1, IL-2, IL-6, interferon-γ, and tumour necrosis factor-α genes), T-cell proliferation, and T-cell-dependent immunity (Almawi *et al.* 1991). Anti-inflammatory effects of corticosteroids include inhibition of dermal oedema and the movement of inflammatory cells within the skin. Suppression of fibroblast, endothelial cell, and leucocyte function also occurs, as well as attenuation of the humoral inflammatory process.

Corticosteroids inhibit vascular permeability and the transmission of leucocytes through the vessel wall, hindering recruitment to sites of inflammation.

Topical corticosteroids may also cause unwanted effects by acting at the sites of other steroid receptors. Binding to androgen receptors may explain the development of acne and hypertrichosis at the site of topical corticosteroid application. Research into new-generation topical corticosteroids needs to be directed towards molecules that have no affinity for other steroid receptors. If corticosteroids could be designed with prolonged receptor occupation time, a prolonged transcription time could lead to an increased interval between doses and improved patient compliance (Wright 1995). A further desirable effect of corticosteroids would be to develop increased activity at the site of application then rapidly break down to inactive metabolites leading to a marked reduction in systemic side-effects.

9.5 Formulations

The vehicle in which the topical corticosteroid is delivered to the skin is important, as it needs to allow adequate release of the active compound and be cosmetically acceptable. The three main vehicles (grease, liquid and powder) are used in varying mixtures for the treatment of psoriasis. The most popular of these include ointments, creams, lotions, gels and foams. Ointments are occlusive, emollient and protective and are divided into two main groups, fatty or water soluble. Fatty bases such as white soft paraffin are more occlusive and therefore hydrating. They enhance percutaneous absorption of topical corticosteroids by increasing the hydration and temperature of the skin (Pershing *et al.* 1992) Creams are semisolid emulsions containing water and oil. Aqueous or vanishing creams (oil in water) are miscible with surface exudation, absorb well and do not retard heat loss. They do not feel greasy, which makes them cosmetically more acceptable to some patients. Oily creams (water in oil) are immiscible with water and are more difficult to wash off. Lotions are a mixture of powder and liquid in an aqueous or alcoholic suspension, and gels are transparent semisolid emulsions that liquefy on contact with warm skin, drying as a greaseless non-occlusive film.

The choice of vehicle for a topical corticosteroid depends on the area of the body where it is to be used. Ointments are best used for the dry, hyperkeratotic, scaly plaques of psoriasis, leading to rehydration of the stratum corneum. They can be used on hairless areas, such as the palms and soles, where they may prove to be more effective because of difficulty in washing them off. Creams are particularly useful for infected and exudative psoriatic plaques and are the treatment of choice on flexural and genital areas. Lotions and gels are suitable for the treatment of scalp psoriasis.

Occluding the skin with an impermeable film, for example plastic, is an effective method for enhancing topical corticosteroid penetration. Penetration may be increased 10-fold and lead to a clinical response in resistant cases; however, occlusion may be uncomfortable, warm and difficult to apply. Unwanted side-effects include bacterial and candidal infections and formation of miliaria. Occlusion of topical corticosteroid should not be maintained for longer than 12 h per day as increased absorption will lead to a higher incidence of local and systemic effects. Occlusive dressings include plastic wraps, for example cling film and plastic gloves. Topical corticosteroid-impregnated adhesive tapes are another means of delivering steroids to the skin and compare well to equivalent-strength ointment formulations (Krueger *et al.* 1998). Broby-Johansen *et al.* (1990) showed that the use of less potent topical corticosteroids under hydrocolloid dressing occlusion could clear or improve psoriatic plaques. The hydrocolloid dressing was applied over the topical corticosteroid (betamethasone valerate 0.1%, triamcinolone acetonide 0.1%, and halcinonide 0.1%) and left in position for 2 days, then removed; and the treatment was repeated at 2-day intervals for a maximum of 3 weeks.

9.6 Dilution of steroid preparations

Dilution of topical corticosteroids may alter their bioavailability, either by physical incompatibility with the diluent or by inadequate dispersion. Release of corticosteroid from its vehicle may be affected and the steroid may be changed. For example, dilution or addition of tar or salicylic acid to betamethasone 17-valerate hastens conversion to the considerably less potent betamethasone 21-valerate. Dilution may also introduce contamination and uncertainty as to the shelf life of the preparation, and so is not recommended. If considered necessary, the manufacturers recommended diluent should be used.

9.7 Strength and frequency of application

Tachyphylaxis or acute tolerance has been observed to develop after repeated applications of topical corticosteroids, which explains why control of psoriasis with these agents is ineffective after constant use. This phenomenon has been demonstrated in experiments using the hairless mouse skin model. Once psoriasis clears following treatment with potent topical corticosteroids, recurrence is usually inevitable given the chronic nature of the disorder; and a more long-term therapeutic approach has to be sought aiming to maintain remission. Clinical trials tend to involve short-term treatment regimens and do not study prolonged use of these agents.

Some groups have advocated long-term intermittent maintenance treatment with topical corticosteroids. Katz *et al.* (1987a) found 38 out of 59 patients with psoriasis noted an 86% or greater improvement in their disease after a 2-week treatment regimen of twice-daily betamethasone dipropionate 0.05% ointment. These 38 patients were then randomly allocated to receive either the same topical corticosteroid or placebo ointment to use on weekends, which consisted of three consecutive doses at 12-h intervals once weekly. Fourteen patients (74%) using the topical corticosteroid achieved remission for 12 weeks, as opposed to four patients (21%) in the placebo group. There was no evidence of hypothalamic–pituitary axis suppression.

A further strategy is to treat chronic plaque psoriasis with a potent steroid, applied twice daily until the disease is controlled. Reducing the potency of the steroid and applying less frequently may lead to a longer remission period.

Recent data have shown that the maximal activity of a topical corticosteroid occurs at midnight, which is when endogenous levels of corticosteroid are at their lowest (Pershing *et al.* 1994). The maximum vasoconstriction occurs 6 h after application; therefore, the optimal time to use a topical corticosteroid may be in the late afternoon.

Newer potent topical corticosteroids may offer treatment advances. Mometasone furoate is a novel (2′) furoate-17 ester with a low percutaneous absorption and rapid biotransformation in the liver. Studies using mometasone under occlusion have found no significant effect on the hypothalamic–pituitary axis (Degreef & Dooms-Goossens 1993).

Medansky *et al.* (1988) studied 823 patients with psoriasis and compared once-daily mometasone furoate ointment 0.1% with twice-daily triamcinolone acetonide 0.1% ointment and three times daily fluocinolone acetonide 0.025% ointment using a single-blind design. Mometasone ointment was shown to be as effective as the triamcinolone ointment and more effective than fluocinolone ointment.

Rosenthal and Duke (1988) also found this preparation compared well to standard potent topical corticosteroids in the treatment of psoriasis. Mometasone furoate ointment 0.1% once daily or betamethasone valerate ointment 0.1% twice daily were used by 108 randomly allocated patients for 3 weeks and 69% of patients in the group treated with mometasone furoate improved compared with 29% of patients in the betamethasone valerate treated group ($P<0.01$). Mometasone ointment used once daily in psoriasis would appear to be as effective and safe as other potent topical corticosteroids, which are applied more frequently; however, long-term studies are needed to assess the safety and side-effect profile of this drug.

Fluticasone propionate is another new generation topical corticosteroid which is highly lipophilic and specific for the glucocorticoid receptor, with minimal binding to the androgen, progestogen, oestrogen and mineralocorticoid receptors thought to decrease undesirable side-effects. Rapid metabolization in the liver to the inactive 17β-carboxylic acid decreases its potential for inhibition of the hypothalamic–pituitary axis (Chu & Munn 1995).

Callen (1996) carried out a 2-week, right–left comparison of fluticasone propionate 0.05% cream vs. betamethasone valerate cream 0.1% in the treatment of psoriasis. No significant differences were found between fluticasone and betamethasone cream, either by investigator observation or by subject preference.

9.8 Cutaneous side-effects

Side-effects of topical corticosteroids are well documented and are directly related to potency.

9.8.1 Epidermal side-effects

Microscopic degenerative changes may be seen in the epidermis with a reduction in cell size and number of cell layers within 3–14 days of using topical corticosteroids. Melanocyte inhibition causing a vitiligo-like appearance may be noted, especially in black skin. At first, these changes are rapidly reversible, but may become permanent with chronic administration.

9.8.2 Dermal and vascular side-effects

Topical corticosteroids have a direct antiproliferative action on fibroblasts causing dermal atrophy (Kerscher & Korting 1992). Collagen and mucopolysaccharide synthesis is reduced, resulting in a loss of dermal support. Striae develop when elastin fibres in the upper layers of the dermis become thin and fragmented and deeper fibres form a compact and dense network. Atrophy is to some extent reversible but striae are permanent. Inadequate support of dermal vasculature leads to easy rupture causing telangiectases and pur-pura. Initial vasoconstriction of the superficial small vessels is followed by rebound vasodilatation which may be permanent in its later stages.

Localized fine-hair growth known as hypertrichosis may occur, although this is usually temporary. Perioral dermatitis or rosacea may develop after the application of potent topical steroids to the face. Steroid acne can occur on the face or elsewhere. The use of topical corticosteroids on the eyelids and periorbital area may result in sufficient conjunctival accumulation equiva-lent to direct ocular application.

Although rare, posterior subcapsular cataracts, glaucoma, increased inci-dence of ocular mycotic infections, and exacerbation of viral infections of the eye may occur. Patients need to be instructed to avoid the eyelids when ap-plying potent topical steroids to the face and to avoid getting any of the medi-cation into the eyes.

Topical corticosteroids have not been shown to increase the incidence of cutaneous infection, either bacterial, viral or fungal; but they may exacer-bate it if infection is already present, for example tinea incognito. Occlusion folliculitis is a relatively common side-effect secondary to the obstruction of hair follicles.

Topical application of corticosteroids may cause allergic contact dermati-tis (Lauerma & Reitamo 1993). Patients with psoriasis who have a flare of their disease after initial improvement, or who develop a superimposed der-matitis, should be patch tested. The allergen may be the vehicle, the pre-servative, or the steroid itself. The incidence of topical corticosteroid allergy has been found to be surprisingly high; Boffa *et al.* (1995) found that 127 patients (5.9%) out of 2123 tested had a contact allergy to at least one topical corticosteroid. Testing for tixocortol pivalate and budesonide allergy picked up 91% of corticosteroid allergic subjects, and the authors suggested that these agents should be included in the European Standard Battery of patch tests. Cross-reactivity between topical corticosteroids may occur and be diffi-cult to predict but Coopman *et al.* (1989) found that most patients who de-veloped a corticosteroid allergy did not react to the older fluorinated topical corticosteroids. They recommended using a betamethasone, flumetasone or halomethasone ester.

9.8.3 Systemic side-effects

Suppression of the pituitary–adrenal axis by excessive application of topi-cally applied corticosteroids is now well documented (Katz *et al.* 1987b). La-belling topical corticosteroids with 14C also showed that systemic absorption occurs. The absorption process may be increased by disruption of the stratum corneum by a disease process or by increasing the permeability of the skin via occlusion. Basal 9 am plasma cortisol, a short synacthen test, and 24-h urine collection for 17-hydroxycorticosteroid and other cortisol metabolites are the most usual way to detect adrenal suppression. If inhibition of the pituitary–adrenal axis is detected during treatment with topical corticosteroids, function tends to return to normal once the integrity of the barrier function of the stratum corneum is restored or after treatment has been stopped, usually by the third day after treatment. In most cases, the presence of minor abnormalities are not of any clinical significance, as long as enough reserve adrenal function exists to respond to added stress such as infection or surgery. There is a risk of developing chronic adrenal insufficiency if very potent topical corticosteroids are used on large areas of the body for longer than 3–4 weeks. The young and elderly are particularly predisposed to increased absorption of topical corticosteroids because of less efficient adrenal reserve capacity and thinner skin, and in babies a high surface area to body volume.

The site and mode of application of topical corticosteroids must also be taken into account, with increased absorption in areas where the stratum corneum is relatively thin such as the face, axillae, genitals and groin. Keratolytics and hydrating agents such as propylene glycol, salicylic acid or urea will enhance the penetration of most topical corticosteroids.

Iatrogenic topical steroid-induced adrenal insufficiency is rare and similar to Addison's disease in that fatigue, generalized weakness, hypotension, weight loss and gastrointestinal disturbances may occur in an insidious fashion.

A distinguishing feature between the two conditions is hyperpigmentation, which occurs in Addison's disease secondary to elevated levels of endogenous adrenocorticotrophic hormone (ACTH) but is not seen in iatrogenic disease. Laboratory findings in topical corticosteroid-induced adrenal insufficiency show a reduced 9 am serum cortisol, decreased 24-h urinary free cortisol, and attenuated cortisol response to a short synacthen test.

Another extremely rare side-effect of systemic absorption of topical corticosteroids is Cushing's syndrome, usually occurring secondary to misuse (Teelucksingh *et al.* 1993). Clinical features are well known and include centripetal truncal obesity, 'buffalo-hump' neck, striae, plethoric 'moon' facies and widespread easy bruising. Serum morning cortisol and 24-h urinary steroids are reduced, whereas they are increased in the endogenous form of Cushing's syndrome.

Other uncommon systemic side-effects secondary to the absorption of topical corticosteroids includes the worsening or unmasking of diabetes and hypertension. Patients with liver failure are particularly prone to pituitary–adrenal axis suppression, therefore caution in prescribing topical corticosteroids in this group is important.

As a working rule, a recommended weekly dose of not more than 50 g of superpotent or 100 g of potent topical corticosteroid should be applied long-term (without occlusion) if systemic absorption is to be avoided.

9.9 Systemic corticosteroids

Systemic corticosteroids are rarely used in the treatment of psoriasis. Cautious use is very occasionally justified in the setting of generalized pustular and erythrodermic psoriasis and is reserved for patients who are unresponsive to other treatment, or when their clinical condition is so severe that a therapeutic trial is justified.

Ryan and Baker (1969) evaluated 104 patients with pustular psoriasis and found that although treatment with systemic steroids could control the pustular phase; the high incidence of side-effects limited their value. Once systemic corticosteroids were withdrawn, increasingly severe pustular relapses were noted.

Occasionally, systemic corticosteroids can prolong generalized pustular and erythrodermic psoriasis. If used to achieve immediate remission of pustular and erythrodermic psoriasis, steroid dosage must be decreased slowly to minimize the risk of a rebound flare. Concurrent administration of a definitive treatment such as methotrexate, acitretin or cyclosporin may help to achieve this. One approach was to use triamcinolone or tetracosactide depot injections for the initial 2 weeks of the disease while the patient was closely monitored in hospital.

Impetigo herpetiformis is a very rare and aggressive form of pustular psoriasis that occurs in pregnancy or with the oral contraceptive pill. It is often treated with systemic corticosteroids because of the extreme debility of the patient and because of the teratogenicity of other therapies (Lotem *et al.* 1989).

Systemic corticosteroid therapy is contraindicated for the treatment of chronic plaque psoriasis because of the high risk of precipitating the pustular and unstable form of the condition.

9.10 Combined therapies

9.10.1 Topical corticosteroids in combination with other topical therapies

Combinations of topical corticosteroids with antibacterial and/or antifungal agents are commonly used in the treatment of flexural psoriasis or facial sebo-psoriasis. These areas are frequently colonized by yeasts, for example *Candida* species and/or bacteria, for example *Staphylococcus aureus*. Care must be taken to avoid long-term treatment and the development of resistance.

Keratolytics such as propylene glycol, salicylic acid or urea increase the absorption of topical corticosteroids; used in combination, they are particularly helpful for the treatment of the acral hyperkeratosis or thickened hyperkeratotic psoriatic plaques on the body (Giannotti & Pimpinelli 1992).

Emollients used in conjunction with topical corticosteroids may reduce scaling and contribute to patient comfort, especially if the corticosteroid dose is being gradually reduced (Gordon 1998).

Studies using a very potent topical corticosteroid in combination with dithranol produced equally satisfactory clearance as dithranol in Lassar's paste. The mixture is clinically very effective in the treatment of psoriasis but is potentially unstable and needs to be made up with care. Addition of 0.25% dithranol to corticosteroid ointments in opaque (usually amber-coloured) glass jars and stored at room temperature creates a stable admixture of up to 28 days with clobetasol propionate and up to 3 months with betamethasone valerate and clobetasone butyrate.

A longer remission period after treatment with a potent topical corticosteroid in comparison with dithranol has been reported, although a more rapid relapse rate after stopping topical corticosteroid treatment compared with dithranol has also been observed.

Coal tar solutions are often added to topical corticosteroids; but it is advisable to use an ointment rather than a cream base, because of its greater stability. Coal tar in any formulation is alkaline, and this could cause changes in steroid structure and potency, creating a steroid preparation weaker than expected.

Lebwohl (1997) reviewed the data on combining calcipotriol formulations with topical corticosteroids and concluded that regimens used in the treatment of psoriasis combining calcipotriol ointment with superpotent steroids such as halobetasol ointment resulted in greater improvement and fewer side-effects than using either therapy alone.

9.10.2 Topical corticosteroids in combination with systemic therapies

Meola *et al.* (1991) reviewed the use of topical corticosteroids as adjunctive therapy for psoriasis in combination with phototherapy showed that there is a benefit if they are used with psoralen and UVA (PUVA) but not with UVB. There may be a faster response to PUVA therapy if topical corticosteroids are used as well, but time to relapse after PUVA was not altered.

Topical corticosteroids have also been used in combination with retinoids for the treatment of psoriasis, and they have been noted to improve both the rate of remission and the time for the plaques to clear (Fritsch 1992).

In practice, topical corticosteroids are used regularly in combination with other antipsoriatic treatments such as methotrexate, cyclosporin and tacrolimus. Clinical experience indicates they are effective as adjunctive treatment but no randomized-controlled trials have confirmed this observation.

References

Almawi, W.Y., Lipman, M.L., Stevens, A.C., Zanker, B., Hadro, E.T. & Strom, T.B. (1991) Abrogation of glucocorticosteroid-mediated inhibition of T-cell proliferation by the synergistic action of 1L-1, 1L-6, and IFN-gamma. *Journal of Immunology* **146**, 3253–3257.

Barry, B.W. (1983). *Dermatological Formulations: Percutaneous Absorption.* Vol 18, Drugs and the pharmaceutical sciences. Marcel Dekker, New York.

Boffa, M.J., Wilkinson, S.M. & Beck M.H. (1995) Screening for corticosteroid hypersensitivity. *Contact Dermatitis* **35**, 149–151.

Broby-Johansen, U., Karlsmark, T., Petersen, L.J. & Serup, J. (1990) Ranking of the antipsoriatic effect of various topical corticosteroids applied under a hydrocolloid dressing—skin thickness, blood flow and colour measurements compared to clinical assessments. *Clinical and Experimental Dermatology* **15**, 343–348.

Callen, J. (1996) Comparison of safety and efficacy of fluticasone propionate cream 0.05% and betamethasone valerate cream 0.1% in the treatment of moderate-to-severe psoriasis. *Cutis* **57**, 45–50.

Chu, A.C. & Munn, S. (1995) Fluticasone propionate in the treatment of inflammatory dermatoses. *British Journal of Clinical Practice* **49**, 131–133.

Coopman, S., Degreef, H. & Dooms-Goossens, A. (1989) Identification of cross-reaction patterns in allergic contact dermatitis from topical corticosteroids. *British Journal of Dermatology* **121**, 27–34.

Cornell, R.C. (1992) Clinical trials of topical corticosteroids in psoriasis: Correlations with the vasoconstrictor assay. *International Journal of Dermatology* **31** (Suppl.), 38–40.

Degreef, H. & Dooms-Goossens, A. (1993) The new corticosteroids: are they effective and safe? *Dermatology Clinics* **11**, 155–160.

Elks, J. (1976) Steroid structure and steroid activity. *British Journal of Dermatology* **94** (Suppl. 12), 3–13.

Fritsch, P.O. (1992) Retinoids in psoriasis and disorders of keratinization. *Journal of the American Academy of Dermatology* **27**, S8–S14.

Giannotti, B. & Pimpinelli, N. (1992) Topical corticoids: Which drug and when? *Drugs* **44**, 65–71.

Gordon, M.L. (1998) The role of clobetasol propionate emollient 0.05% in the treatment of patients with dry, scaly, corticosteroid-responsive dermatoses. *Clinical Therapeutics* **20**, 26–39.

Katchman, S.D., Del Monaco, M., Wu, M., Brown, D., Hsu Wong, S. & Uitto, J. (1995) A transgenic mouse model provides a novel biological assay of topical glucocorticosteroid potency. *Archives of Dermatology* **131**, 1274–1278.

Katz, H.I., Hien, N.T., Prawer, S.E., Scott, J.C. & Grivna, E.M. (1987a) Betamethasone in optimized vehicle. Intermittent pulse dosing for extended maintenance treatment of psoriasis. *Archives of Dermatology* **123**, 1308–1311.

Katz, H.I., Hien, N.T., Prawer, S.E., Mastbaum, L.I., Mooney, J.J. & Samson, C.R. (1987b) Superpotent topical steroid treatment of psoriasis vulgaris—clinical efficacy and adrenal function. *Journal of the American Academy of Dermatology* **16**, 804–811.

Kerscher, M.J. & Korting, H.C. (1992) Comparative atrophogenicity potential of medium and highly potent topical glucocorticoids in cream and ointment according to ultrasound analysis. *Skin Pharmacology* **5**, 7–80.

Krueger, G.G., O'Reilly, M.A., Weidner, M., Dromgoole, S.H. & Killey, F.P. (1998) Comparative efficacy of once-daily flurandrenolide tape versus twice-daily diflorasone diacetate ointment in the treatment of psoriasis. *Journal of the American Academy of Dermatology* **38**, 186–190.

Lauerma, A.I. & Reitamo, S. (1993) Contact allergy to corticosteroids. *Journal of the American Academy of Dermatology* **28**, 618–622.

Lebwohl, M. (1997) Topical application of calcipotriene and corticosteroids: combination regimens. *Journal of the American Academy of Dermatology* **37**, S55–8.

Lotem, M., Katzenelson, V., Rotem, A., Hod, M. & Sandbank, M. (1989) Impetigo herpetiformis: a variant of pustular psoriasis or a separate entity? *Journal of the American Academy of Dermatology* **20**, 338–341.

Mackenzie, A.W. & Stoughton, R.B. (1964) Method for comparing percutaneous absorption of steroids. *Archives of Dermatology* **86**, 608–610.

Medansky, R.S., Bressinck, R. & Cole, G.W. *et al.* (1988) Mometasone furoate ointment and cream 0.1% in treatment of psoriasis: Comparison with ointment and cream formulations of fluocinolone acetonide 0.025% and triamcinolone 0.1%. *Cutis* **42**, 480–485.

Meola, T. Jr, Soter, N.A. & Lim, H.W. (1991) Are topical corticosteroids useful adjunctive therapy for the treatment of psoriasis with ultraviolet radiation? *Archives of Dermatology* **127**, 1708–1713.

Oakley, R.H. & Cidlowski, J.A. (1993) Homologous down-regulation of the glucocorticoid receptor: The molecular machinery. *Critical Review of Eukaryotic Gene Expression* **3**, 63–88.

Pershing, L.K., Silver, B.S., Krueger, G.G., Shah, V.P. & Skelley J.P. (1992) Feasibility of measuring the bioavailability of topical betamethasone dipropionate in commercial formulations using drug content in skin and a skin blanching bioassay. *Pharmacological Research* **9**, 45–51.

Pershing, L.K., Corlett, J.L., Lambert, L.D. & Poncelet, C.E. (1994) Circadian activity of topical 0.05% betamethasone dipropionate in human skin in vivo. *Journal of Investigative Dermatology* **102**, 734–739.

Rosenthal, D. & Duke, E. (1988) A clinical investigation of the efficacy and safety of mometasone furoate ointment 0.1% vs betamethasone valerate ointment 0.1% in the treatment of psoriasis. *Current Therapeutic Research* **44**, 790–800.

Ryan, T.J. & Baker, H. (1969) Systemic corticosteroids and folic acid antagonists in the treatment of generalised pustular psoriasis. Evaluation and prognosis based on the study of 104 cases. *British Journal of Dermatology* **81**, 134–145.

Sulzberger, M.B. & Witten, V.H. (1952) The effect of topically applied Compound F in selected dermatoses. *Journal of Investigative Dermatology* **19**, 101–102.

Teelucksingh, S., Bahall, M., Coomansingh, D., Suite, M. & Bartholomew, C. (1993) Cushing's syndrome from topical glucocorticoids. *West Indian Medical Journal* **42**, 77–78.

Wright, S. (1995) Steroids and their mechanism of action. *Proceedings of the Royal College of Physicians of Edinburgh* **25**, 34–39.

Chapter 10: Dithranol

M.J.P. Gerritsen

10.1 Introduction

Dithranol is among the most effective antipsoriatic modalities for topical treatment in psoriasis. It reaches clearance rates up to 95% in chronic plaque psoriasis, with long remission times. It is still one of the most effective topical drugs in psoriasis. Although dithranol offers a safe approach without severe adverse events, the staining and the, to some extent obligatory, irritation remain major drawbacks in its use. The precise mode of action is unknown, but it may influence a broad spectrum of events in psoriasis by the generation of extracellular oxygen radicals.

10.2 History

For more than 120 years dithranol has been known to have antipsoriatic potential. In 1876 Squire reported the beneficial use of Goa powder in a patient with psoriasis. The psoriasis was mistaken for ringworm and accidentally, but successfully, treated with Goa powder, which was until then known to be only effective in ringworm (Squire 1876). The active ingredient of Goa powder, also known as araroba powder, is chrysarobin (also known as yellow araroba, 3-methyl dithranol) (Liebermann & Seidler 1878). In China and Malaysia this ingredient was called 'poh de Bahia' (named after a province in Brazil). The powder was derived from the medulla of the stem and the branches of the araroba tree, and was exported by the Portuguese from Brazil to Goa in India and Mozambique (Ashton *et al.* 1983; Squire 1876). Araroba means 'tawny coloured'. At this time the adverse events of skin irritation and staining had already been noted, and they remain today the most important disadvantages of dithranol therapy.

The great variation in composition of the naturally derived chrysarobin was a disavantage and led to unpredictable efficacy and irritation. Another drawback was that during the First World War trade with Brazil was disrupted and the supply of chrysarobin became very difficult. As a consequence in Europe many efforts were made to develop a synthetic form of chrysarobin. In Germany, Galewski (1916) developed a synthetic derivate of dithranol or 1,8-dihydroxy-9-anthrone, which lacked the methyl group of chrysarobin at the 3 position (also known as dithranol or cignolin). His formulations contained 0.25–1.0% cignolin in acetone or 0.05–0.1% cignolin

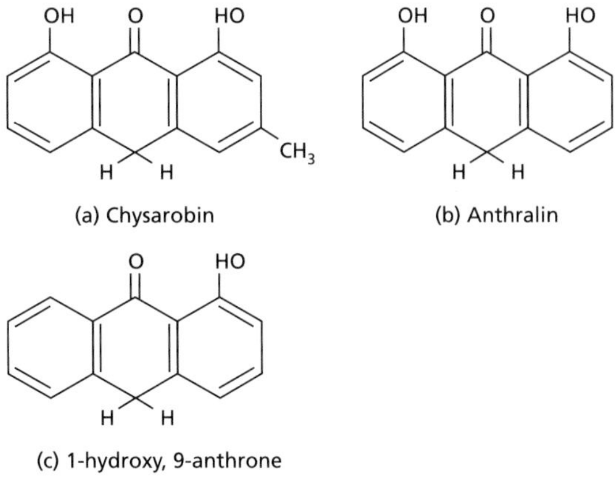

(a) Chysarobin

(b) Anthralin

(c) 1-hydroxy, 9-anthrone

Fig. 10.1 Antipsoriatic anthrones.

in white petrolatum in combination with 0.5% salicylic acid and 5% liquor carbonis detergens. Also in 1916, Unna reported on the antipsoriatic efficacy of dithranol and 1-hydroxy-9-anthrone. Until now, no anthrone derivative has been developed that is more effective (Krebs & Schaltegger 1969; Ashton *et al*. 1983) (Fig. 10.1).

In Europe, dithranol was first used in Germany, but was introduced in Britain in the 1930s. Dithranol never became very popular in America. It took more than 20 years before Ingram reported his experience with this very effective modality. In an inpatient setting or at a day-care unit patients with psoriasis were treated daily with a tar bath (90 L water, 120 mL coal tar in an alcoholic solution and 30 mL Teepol), followed by UVB phototherapy. Afterwards these patients were treated with 0.42% dithranol in stiff Lassar's paste (Ingram 1953). This regimen was extremely effective; however, the costs of the triple therapy, the side-effects of irritation and staining, the time-consuming aspects and the difficulty of using dithranol at home prevent dithranol therapy becoming widely popular.

The development of short-contact therapy with dithranol ointments, which can be washed off easily, has offered new possibilities for outpatient treatment.

10.3 Chemistry, mode of action and pharmacology

1,8-dihydroxy-3-methyl-9-anthrone (chrysarobin) and 1,8-dihydroxy-9-anthrone (dithranol or cignolin) are anthracene derivatives. Anthracene is an aromatic compound with three benzene rings fused together with carbon atoms 1–8 in the two outer rings, and two centre carbon atoms, 9 and 10. Dithranol has two hydroxyl groups at the C-1 and the C-8 position, a carbonyl group at the C-9 position, and a methylene group at the C-10 position. Thus, dithranol is stabilized by hydrogen binding in the ketonic form. The association of the hydroxyl (at C-1) and the carbonyl groups (at C-9) at one end with the methylene group at the other (C-10) is essential for activity. Because of the methylene group, dithranol is easily oxidized by air, light, alkalis or after application onto the skin. This oxidation results in inflammation and staining. The oxidation leads to biologically active free-radical formation and further oxidation in which chrysarobin changes to chrysophanic acid and dithranol to chrysazin. Chrysophanic acid and chrysazin are responsible for the yellow colour. When the anthrone molecules change during the oxidation to dithranol dimers, formed by the addition of two free radicals at the 10 position, they may further oxidize to anthraquinone dimers, which are responsible for the purple–brown staining (Krebs and Schaltegger 1969). The extracellularly generated oxygen radicals are responsible for both the antipsoriatic and irritative effect of dithranol. The extracellularly generated superoxide anion radical induces an active adaptation mechanism resulting in increased tolerance to dithranol upon repeated application, which may explain the requirement for increasing dithranol concentrations to maintain antipsoriatic efficacy (Kemény *et al.* 1990). Although many investigators believe that the inflammation caused by dithranol is necessary for antipsoriatic efficacy, there is one study showing that dithranol-induced inflammation and therapeutic effect can be dissociated (Ramsay *et al.* 1990).

Psoriasis vulgaris is characterized by epidermal hyperproliferation, hyperortho- and parakeratosis, diminishing of the granular layer, acanthosis with elongation of the rete ridges with abnormal keratinization, intraepidermal accumulation of polymorphonuclear leucocytes and cellular inflammation in the upper dermis. During dithranol therapy normalization of these histopathological changes may occur. The interference of dithranol with epidermal hyperproliferation has been investigated by many groups. As described above the biochemical basis for the mode of action at the molecular level is related to the redox activity leading to the production of singlet oxygens, superoxide anion radicals and hydroxyl radicals. The extracellularly generated oxygen radicals are responsible for both the antipsoriatic and irritative effect. Their growth-modulating effects comprise inhibition of DNA synthesis and repair, interference with mitochondria, inhibition of glucose-6-phosphate dehydrogenase (G6PD), ornithine decarboxylase, polyamine synthesis, calmodulin and interference with cyclic nucleotides. However, at certain concentrations dithranol may stimulate epidermal DNA synthesis (Kemény *et al.* 1990). Dithranol may also have an effect on inflammation and abnormal keratinization (Table 10.1).

Although many modes of action have been proposed, the precise working mechanism of dithranol is still unclear. Most influencing effects of dithranol may be rather secondary than primary. In 1966, Swanbeck and Liden demonstrated the inhibitory effect of dithranol on DNA synthesis. They observed an inhibition of thymidine incorporation into the guinea-pig epidermis. The phenomenon appeared not to be a direct action on DNA, but more

Table 10.1 Mode of action of dithranol in psoriasis.

Interference with epidermal growth
Inhibition of DNA synthesis, mitotic rate and repair
Interference with mitochondria
Inhibition of glucose-6-phosphate dehydrogenase
Inhibition of ornithine decarboxylase/polyamine
  biosynthesis
Interference with cyclic nucleotides
Inhibition of calmodulin

Interference with inflammation
Interference with arachidonic acid metabolism
Inhibition of granulocyte function
Inhibition of lymphocyte function
Interference with dendritic cells

Interference with keratinization
Transglutaminase
Involucrin
Acanthosis
Keratin 16
Filaggrin

(Kemény *et al.* 1990; van de Kerkhof 1991; Swanbeck & Liden 1966; Gaudin *et al.* 1972; Fisher & Maibach 1975; Jacques & Reichert 1981; Muller *et al.* 1995; Fuchs *et al.* 1990; Cavey *et al.* 1982; Morlière *et al.* 1985; Bohlen *et al.* 1978; Bisschop *et al.* 1984; Saihan *et al.* 1980; Tucker *et al.* 1986; Black *et al.* 1985; Barr *et al.* 1989; Ternowitz 1987; Anderson *et al.* 1987; Schröder *et al.* 1985; van der Vleuten *et al.* 1996; Morhenn *et al.* 1983; Bacharach Buhles *et al.* 1996; Bedord *et al.* 1983; Muller *et al.* 1991)

likely a consequence of a potent effect on cellular respiration and subsequent energy production (Shroot 1992).

Strong evidence indicates that the target organelle for dithranol is the mitochondrion, resulting in a reduction of the adenosine triphosphatase (ATP) synthesis (Morlière *et al.* 1985; Shroot 1992), which may lead to inhibition of energy-dependent biosynthetic processes, for example DNA replication and repair. The inhibitory effect of dithranol on the elevated activity of G6PD in psoriasis may be related to decomposition products formed by the autoxidation of dithranol (Cavey *et al.* 1982). This mode of action, however, was later thought to be unlikely, because toxicity of dithranol to human fibroblasts decreases during the 5-h period, during which Cavey *et al.* observed an increased inhibition of G6PD, and because the oxidation products of dithranol are ineffective in the treatment (Kemény *et al.* 1990).

Because α-difluoromethylornithine, a highly specific inhibitor of the key enzyme in polyamine synthesis, ornithine decarboxylase (ODC), has no antipsoriatic potential, the inhibition of the activity of ODC by dithranol is more likely to be a secondary than a primary phenomenon (Bohlen *et al.* 1978; Kemény *et al.* 1990).

In psoriasis, dithranol also exerts an inhibitory effect on the elevated epidermal cyclic guanosine monophosphate (cGMP) level, while leaving the decreased cAMP level unaffected (Saihan *et al.* 1980). Tucker *et al.* (1986) demonstrated inhibition of calmodulin activity in psoriatic lesions by dithranol, suggesting another possible therapeutic mode of action in psoriasis. Dithranol causes a reduction in the concentration of arachidonic acid, concurrent with clinical improvement of psoriatic lesions (Barr *et al.* 1989).

Immunohistochemically, a major decrease of keratin 16 and Ki-67-positive nuclei, and virtually complete restoration of filaggrin-positive cell layers was noted following dithranol therapy in psoriasis. The stratum granulosum and keratohyalin granules reappear. Hyperkeratosis decreases with loss of parakeratosis. The number of transglutaminase- and involucrin-positive cell layers was minimally affected. Whereas the epidermal T lymphocytes and the epidermal and dermal polymorphonuclear leucocytes showed no significant changes, the number of dermal T lymphocytes demonstrated a significant reduction (van der Vleuten *et al.* 1996). Other studies, however, reported on an inhibition of mitogen-stimulated lymphocyte proliferation and neutrophil chemotaxis by dithranol (Anderson *et al.* 1987).

There are four principal factors which affect the pharmaceutical formulation of a drug for dermatological use: stability, the drug must be released from its formulation, it must partition into the outer layers of the skin, and it must permeate through the epidermis. The drug must reach the receptor sites in sufficient quantities. Dithranol possesses chemical characteristics that permit rapid penetration through the skin, the molecule has sufficient lipophilicity or oil solubility and in addition the molecule has projecting phenolic hydoxyl groups which can hydrogen bond with proteins within the tissue to increase water solubility (Whitefield 1981).

Dithranol can be prepared in an ointment, paste, cream or stick. The bioavailability is influenced by the vehicle. The penetration of dithranol through the epidermis is faster in lipophilic than in a hydrophilic vehicle (Swanbeck & Liden 1966). Thus, the bioavailability of dithranol in an ointment base is better compared with a cream base. With dithranol, the criteria for penetration are best fulfilled by the established formulations based on white soft paraffin, since the solubility of dithranol in white soft paraffin is sufficient for clinical effectiveness, and partition into the skin is efficient as there is no association between the molecules of the solute and those of the solvent (Whitefield 1981).

Because the paraffin softens at skin temperature, once applied it spreads easily beyond the border of the psoriatic lesions. To avoid this spreading, the ointment may be stiffened by the inclusion of zinc oxide and starch. However, zinc oxide contains alkaline impurities, which will inactivate the dithranol.

By including salicylic acid in the formulation, before the dithranol is added, the alkaline contaminants will be neutralized and oxidation will be prevented (Comaish *et al.* 1971; Dean 1971).

In the absence of air and light, ketonic dithranol in white soft paraffin is relatively stable over short periods. The stability of dithranol also depends on the concentration and the vehicle. In general, the higher the concentration and the greasier the vehicle, the more stable the dithranol becomes. Over longer periods, and to a greater extent in the presence of air, light, water or alkaline environment, dithranol will oxidize. The colour of the dithranol ointment changes to brown, which implicates that the drug has become inactive. Therefore, dithranol should always be freshly prepared and delivered in small tubes (40–50 g). The low concentrations of dithranol, especially the cream forms, must be stored in the refrigerator. Dithranol ointments may be more stabilized by the adding of the antioxidant ascorbic acid. In some cream bases salicylic acid or ascorbic acid can be added to suppress oxidation. It must be kept in mind, however, that the addition of salicylic acid may increase the irritancy properties of the vehicle (Prins *et al.* 1998). Mahrle (1997) gives a clear overview on the stability of dithranol in various vehicles and solvents.

The concentration of dithranol reaches its maximum in the epidermis between 60 and 300 min after application (Kammerau *et al.* 1975; Schalla *et al.* 1981). Schalla *et al.* (1981) demonstrated that when the skin barrier is intact, the rise of concentration in the skin is much slower. Therefore, he states, when penetration kinetics in the skin are much faster in involved skin of psoriatic patients, removal of the excess dithranol after a short time period should diminish the concentration in uninvolved skin. The more delayed the washing off, the smaller the difference was between different states of skin barrier.

On the other hand, if the removal of the excess dithranol is too early, even penetration into the involved skin with the damaged barrier may not reach a desired concentration. The optimal time for washing off is between 30 and 60 min.

10.4 Indications and contraindications

Dithranol may be the first choice therapy in a moderate to severe chronic plaque psoriasis. Depending on the extent of the psoriasis, the condition, motivation and understanding of the patient, the choice may be treatment at an inpatient department or at a day-care unit.

Contraindications for dithranol treatment are acute, instable, generalized pustular and erythrodermic psoriasis. After stabilizing the activity of the psoriasis with bland emollients, dithranol may be applied in low concentrations, if necessary during short treatment schedules. Dithranol is safe for daily long-term treatment.

At the moment it is uncertain whether treatment during pregnancy is harmful. In Germany, dithranol without the addition of salicylic acid is allowed during pregnancy. Salicylic acid in high doses has proven to be teratogenic in animal studies (Zesch 1990).

10.5 Side-effects

No serious side-effects of dithranol have been reported. There is, however, one report by Phillips and Alldrick (1994) who reported skin papillomas in a classical two-stage carcinogenesis protocol when using the combination of coal tar (a tumour initiator) and dithranol (a tumour promotor) at therapeutic doses in mice, while treatment with either topical agent alone did not.

Although dithranol exerts tumour promotor properties in the *in vivo* animal model, there are no reports of an enhanced incidence of skin cancer in psoriatic patients (Boch & Burns 1963; Swanbeck & Hillstrom 1971).

Following topical application, danthrone, an oxidation product of dithranol, is excreted in urine (Ippen 1981). After oral ingestion of Istizin[R] (Chrysazin), danthrone is partially absorbed in the upper gastrointestinal tract and excreted with urine, whereas in the large bowel danthrone is reduced to dithranol and excreted with the faeces. The formation of dithranol in the large bowel can be shown by the so-called 'Istizin-exanthema' due to perianal dithranol irritation, which is comparable with dithranol erythema of the skin after topical application (Ippen 1959). A higher incidence of carcinoma of the colon following systemic treatment with dithranol and anthraquinone as laxatives has not been demonstrated (Ippen 1981).

Gay *et al.* (1972) performed a study on systemic toxicity during 3 months treatment with dithranol paste in psoriatic patients. He found no significant change in blood picture, liver and renal function.

An almost obligatory side-effect is irritation, which may be clinically observed as erythema. Following high concentrations of dithranol or long application time, troublesome irritation may appear, while in severe cases, although rare, even blisters can occur. It may be necessary to interrupt the therapy. Depending on the duration of this interruption, the application time and/or concentration of dithranol should be adjusted. The irritation may be treated with bland preparations or tar ointments.

Kingston and Marks (1983) demonstrated that patients with skin type I are more sensitive to irritation following dithranol.

Maurice and Greaves (1983) found a small significant difference between the erythema dose–response curves from patients with skin type I and IV, but concluded that this was not sufficient to account for the clinical impression of increased dithranol irritancy in fair-skinned subjects.

There have been many studies on factors influencing dithranol erythema. Juhlin (1981) concludes that the most effective way to inhibit dithranol erythema is pretreatment of the skin with UVB irradiation or PUVA. UVA alone does not show this effect. It was assumed that this inhibition could partly be due to a decreased penetration of dithranol through a thickened epidermis. It is also likely that this is mainly due to an altered release of mediators. Whether depletion of Langerhans cells by pretreatment with UVB plays a major role in suppressing dithranol erythema is not known. In the case of known sensitivity for dithranol, patients may start with UVB or PUVA before dithranol treatment.

Pretreatment with histamine releasers, or treatment with antihistamines, aspirin, or oral or topical corticosteroids did not change the inflammatory reaction. Misch et al. (1981) confirms some of these findings. In addition they also observed no effect of indometacin (anti-inflammatory drug and inhibitor of the prostaglandin-forming enzyme cyclo-oxygenase) and scopolamine (acetylcholine antagonist) on dithranol erythema. The formation of free-radical oxygen species could lead to chemical oxidation of arachidonic acid and consequent liberation of pharmacologically active metabolites of arachidonic acid without the involvement of prostaglandin synthetase enzyme activity. Thus, they conclude that it is unlikely that prostaglandins, histamine and acetylcholine are involved in the pharmacogenesis of delayed dithranol erythema and that aspirin and indometacin would not be effective inhibitors of arachidonate metabolites. In contrast to this report, in 1983 an inhibiting effect of indometacin on dithranol inflammation was shown.

Indometacin blocked dithranol-induced skin-temperature increase and it was suggested that prostaglandins may play a role as mediators in dithranol erythema (Kingston & Marks, 1983).

Wemmer et al. (1986) reported that coal tar solution was as effective as coal tar itself in suppressing dithranol erythema. There are many other reports on the beneficial effect of tar on dithranol irritation.

Application of amines may exert an inhibiting effect on dithranol-induced inflammation, which may be related to lipid solubility and transdermal permeability. These amines are lipid soluble and may penetrate cell walls and exert a direct effect on membrane-bound dithranol, which leads to inactivation of dithranol. The application of amines might be of relevance in reducing perilesional inflammation, mainly in short-contact dithranol therapy, without diminishing the therapeutic effect (Ramsay et al. 1990). Table 10.2 gives a summary of several studies on factors that influence dithranol irritation.

Following the use of topical steroids, a wash-out period of about 2 weeks with bland emollients or tar ointments may be necessary, to avoid a rebound from the steroid withdrawal and/or intolerance to dithranol.

Contact allergy to dithranol, although very rare, has been reported (de Grood & Nater 1981). In most cases dithranol allergy may be mistaken for irritation, which is mainly dose dependent.

The side-effects of staining of the skin, clothing, furniture and bathroom are well known. This side-effect is due primarily to oxidation of dithranol.

Table 10.2 Influence on dithranol irritation (Finnen *et al.* 1984; Wemmer *et al.* 1986; Misch *et al.* 1981; Juhlin 1981; Ramsay *et al.* 1990a,b; Lawrence *et al.* 1987; Ramsay *et al.* 1992; Kingston *et al.* 1983; Munro *et al.* 1989).

Treatment	Positive influence	No influence
Antioxidants	X	
Tar	X	
Corticosteroids		X
UVB	X	
PUVA	X	
Pretreatment with histamine releasers		X
Antihistaminica		X
Aspirin		X
Topical corticosteroids		X
Alkaline amines	X	
KOH	X	
Teepol	X	
Indometacin (orally and topically)	X	X
Cyclosporin A	X	

The oxidation products are increased by alkalis. They bind to keratin, and stain natural and synthetic fibers. The staining of the skin with dithranol may be treated with 5% salicylic acid in vaseline. The staining of the tiles of the shower may be prevented by water rinsing these tiles before washing off dithranol ointments.

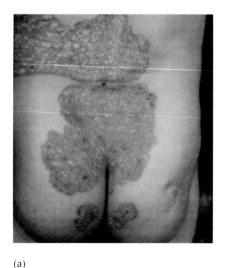
(a)

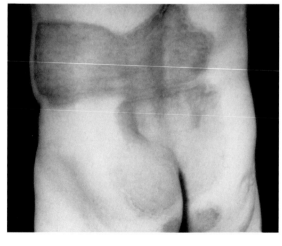
(b)

Fig. 10.2 (a) Psoriasis vulgaris before treatment. (b) Psoriasis vulgaris after treatment with dithranol paste.

The washing off should be done without soap because the alkalis in the soap increase the staining. The stains on white fabrics may be removed with a 10-minute soak in full-strength chlorine bleach, followed by water rinse and air drying. This procedure must be repeated twice to obtain best results. In the case of coloured textiles the bleach should be diluted 1 : 10 and it is recommended to perform a bleach-safe test to assure colour fastness to 1 : 10 bleach. It must be kept in mind that the longer the stain remains on the fabric the more difficult it is to remove. To remove dithranol stains from plastic shower curtains it is advised to wash within 5 min with 95% ethyl alcohol and follow with a water rinse. (Wang *et al.* 1986).

10.6 Clinical effectiveness

Comparing various vehicles and treatment schedules of dithranol, monotherapy with 24-h applications appears to be the most effective. Inpatient treatment results in a significantly faster clearance as compared to outpatient treatment. It is, however, difficult to compare the different dithranol regimens with regard to clearance times and relapse rates. The definition of clearance may vary. Often clearance is described as lack of palpable psoriatic lesions, other authors may consider erythema as residual psoriasis. The surface of involved skin may be of relevance in clearance. Moreover, in different studies, the involved skin at the start of treatment may vary widely. The definition of relapse may also differ, which makes comparison of separate studies difficult. For an extensive overview of the efficacy of the different vehicles and treatment modules the reader is referred to the review by van de Kerkhof (1991).

Despite the longer treatment periods, in some patients the combined day care and home treatment may be more worthwhile, because it gives them the opportunity to stay in their social and economic environment. Another important aspect is that the costs of outpatient treatment compared with inpatient treatment are very low.

Patients can be educated to treat themselves with dithranol at home, which makes even a patient with severe psoriasis more independent. However, careful instruction about the therapy, together with motivation and compliance of the patient, are indispensable.

In a multicentre comparison of outpatient treatment during 8 weeks with calcipotriol ointment and short-contact dithranol therapy in chronic plaque psoriasis, difference in improvement was in favour of calcipotriol (Berth-Jones *et al.* 1992). However, it is known that the efficacy of home treatment is far less compared with the inpatient or combined day care and home treatment with dithranol. Another limitation of this study is that an open-label comparative study may be more biased in favour of the new therapy.

Because of the staining properties of dithranol it is difficult, if not impossible, to carry out blind comparative studies with other topical therapies not containing dithranol. In a double-blind comparison of a dithranol and steroid mixture with a conventional dithranol regimen for chronic psoriasis it was demonstrated that the addition of the topical steroid produced more rapid initial clearance and less burning, but more rapid relapse of the psoriasis (Grattan *et al.* 1988).

10.7 Combination treatment

Although dithranol monotherapy is very effective, in an individual patient it may be necessary to treat with combination therapies (Table 10.3). The combination of dithranol and UV radiation is a time-honoured approach. On the other hand the superiority of this combination above the monotherapies has been debated by various groups. Schauder and Mahrle (1982) compared the effect of UVB combined with short-contact dithranol with that of short-contact dithranol alone in patients with psoriasis. They did not find a significant difference between the two therapies. Boer and Smeenk (1986) demonstrated that the addition of short-contact dithranol to UVB phototherapy in outpatients yielded only moderate improvement in a minority of patients with psoriasis. Paramsothy *et al.* (1988) also noted no significant difference between the clearance effect of the combination of UVB therapy with short-contact dithranol therapy and dithranol only. However, the combined therapy of UVB with dithranol did significantly postpone relapse.

In general, the combination with UV radiation results in longer remission times. Although in general most studies (Elbracht & Landes 1983; Lebwohl *et*

Table 10.3 The effect of combination therapies with dithranol compared to dithranol only (Bunse & Merk 1990; Elbracht & Landes 1983; Grattan *et al.* 1988; Lebwohl *et al.* 1985; Lidbrink *et al.* 1986; Morison *et al.* 1978; Paramsothy *et al.* 1988; Pearlman *et al.* 1984; Reshad *et al.* 1984; Runne & Kunze 1985; Schulze *et al.* 1987; Seville 1976; Storbeck *et al.* 1993; Mahrle *et al.* 1985; Mahrle & Schulze 1990).

Therapy	Dithranol ointment	Dithranol paste
Topical corticosteroids		= remission time shorter/ more sensitive for irritation
Broad-band UVB	=	
Small-band UVB	↑	
Broad-band UVB + topical corticosteroids	↑ remission time shorter	
Broad-band UVB + tar bath	↑ remission time longer	
Tar	↑	↑
UVA	=	
PUVA	↑ remission time longer	
Oral retinoids	↑	
Oral cyclosporin A	↑	
Under occlusion	↑	

=, equally effective; ↑, more effective.

al. 1985) do not show an additional effect of broad-band UVB, in the individual patient this regimen may be more effective. In some cases it may be necessary to pretreat with UVB or PUVA in order to avoid dithranol irritation. The combination with narrow-band UVB, however, has proven to be superior to the combination with broad-band UVB (Storbeck *et al.* 1993). Storbeck *et al.* investigated the therapeutic efficacy of the Philips TL-01 lamp with a 100-W version compared with conventional broad-band lamps (Sylvania UV 6) in a controlled trial. Twenty-three patients with psoriasis were treated with half-body exposures from the UVB sources. In 13 patients, dithranol in a modified Ingram regimen was added, the other patients used emollients. The modified Ingram therapy comprised the following procedure: six patients were treated by a 12-h application schedule of dithranol, seven patients were treated with short-term application of dithranol lasting from 10 to 30 min. In 20 out of 23 patients the TL-01 lamps proved to be significantly more effective. Application of dithranol provided a substantial additional therapeutic effect.

The combination of dithranol and tar reduces dithranol erythema and may increase the antipsoriatic efficacy (Schulze *et al.* 1987). The addition of tar may be particularly beneficial in patients with pruritus and irritation.

In patients with a recalcitrant psoriasis, who are treated with systemic therapy, for example acitretin, PUVA, methotrexate or cyclosporin A, a combination with dithranol may be more effective. In some cases the combination treatment may be necessary to gain dose reduction of the oral treatment. (Orfanos & Runne 1976; Morison *et al.* 1978; Gottlieb *et al.* 1995). On the other hand the combination may lead to shorter inpatient treatments, which may be an advantage for the patient. In the case of a combination with retinoids it may be important to treat with low concentrations of dithranol, because the retinoid may thin the skin, which may lead to a higher sensitivity to dithranol. Gottlieb *et al.* (1995) did a study in which 12 patients with psoriasis were treated with cyclosporin (5 mg/kg/day). These patients were proven to be unresponsive to, and/or considered unsuitable for, standard therapies for psoriasis including topical tar, corticosteroids or dithranol as monotherapy, and at least to one of the following treatments: UVB irradiation, PUVA, methotrexate or etretinate. The patients applied dithranol only to plaques on half of their body. Of the 12 patients, five cleared within 10 weeks irrespective of dithranol use. The other seven (slow responders) continued treatment for a mean of 18 weeks. These slow responders had a significantly lower severity index, a thinner epidermis, fewer CD8+ cells and fewer proliferating keratinocytes on the dithranol treated side than on the other side. They conclude that the combination of cyclosporin and topical dithranol is effective in patients who are slow to respond to cyclosporin alone.

For patients with limited plaque disease, paper-tape occlusion of dithranol paste may be a solution. Pearlman *et al.* (1984), in a study with 12 patients with unresponsive plaque psoriasis, instructed patients to cover the nightly paste application with semipermeable paper tape during home therapy. Six responded with more than 90% clearing and two with 70% clearing, compared with the contralateral control sites. The average duration was 11 weeks. After 3 months none of the patients had relapsed. The expected irritation was manageable, except for three patients.

10.8 Guidelines for treatment

Although time consuming, for a successful treatment it is indispensable to motivate patients and explain the necessity of a safe approach. To avoid discoloration and irritation on the hands, dithranol is applied to the skin using plastic gloves. Contact with the face, especially the eyes and the mucous membranes, should be avoided. However, in some patients it may be necessary to treat the face with dithranol preparations, in which case extra care must be taken to prevent spreading to eyes and mucous membranes. If irritation of eyes has taken place, the patient must be advised to irrigate the eyes thoroughly with running water for at least 10 min. In severe irritation it may be desirable to refer the patient to the ophthalmologist.

In patients with extensive scaling, efficacy may be enhanced by pretreatment with ointments containing salicylic acid.

Dithranol is only effective if given in the right concentration. Because irritation due to dithranol shows a great variation, it is important to start at a low strength. Depending on the base, the initial concentration is 0.01–0.5% dithranol. During treatment the concentration or the application time (in case of short-contact therapy) of dithranol should increase to gain an optimal effect. Repeated application of dithranol results in increased tolerance which explains the necessity for increasing dithranol concentration to maintain efficacy (Kemény et al. 1990). The aim is minimal erythema and warmth at the treated lesions. The irritation due to dithranol has an early phase with oedema (24–48 h) and a late phase with erythema (48–96 h). The erythema is maximal between 48 and 72 h after application. Thus, in a daily treatment one observes a cumulative irritative effect. Consequently, if well tolerated, the concentration or application time should be increased not more frequently than twice weekly.

In case of irritation with erythema and pain, the dithranol treatment should be withheld for several days. If necessary, the irritation may be treated with bland emollients or tar products. Although in clinical practice topical corticosteroids are often used, the benefit for dithranol irritation is disputed. Depending on the duration of the interruption of the dithranol treatment, the concentration or application time should be adjusted.

In a clinical setting 24-h application of dithranol may be the treatment of choice. Because irritation is mainly observed in the uninvolved skin, dithranol in a paste, which has the advantage of staying confined to the psoriatic lesions, gives the opportunity to treat with optimal concentrations. In the case of an extensive psoriasis with many small lesions, the treatment of choice may be dithranol in an ointment, for example soft paraffin, which, because the whole skin can be treated, is less time consuming. After application the skin is allowed to dry, after which a powder with talc will be used and the arms, trunk and legs will be covered with stockinet.

Treatment of the scalp with dithranol is very effective; however, extra care has to be taken when instructing the patient. Dithranol may stain blond hair pink and silver hair mahogany. In patients with dark hair the staining may be no problem. Uninvolved skin behind ear and hair margins must be avoided and it may be necessary to protect these area with bland ointments such as soft paraffin. Care should be taken to avoid eye contact with dithranol during removal, as it may cause irritation and conjunctivitis. Because creams are easy to apply and to remove, they are the first choice for scalp treatment. In the case of extensive scaling it may be necessary to start with keratolytics, for example salicylic acid in ointments, if possible under plastic occlusion. Treatment of the scalp is best done overnight.

To avoid irritation, the body folds may be treated with dithranol in a cream base in a short-contact schedule; after washing off the dithranol cream, treatment may be followed by coal tar solution.

Short-contact therapy of dithranol in creams allows treatment on an out-patient basis. Several studies have shown that shortening the application time does not significantly affect the clinical efficacy of dithranol. Moreover, removal of excess dithranol up to 2 h after application particularly diminishes the skin concentration in uninvolved skin (Schalla et al. 1981). This is an important observation because, although dithranol penetrates more easily into the involved skin, irritation is mainly observed in uninvolved skin, thus if necessary dithranol may be applied for a short time, without having an important influence on efficacy.

The effectiveness of home treatment with dithranol depends on the compliance and insight of the patient. The combination of day care and home treatment allows accurate surveillance and careful instruction. At home, the treatment should be carried out in a warm bathroom. The ointment or cream is left in position or if necessary covered with old clothing. After the advised application time the dithranol is removed by bathing or showering. The patients have to be instructed to prevent staining of the tiles of the shower by water rinsing the tiles before washing off dithranol ointments. The use of soap may enhance the staining property of dithranol. The patients should treat themselves with a 'no-touch technique', thereby taking care that parts of the body do not come in contact with another during treatment. If necessary short-contact therapy may be applied twice daily.

After the lesions have become non-palpable, it is advised to continue therapy for a short period to ensure clearance. The staining of the skin will disappear after about 2 weeks, or may be removed by application of a low concentration of salicylic acid in an ointment.

10.9 Conclusion

Although dithranol still has side-effects with regard to staining and irritancy, it remains a first line of treatment, mainly because of its effectiveness and safety. The biological efficacy is correlated with irritation and staining. Experimental data suggest that extracellularly generated oxygen radicals are responsible for both the antipsoriatic and irritative effect. Moreover, the extracellularly generated superoxide anion radical also induces an active adaptation mechanism resulting in increased tolerance to dithranol upon repeated application, which may explain the requirement for increasing dithranol concentrations to maintain efficacy (Kemény *et al.* 1990).

Several approaches have been tried to limit its staining and irritation properties. The development of new formulations which can be washed off easily and combine adequate efficacy with low irritancy and staining properties enables dithranol therapy on an outpatient basis. For cooperative and compliant patients, short-contact therapy in a combination of day care and home treatment is an effective alternative for the 24-h inpatient treatment. Several investigations have shown an improved cosmetic acceptability of new principles such as the micanol formulation, in which dithranol is microencapsulated in lipid crystals, which will help to further popularize dithranol treatment (Christensen *et al.* 1992; Volden *et al.* 1992).

Combination therapies may lower irritancy and enhance efficacy. Continuing investigations in this respect look promising.

References

Anderson, R., Lukey, P.T., Dippenaar, U. *et al.* (1987) Dithranol mediates pro-oxidative inhibition of polymorphonuclear leukocyte migration and lymphocyte proliferation. *British Journal of Dermatology* **117** (4), 405–418.

Ashton, R.E., Andre, P., Lowe, N.J. & Whitefield, M. (1983) Anthralin, historical and current perspectives. *Journal of the American Academy of Dermatology* **9**, 173–192.

Bacharach Buhles, M., Rochling, A., el Gammal, S. & Altmeyer, P. (1996) The effect of fumaric acid esters and dithranol on acanthosis and hyperproliferation in psoriasis vulgaris. *Acta Dermato-Venereologica* **76** (3), 190–193.

Barr, R.M., Wong, E., Cunningham, F.M., Mallet, A.I. & Greaves, M.W. (1989) Effect of dithranol on arachidonic acid and its lipoxygenase products in psoriasis. *Archives of Dermatological Research* **280** (8), 474–476.

Bedord, C.J., Young, J.M. & Wagner, B.M. (1983) Anthralin inhibition of mouse epidermal arachidonic acid lipoxygenase in vitro. *Journal of Investigative Dermatology* **81** (6), 566–571.

Berth-Jones, J., Chu, A.C., Dodd, W.A. *et al.* (1992) A multicentre, parallel-group comparison of calcipotriol ointment and short-contact dithranol therapy in chronic plaque psoriasis. *British Journal of Dermatology* **127** (3), 266–271.

Bisschop, A., Vankan, P.M., van Uijtewaal, B. & Wijk, R. (1984) Effect of 1,8-dihydroxy-9-anthrone (anthralin) on rat hepatic ornithine decarboxylase activity in vivo. *Cancer Letters* **23** (2), 151–157.

Black, A.K., Barr, R.M., Wong, E. *et al.* (1985) Lipoxygenase products of arachidonic acid in human inflamed skin. *British Journal of Clinical Pharmacology* **20** (3), 185–190.

Boch, F.G. & Burns, R. (1963) Tumor-promoting proporties of anthralin. *Journal of the National Cancer Institute* **30**, 393–397.

Boer, J. & Smeenk, G. (1986) Effect of short-contact anthralin therapy on ultraviolet B irradiation of psoriasis. *Journal of the American Academy of Dermatology* **15**, 198–204.

Bohlen, P., Grove, J., Beya, M.F., Koch-Weser, J., Henry, M.H. & Grosshans, E. (1978) Skin polyamine levels in psoriasis: the effect of dithranol therapy. *European Journal of Clinical Investigation* **8** (4), 215–218.

Bunse, T. & Merk, H. (1990) Effect of an anthralin containing hydrocolloid dressing in psoriasis vulgaris. *Zeitschrift fur Hautkrankheiten* **65** (8), 730–732.

Cavey, D., Caron, J.-C. & Shroot, B. (1982) Anthralin: Chemical instability and glucose-6-phosphate dehydrogenase inhibition. *Journal of Pharmacological Science* **71**, 980–983.

Christensen, O.B., Enstrom, Y., Juhlin, L. *et al.* (1992) A novel dithranol formulation in the over night treatment of psoriasis at home. *Acta Dermato-Venereologica* **172**, 25–27.

Comaish, S., Smith, J. & Seville, R.H. (1971) Factors affecting the clearance of psoriasis with dithranol (anthralin). *British Journal of Dermatology* **84**, 282–289.

Dean, F.D. (1971) The action of zinc oxide on dithranol. *British Journal of Dermatology* **85** (5), 494.

de Grood, A.C. & Nater, J.P. (1981) Contact allergy to dithranol. *Contact Dermatitis* **7**, 5–8.

Elbracht, C. & Landes, E. (1983) Study on the efficacy of a combined treatment of psoriasis with dithranol and UVB (selective ultraviolet phototherapy). *Zeitschrift fur Hautkrankheiten* **58** (6), 387–397.

Finnen, M.J., Lawrence, C.M. & Shuster, S. (1984) Inhibition of dithranol and inflammation by free radical scavengers. *Lancet* **ii**, 1129–1130.

Fisher, L.B. & Maibach, H. (1975) The effect of anthralin and its derivates on epidermal cell kinetics. *Journal of Investigative Dermatology* **64**, 338–341.

Fuchs, J., Milbradt, R. & Zimmer, G. (1990) Multifunctional analysis of the interaction of anthralin and its metabolites anthraquinone and anthralin dimer with the inner mitochondrial membrane. *Archives of Dermatological Research* **282** (1), 47–55.

Galewski, E. (1916) Über Cignolin, ein Ersatz präparat des Chrysarobins. *Dermatologische Wochenschrift* **6**, 113–115.

Gaudin, D., Greggs, R.S. & Yielding, K.L. (1972) Inhibition of DNA repair by cocarcinogens. *Biochemical and Biophysical Research Communication* **48**, 945–949.

Gay, M.W., Moore, W.J., Morgan, J.M. & Montes, L.F. (1972) Anthralin toxicity. *Archives of Dermatology* **105**, 213–215.

Gottlieb, S.L., Heftler, N.S., Gilleaudeau, P. et al. (1995) Short-contact anthralin treatment augments therapeutic efficacy of cyclosporine in psoriasis: a clinical and pathologic study. *Journal of the American Academy of Dermatology* **33**, 637–645.

Grattan, C.E., Christopher, A.P., Robinson, M. & Cowan, M.A. (1988) Double-blind comparison of a dithranol and steroid mixture with a conventional dithranol regimen for chronic psoriasis. *British Journal of Dermatology* **119** (5), 623–626.

Ingram, J.T. (1953) The approach to psoriasis. *British Medical Journal* **2**, 591–594.

Ippen, H. (1959) Aetiologie und Pathogenese des sog. Istizin-Exanthema. *Deutsche Medizinische Wochenschrift* **84**, 1062–1063.

Ippen, H. (1981) Basic questions on toxicology and pharmacology of anthralin. *British Journal of Dermatology* **105** (Suppl. 20), 72–76.

Jacques, Y. & Reichert, U. (1981) Effects of anthralin and analogues on growth and [3H] thymidine incorporation in human skin fibroblasts. *British Journal of Dermatology* **105** (Suppl. 20), 45–48.

Juhlin, L. (1981) Factors influencing anthralin erythema. *British Journal of Dermatology* **105** (20), 87–91.

Kammerau, B., Zesch, A. & Schaefer, H. (1975) Absolute concentrations of dithranol and triacetoxy-dithranol in the skin layers after local treatment; *in vivo* investigations with four different types of pharmaceutical vehicles. *Journal of Investigative Dermatology* **64**, 145–149.

Kemény, L., Ruzicka, T. & Braun-Falco, O. (1990) Dithranol: a review of the mechanism of action in the treatment of psoriasis vulgaris. *Skin Pharmacology* **3**, 1–20.

Kingston, T. & Marks, R. (1983) Irritant reactions to dithranol in normal subjects and psoriatic patients. *British Journal of Dermatology* **108**, 307–313.

Krebs, A. & Schaltegger, H. (1969) Untersuchungen zur Strukturspezifität der Psoriasis-heilmittel Chrysarobin und Dithranol. *Hautarzt* **20**, 204–209.

Lawrence, C.M., Shuster, S., Collins, M. *et al.* (1987) Reduction of anthralin inflamma-tion by potassium hydroxide and Teepol. *British Journal of Dermatology* **116**, 171–177.

Lebwohl, M., Berman, B. & France, D.S. (1985) Addition of short-contact anthralin therapy to an ultraviolet B phototherapy regimen: assessment of efficacy. *Journal of the American Academy of Dermatology* **13**, 780–784.

Lidbrink, P., Johannesson, A. & Hammar, H. (1986) Psoriasis treatment: faster clearance when UVB-dithranol is combined with topical clobetasol propionate. *Dermatologica* **172** (3), 164–168.

Liebermann, C. & Seidler, P. (1878) Über Chrysarobin und die angebliche Chrysophan-säure im Goapulver. *Bericht Deutsche Chemie Gesellschaft* **14**, 1603–1605.

Mahrle, G. (1997) Dithranol. *Clinics in Dermatology* **15**, 677–685.

Mahrle, G. & Schulze, H.J. (1990) The effect of initial external glucocorticoid administra-tion on cignolin treatment of psoriasis. *Zeitschrift fur Hautkrankheiten* **65** (3), 282–287.

Mahrle, G., Schulze, H.J. & Steigleder, G.K. (1985) Dithranol and combined treatment procedures: pro and con. *Hautarzt* **36** (1), 34–39.

Maurice, P.D. & Greaves, M.W. (1983) Relationship between skin type and erythemal response to anthralin. *British Journal of Dermatology* **109** (3), 337–341.

Misch, K., Davies, M., Greaves, M. & Coutts, A. (1981) Pharmacological studies of anthralin erythema. *British Journal of Dermatology* **105** (Suppl. 20), 82–86.

Morhenn, V.B., Orenberg, E.K., Kaplan, J. *et al.* (1983) Inhibition of a Langerhans cell mediated immune respons by treatment modalities useful in psoriasis. *Journal of Investigative Dermatology* **81** (1), 23–27.

Morison, W.L., Parrish, J.A. & Fitzpatrick, T.B. (1978) Controlled study of PUVA and adjunctive topical therapy in the management of psoriasis. *British Journal of Dermatology* **98** (2), 125–132.

Morlière, P., Dubertret, L.S.a.E., Melo, T. *et al.* (1985) The effect of anthralin (dithranol) on mitochondria. *British Journal of Dermatology* **112** (5), 509–515.

Muller, K., Leukel, P., Mayer, K. & Wiegrebe, W. (1995) Modification of DNA bases by anthralin and related compounds. *Biochemical Pharmacology* **49** (11), 1607–1613.

Muller, K., Seidel, M., Braun, C., Zieresi, K. & Wiegrebe, W. (1991) Dithranol, glucose-6-phosphate dehydrogenase inhibition and active oxygen species. *Arzneimittelforschung* **41** (11), 1176–1181.

Munro, C., Ramsay, B., Lawrence, C. *et al.* (1989) Reduction of cutaneous inflammation by cyclosporin A. *Journal of Investigative Dermatology* **92**, 487.

Orfanos, C.E. & Runne, U. (1976) Systemic use of a new retinoid with and without local dithranol treatment in generalised psoriasis. *British Journal of Dermatology* **95**, 101–103.

Paramsothy, Y., Collins, M. & Lawrence, C.M. (1988) Effect of UVB therapy and a coal tar bath on short contact dithranol treatment for psoriasis. *British Journal of Dermatology* **118**, 783–789.

Pearlman, D.L., Burns, J. & Cannon, T.C. (1984) Paper-tape occlusion of anthralin paste. A new outpatient therapy for psoriasis. *Archives of Dermatology* **120** (5), 625–630.

Phillips, D.H. & Alldrick, A.J. (1994) Tumorigenicity of a combination of psoriasis therapies. *British Journal of Cancer* **69** (6), 1043–1045.

Prins, M., Swinkels, O.Q.J., Kolkman, E.G.W. *et al.* (1998) Skin irritation by dithranol cream. A blind study to assess the role of the cream formulation. *Acta Dermato-Venereologica* **78**, 1–4.

Ramsay, B., Lawrence, C.M., Bruce, J.M. & Shuster, S. (1990a) The effect of triethanolamine application on anthralin-induced inflammation and therapeutic effect in psoriasis. *Journal of the American Academy of Dermatology* **23** (1), 73–76.

Ramsay, B., Lawrence, C.M., Shuster, S. & Bruce, J.M. (1990b) Reduction of anthralin-induced inflammation by the application of amines. *Journal of the American Academy of Dermatology* **22**, 765–772.

Ramsay, B., Rice, N. & Lawrence, C. (1992) The effect of indomethacin on anthralin inflammation. *British Journal of Dermatology* **126**, 262–265.

Reshad, H., Barth, J.H., Darley, C.R. *et al.* (1984) Does UV-A potentiate 'short contact' dithranol therapy? *British Journal of Dermatology* **111** (2), 155–158.

Runne, U. & Kunze, J. (1985) Minute therapy of psoriasis with dithranol and its modifications. A critical evaluation based on 315 patients. *Hautarzt* **36** (1), 40–46.

Saihan, E.M., Albana, J. & Burton, J.L. (1980) The effect of steroid and dithranol therapy on cyclic nucleotides in psoriatic epidermis. *British Journal of Dermatology* **102**, 565–569.

Schalla, W., Bauer, E. & Schaefer, H. (1981) Skin permeability of anthralin. *British Journal of Dermatology* **105** (Suppl. 20), 104–108.

Schauder, S. & Mahrle, G. (1982) Kombinierte Einstundentherapie der Psoriasis mit Anthralin und UV-licht. *Hautartz* **33**, 206–209.

Schröder, J.M., Kosfeld, U. & Christophers, E. (1985) Multifunctional inhibition by anthralin in nonstimulated and chemotactic factor stimulated human neutrophils. *Journal of Investigative Dermatology* **85**, 30–34.

Schulze, H.J., Schauder, S., Mahrle, G. *et al.* (1987) Combined tar-anthralin versus anthralin treatment lowers irritancy with unchanged antipsoriatic efficacy. Modifications of short-contact therapy and Ingram therapy. *Journal of the American Academy of Dermatology* **17**, 19–24.

Seville, R.H. (1976) Relapse rate of psoriasis worsened by adding steroids to a dithranol regime. *British Journal of Dermatology* **95**, 643–645.

Shroot, B. (1992) Mode of action of Dithranol, pharmacokinetics/dynamics. *Acta Dermato-Venereologica Supplementum* **172**, 10–12.

Squire, B. (1876) Treatment of psoriasis by an ointment of chrysophanic acid. *British Medical Journal* **2**, 819–820.

Storbeck, K., Holzle, E., Schurer, N. *et al.* (1993) Narrow band UVB (311 nm) versus conventional broad-band UVB with and without dithranol in phototherapy for psoriasis. *Journal of the American Academy of Dermatology* **28** (2), 227–231.

Swanbeck, G. & Hillstrom, L. (1971) Analysis of etiological factors of squamous cell cancer of different locations. *Acta Dermato-Venereologica* **51**, 151–156.

Swanbeck, G. & Liden, S. (1966) The inhibitory effect of dithranol (anthralin) on DNA synthesis. *Acta Dermato-Venereologica* **46**, 228–230.

Ternowitz, T. (1987) The enhanced monocyte and neutrophil chemotaxis in psoriasis is normalized after treatment with psoralens plus ultraviolet A and anthralin. *Journal of the American Academy of Dermatology* **16** (6), 1169–1175.

Tucker, W.F., MacNeil, S., Dawson, R.A., Tomlinson, S. & Bleehen, S.S. (1986) An investigation of the ability of antipsoriatic drugs to inhibit calmodulin activity: a possible mode of action of dithramol (anthralin). *Journal of Investigative Dermatology* **87** (2), 232–235.

Unna, P.G. (1916) Cignolin als Heilmittel der Psoriasis. *Dermatologische Wochenschrift* **6**, 116–137, 151–163, 175–183.

van de Kerkhof, P.C.M. (1991) Dithranol treatment in psoriasis: after 75 years, still going strong. *European Journal of Dermatology* **1**, 79–88.

van der Vleuten, C.J.M., de Jong, E.M.G.J. & van de Kerkhof, P.C.M. (1996) Epidermal differentiation characteristics of the psoriatic plaque during short contact treatment with dithranol cream. *Clinical Experimental Dermatology* **21**, 409–414.

Volden, G., Bjornberg, A., Tegner, E. *et al.* (1992) Short-contact treatment at home with micanol. *Acta Dermato-Venereologica* **172** (Suppl.), 20–22.

Wang, J.C.T., Krazmien, R.J., Dahlheim, C.E. *et al.* (1986) Anthralin stain removal. *Journal of the American Academy of Dermatology* **15**, 951–955.

Wemmer, U., Schulze, H.J., Mahrle, G. & Steigleder, G.K. (1986) Effect of various kinds of tar and tar concentrations on anthralin erythema. *Zeitschrift fur Hautkrankheiten* **61** (12), 849–852.

Whitefield, M. (1981) Pharmaceutical formulations of anthralin. *British Journal of Dermatology* **105** (Suppl. 20), 28–32.

Zesch, A. (1990) Lokaltherapie in der Schwangerschaft. *Hautarzt* **41**, 365–368.

Chapter 11: Photo(chemo)therapy

J. Krutmann

11.1 Introduction

One important element in the long-term management of moderate to severe psoriasis is photo(chemo)therapy. Psoriasis has been known for decades to show favourable responses to both UVB radiation phototherapy as well as photochemotherapy employing 8-methoxypsoralen (8-MOP) plus UVA radiation (PUVA). In this chapter, the current status of UVB phototherapy with special emphasis on 311-nm UVB and of PUVA photochemotherapy including new developments of topical PUVA therapy will be reviewed. In addition, the present knowledge concerning the photocarcinogenic potential of photo(chemo)therapy as well as the mode of action of photo(chemo)therapy for psoriasis will be discussed.

11.2 311-nm UVB: the phototherapy of choice for psoriasis

A direct comparison of PUVA with classical UVB phototherapy for the treatment of psoriasis indicates that PUVA is superior to UVB phototherapy. Within recent years, however, the availability of new fluorescent bulbs with an emission spectrum that closely conforms to the peak of the action spectrum for clearing psoriasis has significantly improved the efficacy of UVB phototherapy for psoriasis, making it as efficient as PUVA therapy (van Weelden *et al.* 1988).

11.2.1 The rationale for developing 311-nm UVB phototherapy

Parrish & Jaenicke (1981) demonstrated that wavelengths shorter than 295 nm displayed no antipsoriatic effect, even if used at erythemogenic doses, whereas wavelengths between 300 and 313 nm caused the greatest remission of skin lesions. These seminal observations provided the rationale for the development of more selective UVB phototherapy (SUP) irradiation devices (Pullman 1978). These units have a spectrum that is still broad-band UVB but is enhanced in the range of 300–320 nm. As predicted, these light sources proved to be superior to conventional UVB phototherapy for clearing psoriasis. A major breakthrough was achieved shortly after with the development of the Philips TL-01 fluorescent lamp, emitting a narrow UVB band at 311–312 nm and thereby matching closely the assumed therapeutic optimum for psoriasis (van Weelden *et al.* 1988) (Fig. 11.1). A large number of clinical trials comparing

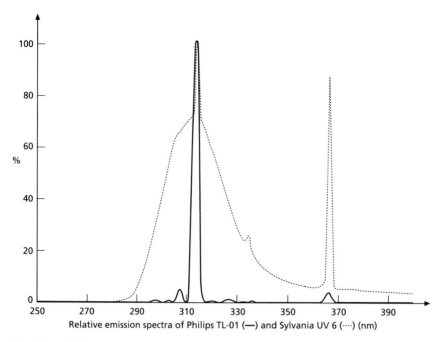

Fig. 11.1 Relative emission spectra of Philips TL-01 and Sylvania UV6.

broad-band vs. 311-nm UVB phototherapy for psoriasis has been conducted since then. Based on these studies, it is now generally accepted that 311-nm UVB therapy is superior to broad-band UVB therapy for psoriasis. Patients treated with a 311-nm spectrum show faster clearance of skin lesions, fewer episodes of excessive erythema, and a longer period of remission (Pullman 1978; Green *et al.* 1988; Larko 1989; Storbeck *et al.* 1991; Picot 1992). Comparative studies of 311-nm UVB phototherapy and PUVA have demonstrated that these two modalities are equally effective (van Weelden *et al.* 1990; Green *et al.* 1992; Tanew *et al.* 1996). This is of particular interest because 311-nm UVB therapy, in comparison to PUVA, does not require psoralens, is cheaper, can be used in pregnancy and childhood, and does not require post-treatment eye protection.

It has also been suggested that 311-nm UVB phototherapy may be less carcinogenic than PUVA (Young 1995). For these reasons, 311-nm UVB therapy currently represents the phototherapeutic modality of choice for the treatment of psoriasis.

11.2.2 Practical aspects

For 311-nm UVB therapy, the Philips TL-01 fluorescence lamps are being used. Prior to phototherapy, the patient's minimal erythema dose (MED) must be determined in order to establish the optimal dosage schedule. For deter-

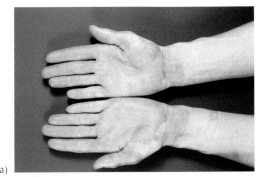

(a)

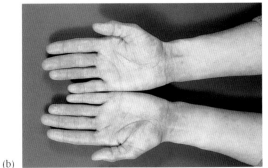

(b)

Plate 11.1 Patient with palmar psoriasis (a) before and (b) after 30 treatments with cream-PUVA-photochemotherapy.

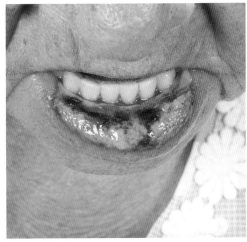

Plate 12.2 Erosive cheilitis following an overdose of methotrexate due to an unobserved decreased renal function.

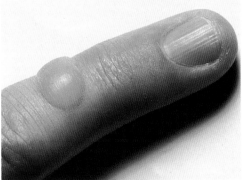

Plate 12.3 Phototoxic bullous reaction in patient treated with methotrexate and PUVA.

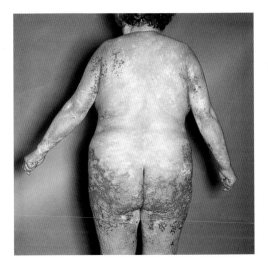

Plate 12.1 Toxic epidermal necrolysis with erosions within the psoriatic lesions, resulting from interaction between methotrexate and sulphonamide.

mination of the MED and subsequent phototherapy, either the same irradiation device or different devices with identical emission spectra must be used. The initial dose is usually set at 0.7 MED, but doses as low as 0.35 MED have been used as well (Hofer *et al.* 1998). The near erythemogenic 311 nm UVB therapy starting with 0.7 MED may clear psoriasis faster than far erythemogenic therapy (initial dose: 0.35 MED) but the latter regimen may be equally effective as it requires slightly more treatment sessions at a lower and possibly less carcinogenic cumulative UV dose. For subsequent exposures a high as well as a low incremental dose regimen have been developed (Wainwright *et al.* 1998). The high increment regimen is based on a 40% and the low increment regimen on a 20% increase of the dose as compared with the previous dose at each visit. When under these conditions a previous treatment results in erythema, no treatment is given the next day or the dose is decreased, depending on whether the erythema is asymptomatic or severe and painful. Recent studies indicate that the low increment regimen achieves a 10% reduction in the median cumulative dose to clearance of psoriasis with one extra treatment in 50% of patients, whereas the duration of treatment was identical for both dose regimens. Patients are being treated either three or five times per week.

When three and five times weekly 311-nm UVB therapy regimens were compared in a randomized, observer-blinded, half-body, within-patient, paired study it appeared that the five times per week regimen cleared psoriasis more rapidly, but no significant difference between regimens could be observed in duration of remission (Dawe *et al.* 1998).

It has therefore been proposed that for the majority of patients the three times per week regimen should be favoured because the more rapid clearance of psoriasis with 5 times weekly phototherapy does not justify the extra exposures.

The end point of phototherapy is complete clearance of all psoriatic skin lesions. Psoriasis is a chronic disease and the remission induced by 311-nm UVB therapy is transient. In a randomized, prospective, multicentre trial, postclearing phototherapy was found to significantly increase the disease-free interval, indicating that patients may profit from maintenance therapy (Stern *et al.* 1986). On the other hand, maintenance therapy with UVB radiation results in a greater cumulative UVB radiation dose and thereby increases the risk of skin cancer and photoaging. It is therefore preferable to maintain remissions with other antipsoriatic modalities if possible. In order to minimize potential carcinogenic risks from chronic UVB phototherapy, a rotational therapeutic approach including a number of primary and secondary agents has been suggested (Mentener *et al.* 1996). Primary agents to treat psoriasis include UVB, PUVA, methotrexate and etretinate. If the primary agents are no longer effective, then secondary agents such as cyclosporin, hydroxycarbamide and low-dose combination regimens (e.g. retinoids plus PUVA) should be considered.

11.3 PUVA therapy for psoriasis

PUVA therapy is based on the interaction between UV radiation and a photo-sensitizing chemical. The acronym PUVA usually refers to the therapeutic use of psoralens and UVA radiation. PUVA therapy is used for psoriasis in several forms, including the oral administration of the psoralens as well as topical administration routes such as bathwater delivery of psoralens or cream–PUVA–photochemotherapy.

Oral PUVA therapy came into use for treatment of moderate to severe psoriasis after a report of its efficacy in a group of patients in 1974 (Parrish *et al*. 1974). Subsequently a multicentre study was started at 16 centres in the United States to further evaluate its efficacy using several clearance and maintenance protocols (Melski *et al*. 1977). In 88% of the patients described in this study, psoriasis was cleared and maintenance treatment was effective in control of disease. Short-term adverse effects were uncommon and generally mild. As a consequence, oral PUVA therapy has become a mainstay in the management of patients with psoriasis (Morison 1991).

11.3.1 Practical aspects

Prior to PUVA therapy a physical examination to assess the extent of psoriasis, to detect skin cancer and to evaluate photoageing is required (Morison 1991). In addition, all patients require a complete eye examination when initiating PUVA therapy, and this has been recommended to be repeated every year. The most widely used photosensitizers for oral PUVA therapy are 8-methoxypsoralen (8-MOP) and 5-methoxypsoralen (5-MOP). 8-MOP (0.6 mg/kg bodyweight) should be given 2 h and 5-MOP (1.2 mg/kg bodyweight) 1 h prior to UVA radiation exposure.

UVA radiation dosimetry is not determined by the skin type of the patient, but by the individual sensitivity toward UVA irradiation, which is defined by the minimal phototoxic dose (MPD) (Hönigsmann & Krutmann 1998). According to the European PUVA-Protocol, the initial dose used is about 75% of the MPD. Since the maximum of the PUVA-induced erythema response requires at least 48 h, and sometimes even 72 h to develop, PUVA therapy should not be started prior to a 72-h period after phototesting.

In order to exclude the possibility of a cumulation of PUVA toxicity, a 11011 treatment schedule, i.e. treatment on Monday, Tuesday, Thursday and Friday, has been developed (Morison 1991). In general, the UVA dose should not be increased before the end of the first week. Subsequent increments (usually by $0.5–1 \, \text{J/cm}^2$ UVA) can be done every third treatment and about 15 treatments are necessary for clearing. It should be noted that the European PUVA-Protocol does not provide a fixed schedule to increase dosage (Hönigsmann & Krutmann 1997). The decision to vary the dose depends on the presence or absence of an erythema during therapy as well as the therapeutic response. Once clearing of psoriasis has been achieved the frequency of treatments will be reduced. For maintenance therapy the last UVA dose is used, and patients are treated twice a week for one month and once a week for another month.

11.3.2 New forms of topical PUVA

Oral PUVA therapy is associated with systemic side-effects such as nausea (in up to 20% of patients treated with 8-MOP), long-lasting photosensitization and the requirement for post-treatment eye protection (Morison 1993). These disadvantages can be avoided when psoralens are topically applied to the skin.

Within recent years, bathwater delivery of psoralens in combination with UVA irradiation (bath-PUVA photochemotherapy) (Fischer & Alsins 1976) or topical application of 8-MOP in a oil-in-water ointment (cream-PUVA photochemotherapy) (Stege *et al.* 1997) are therefore being increasingly used to treat patients with psoriasis.

Bath-PUVA photochemotherapy

For bath-PUVA photochemotherapy, patients are immersed for 20 min in 0.5 mg/L water solution of 8-MOP at a constant temperature of 37.5°C (Gruss *et al.* 1998). Immediately after the bath the skin is dried gently and exposed to UVA radiation. A number of recent studies indicate that bath-PUVA photochemotherapy, compared with oral PUVA photochemotherapy, has an equal therapeutic efficiency for psoriasis, but that it yields fewer adverse effects and completely avoids systemic side-effects. Studies on the phototoxic reactions after bath-PUVA photochemotherapy indicate that for optimal effects UVA radiation has to be administered immediately after the psoralen bath. The photosensitization rapidly decreases over time (about 20-fold after 2 h), indicating that in contrast to oral PUVA photochemotherapy, bath-PUVA photochemotherapy does not have a prolonged risk of phototoxic reactions and thus does not require any restrictive behaviour of the patient.

Cream-PUVA photochemotherapy

A major disadvantage of bath-PUVA photochemotherapy is the logistical requirement for bath tubs in a practice. An alternative form of topical PUVA therapy has therefore recently been developed using a lipophilic emulsion vehicle for the photosensitizer 8-MOP (cream-PUVA photochemotherapy) (Stege *et al.* 1997). A 0.0006% 8-MOP containing water-in-oil emulsion (30% H_2O) was found to be optimal for inducing photosensitivity without increasing 8-MOP plasma levels. Increased skin photosensitivity was maximal 1 h after cream application and persisted for 3 h. In subsequent studies, cream-PUVA photochemotherapy proved to be effective for the treatment of patients with psoriasis, in particular of the palms and soles (Plate 11.1, facing p. 180).

Cream-PUVA photochemotherapy, which is easier to perform than bath-PUVA photochemotherapy, is an effective, safe and low-cost modality that allows the treatment of single skin lesions. A recent survey among German dermatologists indicates that for these reasons cream-PUVA photochemotherapy is in the process of becoming the topical PUVA therapy of choice for dermatological practitioners.

11.4 Photocarcinogenic risk of photo(chemo)therapy

There is currently no doubt that PUVA therapy increases the risk of patients with psoriasis to develop skin cancer. In the United States, the photocarcinogenic risk of PUVA has been assessed in a prospective study of 1308 patients with psoriasis. Squamous cell carcinoma of the skin was first reported as an adverse effect in this group in 1979 (Stern *et al.* 1979). A causal relationship with PUVA therapy was suggested by a strong dose–response relationship, a high incidence on non-sun-exposed skin and a continued increase of risk in patients who have discontinued treatment (Stern & Laird 1994).

These observations were corroborated in other studies (Lobel *et al.* 1981; Bruynzeel *et al.* 1991; Chunag *et al.* 1992). In addition, PUVA was found to be carcinogenic in experimental animal models. It should be noted, however, that not all studies conducted in other countries have confirmed that PUVA therapy is associated with an increased risk of non-melanoma skin cancer (Tanew *et al.* 1986; Henseler *et al.* 1987). This variability is thought to be due to differences in the amount of exposure to PUVA therapy, ethnic background, treatment protocols, and prior exposure to other carcinogens such as arsenic and X-irradiation. In addition, exposure to immunosuppressive therapy after cessation of PUVA may lead to a significant increase in the risk of development of squamous cell carcinoma.

In contrast to squamous cell carcinoma, there has been only a modest, but significant, increase in the incidence of basal cell carcinoma in patients receiving a high number of PUVA treatments, which is most notably for lesions on the trunk (Stern & Laird 1994). This observation has not been confirmed by other studies. A very recent report indicates the possibility that there is an increased risk of melanoma in patients with psoriasis treated with PUVA (Stern *et al.* 1997). This has raised the concern on the part of physicians and patients about the long-term safety of PUVA therapy.

In response to this concern, the National Psoriasis Foundation has sponsored a workshop which has served to prepare a consensus paper on the toxic effects of long-term PUVA (Morison *et al.* 1998). It has been stated that a modest but noticeable increase in the incidence of melanoma has been observed in the US multicentre study, because 11 out of 1380 patients developed malignant melanoma. It should be noted that this increase was only observed in patients receiving the highest doses of therapy and the longest follow-up, and that the overall number of patients treated with PUVA who developed melanoma is small and may return to baseline upon future observation of the cohort.

Squamous cell carcinoma thus remains the primary cause of cancer morbidity and mortality in patients with psoriasis treated with PUVA. The risk of developing melanoma is about the same as the risk of developing metastatic squamous cell carcinoma. In order to reduce the long-term toxic effects of PUVA therapy a number of preventive measures should be used. These include: (i) protection of genitalia in males; (ii) protection of the face unless there is significant psoriasis present; (iii) the use of an opaque protection for the lips; and (iv) the use of protective eye wear (Morison *et al.* 1998).

As with any form of UVB exposure, chronic 311-nm UVB irradiation is likely to increase the risk of skin cancer. Data obtained from a mouse photocarcinogenic model suggest that 311-nm UVB irradiation is two to three times more carcinogenic per MED than broad-band UVB irradiation (Flindt-Hansen *et al.* 1991; Wulf *et al.* 1994). In clinical use, the number of 311-nm UVB MEDs required to clear psoriasis is less than one-third of that needed with broad-band UVB. It has therefore been suggested that the long-term skin cancer risk of 311-nm UVB phototherapy is no more, and most likely less, than would be expected with broad-band UVB sources (Young 1995). There is also current evidence that chronic narrow-band UVB phototherapy is less carcinogenic than PUVA (De Gruijl 1989).

By taking into account the observation that 311-nm UVB therapy is more effective than broad-band UVB and equally effective to PUVA therapy it seems reasonable to assume that within the near future 311-nm UVB phototherapy will not only replace broad-band UVB phototherapy, but will also significantly reduce PUVA use.

11.5 Mode of action of photo(chemo)therapy

Both UVB radiation and PUVA are capable of inducing DNA photoproducts and thereby inhibit cell proliferation (Epstein 1968; Epstein *et al.* 1969; Kramer *et al.* 1974; Bevilaqua *et al.* 1991). It has therefore been thought that the therapeutic effectiveness of these modalities in psoriasis is due mainly to its antiproliferative effects. Since the introduction of photo(chemo)therapy into dermatologic therapy, however, the number of skin diseases showing a favourable response to phototherapy has grown substantially (Volc-Platzer & Hönigsmann 1995). The vast majority are immunological in nature.

In previous years it has been demonstrated that both UVB and PUVA exert profound effects on the skin immune system, and photo(chemo)-therapeutic modalities are therefore currently regarded as immuno-interventive (Krutmann & Elmets 1995). Most of the immunomodulatory effects are not specific for a single modality, but may be observed *in vitro* after

UVB or PUVA treatment as well. Despite exhibiting similar or even identical immunomodulatory effects, UVB radiation and PUVA greatly differ when their underlying photobiological mechanisms are compared.

Photoimmunological effects of therapeutic relevance fall into three major categories: (i) effects on production of soluble mediators; (ii) modulation of the expression of cell-surface-associated molecules (e.g. adhesion molecules, cytokine receptors); and (iii) the induction of apoptosis in pathogenetically relevant cells (Krutmann 1998).

Effects on the production of soluble mediators include UVB- and/or PUVA-inducible factors with anti-inflammatory and/or immunosuppressive properties, such as selected cytokines (e.g. interleukin 10), prostanoids (e.g. prostaglandin E_2) and neuropeptides (e.g. α-melanocyte stimulating hormone) (Grewe *et al.* 1993; Grewe *et al.* 1994; Schauer *et al.* 1994; Grewe *et al.* 1995; Luger & Schwarz 1995; Morita *et al.* 1996; Morita *et al.* 1997).

In addition, UVB radiation and PUVA treatment can directly affect the expression and function of cell-surface receptors, including adhesion molecules, cytokine and growth-factor receptors (Laskin *et al.* 1985; Lisby *et al.* 1989; Krutmann *et al.* 1990; Norris *et al.* 1990; Simon *et al.* 1992; Trefzer *et al.* 1993; Krutmann & Grewe 1995; Grewe *et al.* 1996; Roza *et al.* 1996). Examples are the UVB radiation-induced inhibition of cytokine-mediated upregulation of the expression of intercellular adhesion molecule 1 (ICAM-1) on epidermal keratinocytes as well as antigen-presenting cells, the UVB radiation-induced increased expression of the type II interleukin 1 (IL-1) receptor in keratinocytes, which serves as a decoy receptor to limit IL-1-mediated, proinflammatory effects, and the PUVA-induced modulation of the expression and function of the epidermal growth factor receptor in epidermal keratinocytes. More recent studies have provided compelling evidence that UVB radiation and PUVA are highly efficient in inducing apoptosis in human T cells (Krueger *et al.* 1995; Godar 1996; Yoo *et al.* 1996; Morita *et al.* 1997). T cells, as compared to other cells such as keratinocytes or monocytes, have an increased susceptibility towards UVB- or PUVA-induced apoptosis.

Induction of apoptosis is therefore of particlar importance for T-cell-mediated skin diseases such as psoriasis. Accordingly, successful UVB phototherapy of psoriatic patients induced a reduction in the number of skin-infiltrating T cells, which was followed by normalization of keratinocyte morphology (Krueger *et al.* 1995). *In vitro* UVB irradiation induced T-cell apoptosis, indicating the possibility that the reduction of the inflammatory infiltrate may result from UVB radiation-induced T-cell apoptosis. This hypothesis has recently been proven by the demonstration of apoptotic T cells in lesional psoriatic skin of patients undergoing UVB phototherapy. Induction of T-cell apoptosis was observed regardless of whether broad-band UVB or 311-nm UVB phototherapy was employed.

It should be noted, however, that because of its physical properties, 311-nm UVB radiation penetrates at much higher intensities into human dermis, and T-cell apoptosis therefore did not only occur in epidermal, but also in significant numbers of dermal T cells (J.G. Krueger, personal communication). This difference may at least partially explain the clinical observation that 311-nm UVB phototherapy is superior to broadband UVB phototherapy for the treatment of psoriasis.

11.6 Combination therapy

Phototherapy, and to some extent also photochemotherapy of psoriasis is frequently used in combination regimens in order to achieve higher clearance rates, longer disease-free intervals, and a lower carcinogenic risk (Mentener *et al.* 1996). Photo(chemo)therapy may be combined with topical or systemic agents.

Topical agents include anthralin, vitamin D analogues, corticosteroids, emollients, salt-water baths and tar. Among these, anthralin, vitamin D analogues and topical retinoids constitute the most relevant agents for combination with phototherapy.

Anthralin or dithranol was synthesized by Gallewsky in 1916 and subsequently shown to be effective in the treatment of psoriasis by Unna (Gallewski 1916; Unna 1916). Anthralin is administered in a petrolatum base containing salicylic acid (concentration should not exceed 3%) in order to stabilize anthralin. Salicylic acid may act as a sunscreen (Kristensen & Kristensen 1990), and anthralin application should therefore follow, but not precede, UVB irradiations. Anthralin preparations cause dose-dependent skin irritation (anthralin erythema), which is additive to UVB radiation-induced erythema, and which may be followed by induction of Koebner's phenomenon and pigmentation of treated skin areas. In addition, the generation of oxidation products from anthralin may stain clothes and bathtubs. For these reasons, the use of anthralin is mainly limited to the treatment of inpatients in hospitals (Farber & Harris 1970). Attempts have been made to develop a short-term application of anthralin (0.1–3% dithranol plus 2% salicylic acid in petrolatum for 10–20 min daily), which is suitable for treating outpatients or patients in day-care centres (Runne & Kunze 1982).

The combination of phototherapy and administration of anthralin for the treatment of psoriasis was first proposed by Ingram in 1953 (Ingram 1953).

This concept has since been confirmed by numerous studies including more recent ones, in which topical anthralin treatment was found to enhance the efficacy of either broad-band UVB or 311-nm UVB phototherapy for psoriasis (Karvonen *et al.* 1989; Storbeck *et al.* 1993). In contrast, the combination of UVB irradiation with anthralin short-contact therapy was significantly less effective than the classic Ingram regimen and did not offer an advantage over UVB therapy alone (Lebwohl *et al.* 1985; Staham *et al.* 1993).

Antipsoriatic vitamin D analogues include calcipotriol and tacalcitol, which have antiproliferative as well as anti-inflammatory effects (Berth-Jones &

Hutchinson 1992; Menne & Larsen 1992). Local side-effects are limited to moderate skin irritation (Kragballe 1995). In order to avoid systemic side-effects, which can be expected if more than 100 g calcipotriol ointment or cream is used per week, in particular hypercalcemia with consequent nephrocalcinosis, from percutaneous absorption, the treated body surface should not exceed 30%. Under these conditions, long-term safety may be assured (Ramsay *et al.* 1994). Main indications are psoriatic plaques of limited extent and lesions on the scalp, face, palms, soles and in the intertriginous areas (Berth-Jones & Hutchinson 1992; Menne & Larsen 1992; Klaber *et al.* 1994). The combination of either broad-band UVB or 311-nm UVB therapy with calcipotriol was shown to increase the therapeutic efficacy of phototherapy alone (Kragballe 1990; Kerscher *et al.* 1993). This observation is of particular interest because at the same time UVB therapy reduced the irritation caused by calcipotriol. In contrast to UVB irradiation, a combination of calcipotriol with UVA radiation or a combined UVA/UVB regimen should be avoided, because UVA radiation leads to degradation of vitamin D_3. Vitamin D analogues should therefore be applied after, and not before phototherapy.

Several studies have addressed the question of whether the efficacy of UVB phototherapy for psoriasis may be enhanced through combination with topical corticosteroids. Data from these studies are conflicting and the beneficial effects seem to be limited (Petrozzi 1983; Larko *et al.* 1984; LeVine & Parrish 1989). Topical steroids are useful, however, for treating psoriatic lesions in skin areas not reached by UV irradiation during phototherapy (e.g. scalp, groin, rima ani, perianal area, umbilicus), or for the treatment of lesions recalcitrant to standard phototherapy. They may also be used in the early, highly inflammatory state of psoriasis to achieve a quick improvement.

Topical application of emollients alters the optical properties of psoriatic lesions (Anderson & Parrish 1980). Lubricants improve transmission of UVB and a combination of topical lubricants with UVB therapy was shown to have an increased efficacy (Lebwohl 1995). This is in contrast to thick applications of petrolatum and water-in-oil type creams and salicylic acid, which act as sunscreens.

Balneophototherapy comprises the combination of salt-water baths with UVB phototherapy, which, under natural conditions, has been successfully employed at the Dead Sea for the treatment of patients with recurrent severe psoriasis (Abels *et al.* 1985; Abel *et al.* 1988). Modern approaches to balneophototherapy employing synthetically generated Dead Sea salt or sodium chloride solutions for salt-water baths (usually between 5 and 15%) are hampered by logistic (the requirement for bathtubs) and environmental problems (caused by the salt consumption). The beneficial effects of saline solutions on psoriasis are thought to involve elution of leucocyte elastase from psoriatic skin (Wiedow *et al.* 1989) and anti-inflammatory effects of magnesium ions (Ludwig *et al.* 1995). Controlled studies demonstrating a synergistic effect between salt-water baths and phototherapy are still lacking.

Similarly, the efficacy of balneophototherapy in comparison with established combination regimens for psoriasis remains to be assessed.

The combination of crude coal tar plus UV irradiation has been used in the treatment of generalized psoriasis since 1925 (Goeckermann 1925). Today, the Goeckerman regimen is no longer considered as a standard therapy for psoriasis. Tar has an unpleasant smell, it may lead to discoloration of skin and clothes, it can cause acneiform lesions, and, most importantly, the combination of tar and UVB irradiation may have an increased carcinogenic risk (Stern *et al.* 1980; Pittlekow *et al.* 1981; Wheeler *et al.* 1981; Larko & Swanbeck 1982; Olsen *et al.* 1992). For these reasons, tar should no longer be used in combination with phototherapy.

Systemic agents, which may be used to treat psoriasis, include retinoids, corticosteroids, cyclosporin A and methotrexate. Retinoids are the most widely used agents for systemic treatment in combination with phototherapy. In contrast, the systemic use of steroids in combination with photo(chemo)-therapy is limited to special indications such as generalized pustular psoriasis. Also, combination regimens of UVB therapy with methotrexate or cyclosporin A are not advisable, because both substances increase the possibility of UV-induced skin tumours.

From a theoretical point of view, there are two advantages of combining retinoids and UVB irradiation: (i) retinoids exert antipsoriatic effects, which might act synergistically with UVB phototherapy; and (ii) they have anticarcinogenic effects and thereby could lower the increased skin-cancer risk resulting from long-term UVB therapy. Because of potentially severe side-effects, the use of retinoids as monotherapy should be limited to pustular or erythrodermic variants of psoriasis. Combination regimens with broad-band UVB or SUP therapy together with etretinate induced improvement in psoriatic patients more quickly than with phototherapy alone and reduced the number of treatments and cumulative UV doses (Orfanos *et al.* 1979; Steigleder *et al.* 1979; Marghescu *et al.* 1982).

Similar results were obtained when acitretin, the major metabolite of etretinate, was used in combination with broad-band UVB or 311-nm UVB therapy (Lest & Boer 1989; Ruzicka *et al.* 1990; Lowe *et al.* 1991).

The availability of the topical retinoid tazarotene has offered the possibility of combining UVB phototherapy with retinoid therapy without any systemic side-effects. Recent studies indicate that the combination of broad-band UVB as well as 311-nm UVB phototherapy with tazarotene therapy is well tolerated (Koo 1998; Stege *et al.* 1998). Treatment success was achieved significantly quicker in psoriatic skin treated with the combination regimen, as compared to UVB alone. The combination of broad-band UVB and, in particular, 311-nm UVB phototherapy and tazarotene may prove to become the therapy of choice for patients with moderate to severe psoriasis.

References

Abel, E.A., Barnes, S., Le Vine, M.J., Seidman, D.R. & Wallk, S (1988) Psoriasis treatment at the Dead Sea: second international study tour. *Journal of the American Academy of Dermatology* **19**, 362–366.

Abels, D.J. & Kattan, B.J. (1985) Psoriasis treatment at the dead sea: a natural selective ultraviolet phototherapy. *Journal of the American Academy of Dermatology* **12**, 639–643.

Anderson, R.R. & Parrish, J.A. (1980) Optical properties of human skin. In: *The Science of Photomedicine* (eds Regan, J.D. & Parrish, J.A.), pp. 147–158. Plenum Press, New York.

Berth-Jones, J. & Hutchinson, P.E. (1992) Vitamin D analogues and psoriasis. *British Journal of Dermatology* **127**, 71–75.

Bevilaqua, P.M., Edelson, R.L. & Gasparro, F.P. (1991) High performance liquid chromatography analysis of 8-methoxypsoralen monoadducts and crosslinks in lymphocytes and keratinocytes. *Journal of Investigative Dermatology* **97**, 151–155.

Boer, J. & Smeenk, G. (1986) Effect of short-contact anthralin therapy on ultraviolet B irradiation of psoriasis. *Journal of the American Academy of Dermatology* **15**, 198–202.

Bruynzeel, I., Bergman, W., Hartevelt, H.M. *et al.* (1991) High single-dose European PUVA regimen also causes an excess of non-melanoma skin cancer. *British Journal of Dermatology* **124**, 49–55.

Chunag, T.Y., Heinrich, L.A., Scvhultz, M.D., Reizner, G.T. & Cripps, D.J. (1992) PUVA and skin cancer. *Journal of the American Academy of Dermatology* **26**, 173–177.

Dawe, R.S., Wainwright, N.J., Cameron, H. & Ferguson, J. (1998) Narrow-band (TL-01) ultraviolet B phototherapy for chronic plaque psoriasis: three times or five times weekly treatment ? *British Journal of Dermatology* **138**, 830–839.

De Gruijl, F.R. (1989) Long-term side effects and carcinogenesis risk in UVB therapy. In: *Are Topical Corticosteroids Useful in Phototherapy for Psoriasis?* (eds Dover, J.S. *et al.*). *Journal of the American Academy of Dermatology* **20**, 748–752.

Epstein, J.H. (1968) UVL-induced stimulation of DNA synthesis in hairless mouse epidermis. *Journal of Investigative Dermatology* **52**, 445–448.

Epstein, W.L., Fukuyama, K. & Epstein, J.H. (1969) Early effects of ultraviolet light on DNA synthesis in human skin in vivo. *Archives of Dermatology* **100**, 84–89.

Farber, E.M. & Harris, D.H. (1970) Hospital treatment of psoriasis: a modified anthralin program. *Archives of Dermatology* **101**, 381–384.

Fischer, T. & Alsins, J. (1976) Treatment of psoriasis with trioxsalen baths and dysprosium lamps. *Acta Dermato-Venereologica* **563**, 383–390.

Flindt-Hansen, H., McFadden, N., Eeg-Larsen, T. & Thune, P. (1991) Effect of a new narrow-band UVB lamp on photocarcinogenesis in mice. *Acta Dermato-Venereologica* **71**, 245–248.

Gallewski, E. (1916) Über Cignolin, ein Ersatzpräparat des Chrysarobins. *Dermatologische Wochenschrift* **62**, 113–114.

Godar, D.E. (1996) Preprogrammed and programmed cell death mechanisms of apoptosis: UV-induced immediate and delayed apoptosis. *Photochemistry and Photobiology* **63**, 825–830.

Goeckermann, W.H. (1925) The treatment of psoriasis. *Northwest Medicine* **24**, 229.

Green, C., Ferguson, J., Laksmipathi, T. & Johnson, B.E. (1988) 311 nm UVB phototherapy – an effective treatment for psoriasis. *British Journal of Dermatology* **119**, 691–696.

Green, C., Laksmipathi, T., Johnson, B.E. & Ferguson, J.A. (1992) Comparison of the efficacy and relapse rates of narrow band UVB (TL01) monotherapy vs. etretinate (re-TL-01) vs. etretinate-PUVA (re-PUVA) in the treatment of psoriasis. *British Journal of Dermatology* **127**, 5–9.

Grewe, M., Gyufko, K., Budnik, A. *et al.* (1996) Interleukin-1 receptors type I and type II are differentially regulated in human keratinocytes by ultraviolet B radiation. *Journal of Investigative Dermatology* **107**, 865–871.

Grewe, M., Gyufko, K. & Krutmann, J. (1995) Interleukin-10 production by cultured human keratinocytes: regulation by ultraviolet B and ultraviolet A1 radiation. *Journal of Investigative Dermatology* **104**, 3–6.

Grewe, M., Gyufko, K., Schöpf, E. & Krutmann, J. (1994) Lesional expression of interferon-γ in atopic eczema. *Lancet* **343**, 25–26.

Grewe, M., Krefzer, U., Ballhorn, A. *et al.* (1993) Analysis of the mechanism of ultraviolet B radiation induced prostaglandin E2 synthesis by human epidermoid carcinoma cells. *Journal of Investigative Dermatology* **101**, 528–531.

Gruss, C., Behrens, S., Reuther, T., Husebo, L. *et al.* (1998) Kinetics of photosensitivity in bath-PUVA photochemotherapy. *Journal of the American Academy of Dermatology* **39**, 443–446.

Henseler, T., Christophers, E., Hönigsmann, H. *et al.* (1987) Skin tumors in the European PUVA study. *Journal of the American Academy of Dermatology* **16**, 108–116.

Hofer, A., Fink-Puches, R., Kerl, H. & Wolf, P. (1998) Comparison of phototherapy with near vs. far erythemogenic doses of narrow-band ultraviolet B in patients with psoriasis. *British Journal of Dermatology* **138**, 96–100.

Hönigsmann, H. & Krutmann, J. (1997) Vorschlag für Standardrichtlinien zur praktischen Durchführung der PUVA, Breitband-UVB, 311/nm-UVB und UVA/1-Phototherapie. In: *Handbuch der Dermatologischen Phototherapie und Photodiagnostik* (eds Krutmann, J. & Hönigsmann, H.), pp. 359–366. Springer-Verlag, Heidelberg.

Hönigsmann, H., Jori, G. & Young, A.R. (1996) *The Fundamental Bases of Phototherapy*, pp. 153–170. OEMF SpA, Milano.

Ingram, J.T. (1953) The approach to psoriasis. *British Medical Journal* **2**, 591–593.

Karvonen, J., Kokkonen, E.-L. & Ruotsalainen, E. (1989) 311 nm UVB lamps in the treatment of psoriasis with the Ingram regimen. *Acta Dermato-Venereologica* **69**, 82–85.

Kerscher, M., Plewig, G. & Lehmann, P. (1993) Combination phototherapy of psoriasis with calcipotriol and narrow-band UVB. *Lancet* **342**, 923 (letter).

Klaber, M.R., Hutchinson P.E., Pedvis Leftick, A. *et al.* (1994) Comparative effects of calcipotriol solution (50 micrograms/ml) and bethamethasone 17 valerate solution (1 mg/ml) in the treatment of scalp psoriasis. *British Journal of Dermatology* **131**, 678–682.

Koo, J.Y. (1998) Tazarotene in combination with phototherapy. *Journal of the American Academy of Dermatology* **39**, 144–148.

Kragballe, K. (1990) Combination of topical calcipotriol (MC903) and UVB radiation for psoriasis vulgaris. *Dermatologica* **181**, 211–214.

Kragballe, K. (1995) Efficacy, tolerability, and safety of calcipotriol ointment in disorders of keratinization. Results of a randomized, double-blind, vehicle-controlled, right/left comparative study. *Archives of Dermatology* **131**, 556–560.

Kramer, D.M., Pathak, M.A., Kornahauser, A. & Wiskemann, A. (1974) Effect of ultraviolet irradiation on biosynthesis of DNA in guinea pig skin. *Journal of Investigative Dermatology* **62**, 388–393.

Kristensen, B. & Kristensen, O. (1990) Topical salicylic acid interferes with UVB therapy for psoriasis. *Acta Dermato-Venereologica* **71**, 37–41.

Krueger, J.G., Wolfe, J.T., Nabeja, R.T. *et al.* (1995) Successful ultraviolet B treatment of psoriasis is accompanied by a reversal of keratinocyte pathology and by selective depletion of intraepidermal T cells. *Journal of Experimental Medicine* **182**, 2057–2068.

Krutmann, J. (1998) Therapeutic photoimmunology: photoimmunological mechanisms in photo(chemo)therapy. *Journal of Photochemistry and Photobiology B* **44**, 159–164.

Krutmann, J. & Elmets, C.A. (eds) (1995) *Photoimmunology*. Blackwell Science, Oxford.

Krutmann, J. & Grewe, M. (1995) Involvement of cytokines, DNA damage, and reactive oxygen intermediates in ultraviolet radiation-induced modulation of intercellular adhesion molecule-1 expression. *Journal of Investigative Dermatology* **105**, 67S–70S.

Krutmann, J., Khan, I.U., Wallis, R.S. *et al.* (1990) The cell membrane is a major locus for ultraviolet-B-induced alterations in accessory cells. *Journal of Clinical Investigation* **85**, 1529–1536.

Larkö, O. (1989) Treatment of psoriasis with a new UVB-lamp. *Acta Dermato-Venereologica* **69**, 357–359. Stockholm.

Larkö, O. & Swanbeck, G. (1982) Is UVB treatment safe? A study of extensively UVB treated psoriasis patients compared with a matched control group. *Acta Dermato-Venereologica* **62**, 507–511.

Larkö, O., Swanbeck, G. & Svartholm, H. (1984) The effect on psoriasis of clobetasol propionate used alone or in combination with UVB. *Acta Dermato-Venereologica* **64**, 151–156.

Laskin, J.D., Lee, E., Yurkow, E.J., Laskin, D.L. & Gallo, M.A. (1985) A possible mechanism of psoralen phototoxicity not involving direct interaction with DNA. *Proceedings of the National Academy of Sciences of the USA* **82**, 6158–6162.

Lebwohl, M. (1995) Effects of topical preparations on the erythemogenicity of UVB: implications for psoriasis therapy. *Journal of the American Academy of Dermatology* **32**, 469–474.

Lebwohl, M., Berman, B. & France, D.S. (1985) Addition of short-contact anthralin therapy to an ultraviolet B phototherapy regimen: assessment of efficacy. *Journal of the American Academy of Dermatology* **13**, 780–785.

Lest, J. & Boer, J. (1989) Combined treatment of psoriasis with acitretin and UVB phototherapy compared with acitretin alone and UVB alone. *British Journal of Dermatology* **120**, 665–670.

LeVine, M.J. & Parrish, J.A. (1989) The effect of topical fluocinonide ointment on phototherapy of psoriasis. *Journal of Investigative Dermatology* **78**, 157–162.

Lisby, S., Ralfkier, E., Rothlein, R. & Veijsgard, G.L. (1989) Intercellular adhesion molecule-1 (ICAM-1) expression correlated to inflammation. *British Journal of Dermatology* **120**, 479–484.

Lobel, E., Paver, K., King, R. *et al.* (1981) The relationship of skin cancer to PUVA therapy in Australia. *Australian Journal of Dermatology* **22**, 100–103.

Lowe, N.J., Prystowsky, J.H., Bourget, T., Edelstein, J., Nychay, S. & Armstrong, R. (1991) Acitretin plus UVB therapy for psoriasis. Comparisons with placebo plus UVB and acitretin alone. *Journal of the American Academy of Dermatology* **24**, 591–596.

Ludwig, P., Petrich, K., Schowe, T. & Diezel, W. (1995) Inhibition of eicosanoid formation in human polymorphonuclear leukocytes by high concentrations of magnesium ions. *Biological Chemistry Hoppe-Seyler* **376**, 739–744.

Luger, T.A. & Schwartz, T. (1995) Effects of UV light on cytokines and neuroendocrine hormones. In: *Photoimmunology* (eds Krutmann, J. & Ellmets, C.A.), pp. 55–76, Blackwell Science, Oxford.

Marghescu, S., Lubach, D. & Rudolph P.O. (1982) Die Therapie der Psoriasis mit Retinoiden. *Zeitschrift fur Hautkrankheiten* **57**, 1410–1412.

Melski, J.W., Tannenbaum, L., Parrish, J.A., Fitzpatrick, T.B. & Belich, H.L. and 28 participating investigators (1977) Oral methoxsalen photochemotherapy for the treatment of psoriasis: a cooperative clinical trial. *Journal of Investigative Dermatology* **68**, 328–335.

Menne, T. & Larsen, K. (1992) Psoriasis treatment with vitamin D derivatives. *Seminars in Dermatology* **11**, 278–283.

Mentener, M.A., See, J.-A., Amend, W.J.C. *et al.* (1996) Proceedings of the psoriasis combination and rotation therapy conference. *Journal of the American Academy of*

Dermatology **34**, 315–321.

Morison, W.L. (1991). *Phototherapy and Photochemotherapy of Skin Disease*, 2nd edn. Raven Press, New York.

Morison, W.L. (1993) Photochemotherapy. In: *Clinical Photomedicine* (eds Lim, H.W., Soter N.A.), pp. 327–345. Marcel Dekker, New York.

Morison, W.L., Baughman, R.D., Day, R.M. *et al.* (1998) Consensus workshop on the toxic effects of long-term PUVA therapy. *Archives of Dermatology* **134**, 595–598.

Morita, A., Grewe, M., Werfel, T., Kapp, A. & Krutmann, J. (1996) Ultraviolet A1 radiation differentially affects cytokine production by atopen-specific human T-helper cells. *Journal of Investigative Dermatology* **106**, abstract 932.

Morita, A., Werfel, T., Stege, H. *et al.* (1997) Evidence that singlet oxygen-induced human T helper cell apoptosis is the basic mechanism of ultraviolet-A radiation phototherapy. *Journal of Experimental Medicine* **186**, 1763–1768.

Norris, D.A., Lyons, B., Midleton, M.H., Yohn, J.Y. & Kashiara-Sawami, M. (1990) Ultraviolet radiation can either suppress or induce expression of intercellular adhesion molecule-1 (ICAM-1) on the surface of cultured human keratinocytes. *Journal of Investigative Dermatology* **95**, 132–138.

Olsen, J.H., Moller, H. & Frentz, G. (1992) Malignant tumors in patients with psoriasis. *Journal of the American Academy of Dermatology* **27**, 716–722.

Orfanos, C.E., Steigleder, G.K., Pullman, H. & Bloch, P.H. (1979) Oral retinoid and UVB radiation: a new alternative treatment for psoriasis on an outpatient basis. *Acta Dermato-Venereologica* **59**, 241–246.

Parrish, J.A. & Jaenicke, K.F. (1981) Action spectrum for phototherapy of psoriasis. *Journal of Investigative Dermatology* **76**, 359–361.

Parrish, J.A., Fitzpatrick, T.B., Tannebaum, L. & Pathak, M.A. (1974) Photochemo-therapy of psoriasis with oral methoxsalen and longwave ultraviolet light. *New England Journal of Medicine* **291**, 1207–1211.

Petrozzi, J.W. (1983) Topical steroids and UV radiation in psoriasis. *Archives of Dermatology* **119**, 207–211.

Picot, E. (1992) Treatment of psoriasis with a 311-UVB lamp. *British Journal of Dermatology* **127**, 509–512.

Pittelkow, M.R., Perry, H.O., Muller, S.A., Maughan, W.Z. & O'Brien, P.C. (1981) Skin cancer in patients with psoriasis treated with coal tar. *Archives of Dermatology* **117**, 465–470.

Pullmann, H. (1978) Praktische Erfahrungen mit verschiedenen Phototherapieformen der Psoriasis—PUVA, SUP, Teer-UV-Therapie. *Zeitschrift fur Hautkrankheiten* **53**, 641.

Ramsay, C.A., Berth-Jones, J., Brundin, D. *et al.* (1994) Long-term use of topical calcipotriol in chronic plaque psoriasis. *Dermatology* **189**, 260–264.

Roza, L., Stege, H. & Krutmann, J. (1996) Role of UV-induced DNA damage in photo-therapy. In: *The Fundamental Bases of Phototherapy* (eds Hönigsmann, H. Jori, G. & Young, A.R.), pp. 145–152, OEMF spa, Milano.

Runne, U. & Kunze, J.J. (1982) Short-duration ('minutes') therapy with dithranol for psoriasis: a new out-patient regimen. *British Journal of Dermatology* **106**, 135–140.

Ruzicka, T., Sommerburg, C., Braun-Falco, O. *et al.* (1990) Efficiency of acitretin in combination with UVB in the treatment of severe psoriasis. *Archives of Dermatology* **126**, 482–486.

Schauer, E., Trautinger, F. & Köch, A. (1994) Proopiomelanocortin derived peptides are synthesized and released by human keratinocytes. *Journal of Clinical Investigation* **93**, 2258–2261.

Simon, J.C., Krutmann, J., Elmets, C.A., Bergstresser, P.R. & Cruz, P.D. (1992) Ultraviolet B irradiated antigen presenting cells display altered accessory signaling for T cell activation: relevance to immune responses initiated in the skin. *Journal of Investigative*

Dermatology **98**, 66S–69S.

Stege, H., Berneburg, M., Ruzicka, T. & Krutmann, J. (1997) Creme-PUVA-Photochemo-therapie. *Der Hautarzt* **48**, 89–93.

Stege, H., Reifenberger, J., Ruzicka, T. & Krutmann, J. (1998) Combination therapy of psoriasis with 311 nm UVB phototherapy plus tazarotene. *Journal of the European Academy of Dermatology and Venereology* **11**, S101–S102.

Steigleder, G.K., Orfanos, C.E. & Pullman, H. (1979) Retinoid-SUP-Therapie der Psoriasis. *Zeitschrift für Hautkrankheiten* **54**, 19–24.

Stern, S. & Laird, N. (1994) For the Photochemotherapy Follow-up Study. The carcinogenic risk of treatments for severe psoriasis. *Cancer* **73**, 2759–2764.

Stern, R.S., Armstrong, R.B., Anderson, T.F. *et al.* (1986) Effect of continued ultraviolet B phototherapy on the duration of remission of psoriasis: a randomized study. *Journal of the American Academy of Dermatology* **15**, 546–552.

Stern, R.S., Nichols, K.T. & Vakeva, L.H. (1997) Malignant melanoma in patients treated for psoriasis with methoxsalen (psoralen) and ultraviolet A radiation (PUVA). *New England Journal of Medicine* **336**, 1041–1045.

Stern, R.S., Thibodeau, L.A., Kleinerman, R.A., Parrish, J.A. & Fitzpatrick, T.B. and 22 participating investigators (1979) Risk of cutaneous carcinoma in patients treated with oral methoxsalen photochemotherapy for psoriasis. *New England Journal of Medicine* **300**, 809–813.

Stern, R.S., Zierler, S. & Parrish, J.A. (1980) Skin carcinoma in patients with psoriasis treated with topical tar and artificial ultraviolet radiation. *Lancet* **1**, 732–735.

Storbeck, K., Holzle, E., Lehmann, P., Schurer, N. & Plewig, G. (1991) Die Wirksamkeit eines neuen Schmalspektrum-UV-B-Strahlers (Philips TL 01, 100 W, 311 nm) im Vergleich zur konventionellen UV-B-Phototherapie der Psoriasis. *Zeitschrift für Hautkrankheiten* **66**, 708–712.

Storbeck, K., Hölzle, E., Lehmann, P., Schurer, N. & Plewig, G. (1993) Narrow-band UVB (311 nm) versus conventional broad band UVB with and without dithranol in phototherapy for psoriasis. *Journal of the American Academy of Dermatology* **28**, 227–231.

Tanew, A., Fijan, S. & Honigsmann, H. (1996) Halfside comparison study on narrowband UVB phototherapy versus photochemotherapy (PUVA) in the treatment of severe psoriasis. *Journal of Investigative Dermatology* **106**, abstract 841.

Tanew, A., Hönigsmann, H., Ortel, B., Zuessner, C. & Wolff, K. (1986) Nonmelanoma skin tumors in long-term photochemotherapy treatment of psoriasis. *Journal of the American Academy of Dermatology* **15**, 960–965.

Trefzer, U., Brockhaus, M., Lötscher, H. *et al.* (1993) The human 55-kd tumor necrosis factor receptor is regulated in human keratinocytes by TNFa and by ultraviolet B radiation. *Journal of Clinical Investigations* **92**, 462–470.

Unna, P.G. (1916) Cignolin als Heilmittel der Psoriasis. *Dermatologische Wochenschrift* 62, 116–118.

van Weelden, H., Baart de la Faille, H., Young, E. & van der Leun, J.C. (1988) A new development in UVB phototherapy for psoriasis. *British Journal of Dermatology* **119**, 11–19.

van Weelden, H., Baart de la Faille, H., Young, E. & van der Leun, J.C. (1990) Comparison of narrow-band UVB phototherapy and PUVA photochemotherapy in the treatment of psoriasis. *Acta Dermato-Venereologica* **70**, 212–215.

Volc-Platzer, B. & Hönigsmann, H. (1995) Photoimmunology of PUVA and UVB therapy. In: *Photoimmunology* (eds Krutmann, J. & Elmets, C.A.), pp. 265–273. Blackwell Science, Oxford.

Wainwright, N.J., Dawe, R.S. & Ferguson, J. (1998) Narrowband ultraviolet B (TL01) phototherapy for psoriasis: which incremental regimen? *British Journal of Dermatology*

139, 410–414.

Wheeler, L.A., Saperstein, M.D. & Lowe, N.J. (1981) Mutagenicity of urine from psoriatic patients undergoing treatment with coal tar and ultraviolet light. *Journal of Investigative Dermatology* **77**, 181–185.

Wiedow, O., Streit V., Christophers, E. & Stander, M. (1989) Freisetzung humaner Leukozytenelastase durch hypertone Salzbäder bei Psoriasis. *Hautarzt* **40**, 518–523.

Wulf, H.C., Hansen, A.B. & Bech-Thomsen, N. (1994) Differences in narrow-band ultraviolet-B and broad-spectrum ultraviolet photocarcinogenesis in lightly pigmented hairless mice. *Photodermatology, Photoimmunology and Photomedicine* **10**, 192–197.

Yoo, E.K., Rook, A.H., Elenitas, R., Gasparro, F.P. & Vowels, B.R. (1996) Apoptosis induction by ultraviolet light A and photochemotherapy in cutaneous T-cell lymphomas: relevance to mechanism of therapeutic action. *Journal of Investigative Dermatology* **107**, 235–242.

Young, A. (1995) Carcinogenicity of UVB phototherapy assessed. *Lancet* **346**, 1431–1432.

Chapter 12: Methotrexate

H. Zachariae

12.1 Introduction

Methotrexate (MTX) is a cytostatic agent that is well established in the treatment of various malignancies. It is also the oldest of the drugs used today for systemic therapy of psoriasis and psoriatic arthritis. For these diseases MTX has been employed for about 40 years. In rheumatoid arthritis the drug has been widely used since the mid 1970s.

MTX or amethopterin is a folic acid antagonist. In psoriasis the drug was preceded by another folic acid antagonist, aminopterin, prescribed by Gubner in 1951 (Gubner 1951). Rees *et al.* (1955) improved the therapeutic index of aminopterin by diminishing the dose. However, following the introduction of MTX by Edmundson and Guy (1958), this more stable derivative soon took over due to a lower toxicity. Originally MTX was prescribed daily for 5–10 days followed by a rest period of a few days, and then repeated; but since the early 1970s weekly oral or weekly parenteral doses have been the established way to treat psoriasis. This was mainly on account of a proven reduction in liver toxicity (Weinstein *et al.* 1973). The divided weekly oral 'Weinstein schedule' is still one of the most popular schedules. It was introduced by Weinstein and Frost (1971) based on cell-cycle kinetics. It is given in three subdoses at 12-h intervals.

The introduction of psoralen and UVA (PUVA), retinoids and cyclosporin A has undoubtedly reduced its use, but MTX is still widely employed because of its efficacy and a high degree of patient compliance. The drug leads to more than 75% improvement in 90% of psoriatic patients (Nyfors 1978); and among patients with psoriatic arthritis 60% are greatly improved and 30% moderately improved (Kragballe *et al.* 1982).

The main reason for the decline in popularity of MTX is without doubt the 'liver scare', and in particular the recommendations that liver biopsies be performed to monitor treatment (Roenigk *et al.* 1988). Although it is well established that long-term MTX usage may induce liver damage, which in turn leads to fibrosis or cirrhosis in some patients (Weinstein *et al.* 1973; Rees *et al.* 1974; Zachariae *et al.* 1975; Nyfors 1978; Robinson *et al.* 1980; Zachariae & Søgaard 1987), other studies have documented that such a cirrhosis in general is not aggressive (Zachariae & Søgaard 1987; Newman *et al.* 1989). At present histological evaluation of liver biopsies is still the rule of the 'guidelines for the use of MTX for psoriasis' as the way to assess liver damage

196

(Roenigk *et al.* 1988). Today, however, two techniques are available, which seem to be able to reduce the number of liver biopsies necessary in order to control MTX-induced liver fibrosis: serum amino-terminal propeptide of type III procollagen (PIIINP) (Risteli *et al.* 1988) and dynamic hepatic scintigraphy (van Dooren-Greebe *et al.* 1996).

12.2 Pharmacology and pharmacodynamics

12.2.1 Chemistry and biochemistry

The folic acid analogue MTX, which is 4-amino-N^{10}-methyl pterylglutamic acid, is a weak bicarboxylic organic acid, with a molecular weight of 454 Da, negatively charged at neutral pH, and with limited lipid solubility (Bleyer 1978).

  The structure of MTX and folic acid can be seen in Fig. 12.1. In general MTX is actively transported into cells. Three main transport systems have been described for folate compounds. One of these, the reduced folate carrier (RFC-1), may be of particular importance, as it displays a low affinity for folic acid and a high affinity for MTX and reduced folates (Moscow *et al.* 1995). Once intracellular MTX competitively binds to dihydrofolate reductase resulting in a decreased formation of reduced folate cofactors, which are necessary in the metabolic transfer of 1-carbon units, MTX will diminish the rate of synthesis of thymidylic acid essential for DNA synthesis. MTX also diminshes inosinic acid essential for both DNA and RNA synthesis. However, the drug appears to inhibit DNA synthesis to a greater extent than RNA synthesis. When present during the S-phase of the cell cycle, it can lead to apoptosis or cell death. MTX treatment is therefore described as an S-phase-specific chemotherapy.

  MTX and folates are metabolized intracellularly to polyglutamates by folyl polyglutamate synthetase (Calabresi & Parks 1985). These are preferentially retained intracellularly, and for MTX allows accumulation of the free intracellular drug far above what could be achieved if the drug were in equilibrium with the extracellular concentration. MTX-polyglutamate has equal affinity with MTX for dihydrofolate reductase but dissociates at a slower rate and crosses cellular membranes less easily (Bleyer 1978; Calabresi & Parks 1985).

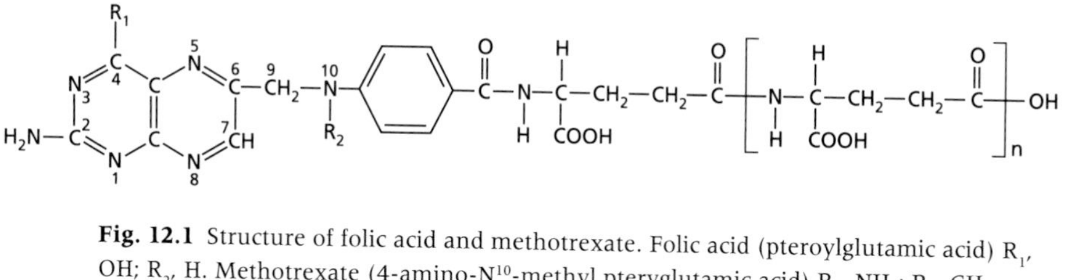

Fig. 12.1 Structure of folic acid and methotrexate. Folic acid (pteroylglutamic acid) R_1, OH; R_2, H. Methotrexate (4-amino-N^{10}-methyl pteryglutamic acid) R_1, NH_2; R_2, CH_3.

12.2.2 Working mechanisms

Despite the many years of MTX use, there are still some uncertainties concerning the mechanism of action of MTX in psoriasis. For a number of years it was generally accepted that interference with epidermal and epithelial cell kinetics, presumably by a temporary reduction in DNA synthesis, was the main factor for the antipsoriatic activity. The construction of the weekly divided oral dose was based upon this assumption (Weinstein & Frost 1971).

Tissue drug exposure for 36 h should theoretically affect the entire population of psoriatic cells, while only partially affecting other proliferating tissues with a longer cell cycle. More recently it was shown that MTX *in vitro* causes differentiation of keratinocytes (Schwartz *et al.* 1995), which could also be of interest. Several observations, however, indicate that mechanisms of action other than a direct effect on keratinocytes could be more important. The effect on psoriatic arthritis (Kragballe *et al.* 1982) is difficult to explain in this manner, and so is the well-known effect on a number of other non-proliferative inflammatory diseases like rheumatoid arthritis (Kremer 1996), systemic lupus erythematosus (Rothenberg *et al.* 1988) and systemic sclerosis (van den Hoogen *et al.* 1996). The lack of clinical and histological responses to topically administered MTX in spite of accumulation of the drug in the psoriasis plaques (Bjerring *et al.* 1986) also indicates other cells as targets for the antipsoriatic effect. Even intralesional injections of MTX, which cause a dramatic response in the cell-cycle kinetics, have shown no clinical effect (Comaish & Juhlin 1969).

The immune system could very well be significant in the working mechanism. *In vitro* studies have shown MTX inhibiting proliferating lymphoid tissue (Jeffes *et al.* 1995) with little effect on epidermal cells, and MTX inhibits interleukin 1 (IL-1) activity (Chang *et al.* 1990; Segal *et al.* 1995) as well as IL-6 production (Straub *et al.* 1997). Also, a number of anti-inflammatory properties of MTX deserve to be mentioned. These include decreases in neutrophil and monocyte chemotaxis (Cream & Poll 1980), inhibition of leukotriene B4-induced penetration of granulocytes (Lammers & van de Kerkhof 1987) and C5a-induced skin responses (Ternowitz *et al.* 1987). It has also been shown that MTX inhibits leucocyte accumulation at inflamed sites by increasing adenosine release due to inhibition of 5-aminoimidazole-4-carboxamide ribonucleotide transformylase (Cronstein 1996).

Other effects which have been addressed are inhibition of endothelial cell growth, inhibition of polyamine synthesis and the generation of a number of 5-lipoxygenase pathway products (Zachariae 1996). In summary, MTX has been suggested to exert its antipsoriatic effect by immunomodulation, inhibition of epidermal proliferation, induction of epidermal differentiation, and/or via interference with a number of aspects of cutaneous inflammation. However, it is still unknown which of these suggested mechanisms is the most valid for the clinical response.

12.2.3 Absorption, metabolism and excretion

The absorption of MTX following oral or intramuscular administration is rapid with peak serum concentrations reached after 1.6 and 1 h (Anderson *et al.* 1970). However, interpatient differences are considerable after oral administration (Hendel *et al.* 1982), and in some patients the absorption may be significantly impaired following long-term treatment (Boomla *et al.* 1979). Food decreases absorption (Evans & Christensen 1985), especially dairy products. For this reason MTX should be taken between meals in order to obtain reproducible and stable absorption. It is not uncommon that a shift from oral to parenteral administration leads to a beneficial clinical response in a poor responder to oral MTX.

Fifty to seventy per cent of MTX is protein bound, especially to albumin (Bleyer 1978). Concomitant drugs that decrease MTX plasma protein binding by competitive displacement or by altering albumin binding affinity to MTX may increase free MTX and toxicity (see later under interaction). Fifty to ninety per cent of MTX is excreted unchanged in the urine within 24 h (Calabresi & Parks 1985), the higher percentages with the lower dosages. The tubular reabsorption process becomes saturated at plasma concentrations well within the range achievable with treatment of psoriasis (Hendel & Nyfors 1984) resulting in increased renal clearance of the drug, while saturation of the tubular secretory mechanism is unlikely to occur at these dosages. Any drug interfering with renal elimination of MTX will increase toxicity (see later under interaction). Most MTX excreted in the bile is reabsorbed, and in total only about 2% MTX is excreted in faeces (Hendel & Nyfors 1984). The amount of metabolites formed after oral administration is about 35% of the absorbed dose, in contrast to only 6% following intravenous administration. Also, after intravenous injection the predominant metabolite has been shown to be 7-hydroxy MTX, which is four times less soluble in acid urine than MTX, and thus in higher dosages may contribute to a renal toxicity not to be found during the low-dose psoriasis treatment (Bleyer 1978).

12.2.4 Drug–drug interaction

MTX interaction can occur with a number of other drugs (Table 12.1). In our experience, the most serious problems have arisen with the concomitant use of sulphonamides—especially when combined with trimethoprim, and with salicylates. In addition, non-steroidal anti-inflammatory agents are best avoided and at the very least should not be given on MTX treatment days. Although a number of patients have clearly benefited from the combination of MTX and retinoids, a warning may be appropriate. In our department at the Marselisborg Hospital in Aarhus, Denmark, two out of 10 patients treated with MTX+etretinate developed life-threatening drug-induced hepatitis, a condition that had not been seen in any of 531 patients taking MTX as

Table 12.1 Drug interactions that may increase methotrexate toxicity.

Mechanism	Drugs
Pharmacological enhancement of MTX-toxic effect	Trimethoprim-sulphamethoxasole Phenylbutazone Ethanol
Decreased renal elimination	Nephrotoxins Salicylates NSAIDs
Reduced tubular secretion	Salicylates Sulphonamides Probenecid Cephalosporin Penicillins Colchicine
Displacement of MTX from plasma protein binding	Salicylates Probenecid Barbiturates Phenytoin
Intracellular accumulation of MTX	Probenecid Dipyridamole
Hepatotoxicity	Retinoids
Additive antihaematopoietic effect	Cytotoxic drugs Chloramphenicol

monotherapy, or in any of 110 patients receiving etretinate alone (Zachariae 1993). Whether this potential hepatotoxicity can be due to an increase of maximum plasma concentration for MTX (Larsen *et al.* 1990) cannot be excluded. The other interactions mentioned can be the result of a direct pharmacological enhancement of MTX toxic effects (additive antifolate or antihaematopoietic effects), decreased renal elimination, especially when due to reduced tubular secretion, displacement of MTX from plasma protein binding, and intracellular accumulation of MTX.

In all these cases the drug–drug interaction may lead to symptoms of MTX overdosage (Plate 12.1, facing p. 180). It should be remembered that concomitant use of systemic corticosteroids will give an increased immunosuppressive effect, and that concomitant use of radiotherapy like concomitant use of other cytotoxic agents may lead to a depression of the haematopoietic system.

12.2.5 Dosage schedules

Three different dosage schedules are in common use for psoriasis, as follows.

1 *The divided weekly oral dosage schedule.* Based upon cell-cycle kinetic studies the schedule was proposed by Weinstein and Frost (1971). MTX is given in three doses at 12-h intervals once weekly. A total weekly dose of 15 mg has been recommended with adjustments up to 22.5 mg to increase efficacy, and lowering dosages according to toxicity. Rheumatologists usually recommend 7.5 mg weekly for treatment of arthritis.

2 *The weekly oral single dosage schedule.* Once a week a single dose of MTX is administered orally. A total weekly dose of 25 mg has been recommended (Collins & Rogers 1992), but some centres regard a dosage of 37.5 mg per week as safe. Dosages should be adjusted according to safety and efficacy.

3 *Intermittent weekly parenteral dosage schedule.* Once a week a single dose of MTX is injected parenterally (i.m. or i.v.). In general the intramuscular route is preferred. A starting dose of 15 mg MTX is common. The maximum dosage varies between different centres, but 50 mg weekly is regarded as safe.

Clinical results and side-effects of each dosage schedule are discussed in Sections 12.3 and 12.4. A true comparison between the different schedules has, however, never been performed, and the superiority of one or the other is therefore difficult to claim.

12.3 Results of methotrexate therapy

The results will be discussed in relation to clearing as well as to maintenance, as previously done by van de Kerkhof (1986), with a section related specifically to results in psoriatic arthritis. It should be noted that the original placebo-controlled studies by Black *et al.* (1964) did not use any of the present low-dose schedules. However, they clearly demonstrated the efficacy of MTX in psoriasis and psoriatic arthritis, and clinical practice and a number of surveys have since, as will be shown below, contributed to the acceptance of MTX as one of the most valuable drugs for severe psoriasis and active psoriatic arthritis.

12.3.1 Clearing phase

Data on clearing rates are sparse in the literature (van de Kerkhof 1986). The first improvement is observed between 1 and 7 weeks, and maximal improvement can be expected between 8 and 12 weeks of treatment. An improvement of more than 75% was found in 31–90% of patients in the literature reviewed by van de Kerkhof (1986). In the largest study, which was performed by Nyfors (1978) excellent results (more than 75% clearing) was found in 90% of 248 patients. More recently Collins and Rogers (1992) claimed a good to excellent result in 85% of 40 patients. In their study, patients with erythroderma or generalized pustular psoriasis did better than patients with plaque psoriasis. Baker (1976) claims a significantly lower success rate in palmoplantar pustulosis than all the other groups he studied.

This was not the experience of the Nijmegen group (van Dooren-Greebe *et al*. 1994); however, their investigation only carried five cases with this entity against Baker's 21. In our hands only patients with the acrodermatitis continua variation of pustular psoriasis have been difficult to treat with MTX.

Nail changes, which often accompany severe psoriasis, can be disfiguring and bothersome. Out of the 141 patients with nail changes treated by Nyfors (1978) a complete resolution occurred in 63 and a definitive improvement was found in 53.

Failure to obtain clearing can be due to too low a dose. Dosages should be adjusted according to clinical effect and side-effects. Dose reductions for subjective side-effects can in many instances be avoided by co-administration of folinic acid, which may counter antifolate actions of MTX without reducing the antipsoriatic effect (Hills & Ive 1992). Decreased absorption from the gut or non-compliance can be other reasons. A change to parenteral treatment may be helpful in both cases.

12.3.2 Maintenance phase

The long-term study by van de Kerkhof & Mali (1982) gives a very good picture (Fig. 12.2) of the remissions to be expected. Following a clearance phase induced by MTX and the Ingram regimen (98 patients) the lesion-free period was extended from approximately 1 month to approximately 1 year by offering a maintenance regimen of oral MTX using the Weinstein regimen. The period before readmission to hospital was extended to more than 3 years. In the more recent study by the Nijmegen group (van Dooren-Greebe *et al*. 1994) on 113 patients with severe psoriasis treated with long-term MTX in a maximum weekly oral dosage of 15 mg, the frequency of hospital admissions during treatment decreased by a factor of 10 compared with the pre-treatment period, from 0.4 per patient per year to 0.04. The estimated mean

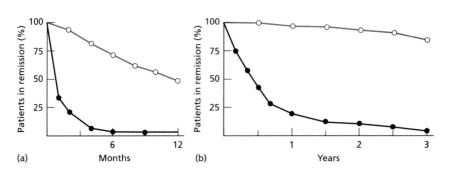

Fig. 12.2 Actuarial remission curves during long-term methotrexate therapy following Ingram therapy. (a) Criterion for relapse is the first indication of new lesions. (b) Criterion for relapse is readmission for Ingram therapy. ○, on methotrexate; ●, without methotrexate. (From van de Kerkhof & Mali 1982.)

treatment period was 8 years and 11 months. The estimated mean cumulative dose was 4803 mg.

The rebound phenomenon is not characteristic for discontinuation of MTX. However, psoriasis can reappear fast, when MTX has been used for a very active and widespread disease, and in these cases a gradual reduction in dosage should be recommended before stopping the drug.

12.3.3 Results in psoriatic arthritis

This extracutaneous manifestation is considered in detail elsewhere. Several disease-modifying drugs are at the clinician's disposal. MTX is one of the most important, not only because it has a dual effect on both skin and joints. The efficacy on the arthritis was demonstrated in 1964 in a double-blind study by Black *et al.* (1964). More recently rheumatologists have overcome the fear provoked by this report due to a high incidence of side-effects, which were the results of the much higher doses than are now used. Black *et al.* gave 1–3 mg/kg bodyweight parenterally with 10 days' interval. The doses today are 7.5–15 mg in weekly oral schedules. The effect of 15 mg weekly by the Weinstein schedule can be seen in Table 12.2. The improvement could be found after 1–3 months (Zachariae & Zachariae 1987) on all of the following parameters: swelling, joint tenderness, morning stiffness, grip strength and pain. Also, erythrocyte sedimentation rate (ESR) improved significantly during this study. After discontinuation the arthritis often flares up. However, it is usually possible to reduce the dose, and continue on a long-term basis at the lowest dose that will control the complaints.

12.4 Side-effects

Serious acute toxic reactions have been recognized, but can be avoided if the drug is correctly used (Roenigk *et al.* 1988; Said *et al.* 1997). MTX may lead to long-term side-effects, mainly in the form of liver toxicity. Liver damage will

Table 12.2 ESR and clinical evaluation in 28 patients with psoriatic arthritis, before and after 3 months and 6 or twelve months with methotrexate (Zachariae & Zachariae 1987).

Evaluation ± SE	Before	3 months	6 or 12 months
ESR	43±6	17±3	17±4
No. of swollen joints	8.5±0.7	2.9±0.7	2.3±0.6
Joint tenderness score	11.5±1.3	3.5±0.6	2.0±0.5
Morning stiffness	12.5±2.4	3.4±1.2	2.4±0.9
Grip strength	10.8±1.6	6.0±1.6	6.8±1.6
Analgesic consumption	9.6±1.5	4.1±1.4	3.6±1.4
Pain assessment	3.8±0.3	1.6±0.3	1.3±0.3
General condition	3.2±0.2	2.3±0.2	1.4±0.2

Table 12.3 Side-effects of methotrexate in psoriasis.

Common and mild	Uncommon	Rare
Nausea	Fatigue	Stomatitis
Abdominal discomfort	Headache	Burning sensation
Leukopenia	Vomiting	Chills
Hepatotoxicity	Thrombocytopenia	Fever
	Liver cirrhosis (see p. 208)	Anaemia
		Dizziness
		Depression
		Hair loss
		Anorexia
		Gastrointestinal ulceration
		Agranulocytosis
		Pneumonitis
		Toxic epidermal necrolysis
		Diffuse fibrosis

be dealt with in detail. A list of side-effects is shown in Table 12.3. The most common are the subjective side-effects.

12.4.1 Subjective side-effects

These effects can be seen from the first week as well as later during treatment. Typically the symptoms arise on the day of MTX administration and within the following few days. Nausea and abdominal discomfort are common and usually mild. Fatigue, headache, dizziness, a slight loss of appetite, and vomiting are uncommon, and depression and anorexia are rare. Other rare side-effects are loss of libido and impaired memory. Decreasing the dosage is often followed by resolution, and discontinuation always gives a total disappearance of symptoms. In our hands, however, most patients can manage with metoclopramide for nausea or by taking folic acid 5 mg twice weekly. The latter may be helpful against most of the subjective side-effects. Nevertheless, there are patients with whom it is necessary to discontinue MTX permanently due to disabling subjective symptoms.

12.4.2 Haematopoietic side-effects

Haematopoietic suppression may occasionally occur, but with the dosages used in psoriasis it is not frequently encountered. Leukopenia is more frequent than thrombocytopenia. Anaemia rarely arises and agranulocytosis is an extremely rare occurrence. All haematopoietic side-effects, however, may arise as a result of overdosing with MTX, which may be the result of an unobserved decreased renal function, interaction with other drugs, or poor patient instruction. Good control of blood counts and in particular of leucocyte and thrombocyte counts is mandatory during MTX treatment.

12.4.3 Skin and mucosal complaints

Oral lesions of stomatitis are to be considered a warning sign of an overdose (Plate 12.2, facing p. 180) as is a burning sensation of the skin. The severe reaction of a toxic epidermal necrolysis is associated with overdoses brought forward by interactions (Plate 12.1).

Hair loss has been considered rare, but was found in seven of the 113 patients studied by the Nijmegen group (van Dooren-Greebe *et al.* 1994). Increased photosensitivity is not uncommon following MTX in high-dose regimens, but in general this is not a problem with the use of MTX as monotherapy in psoriasis. Roenigk *et al.* (1969) found photosensitivity in 5% of patients receiving MTX together with Goeckerman therapy.

12.4.4 Pulmonary complications

Pulmonary complications are well-known side-effects of MTX as cancer chemotherapy. Pneumonitis is feared under these circumstances, but MTX pneumonitis is rare in the treatment of psoriasis. We have reported one case (From 1975) in 531 patients. The respiratory illness is characterized by an acute onset with fever, cough, dyspnoea, cyanosis and bilateral pulmonary infiltrates. Radiography shows bilateral, diffuse, interstitial pulmonary infiltrates, which are most marked at the basis (Fig. 12.3). The histological picture is that of an allergic granulomatous pneumonitis. This MTX-induced pneumonitis can be life-threatening, but it resolves rapidly after discontinuation of the drug and treatment with glucocorticoids. MTX-induced pneumonitis appears to be far more of a risk factor in rheumatoid arthritis (Golden *et al.* 1995), especially in patients with pre-existing lung disease. Nyfors reported pulmonary infiltrates at routine chest X-rays in six out of 248 MTX-treated patients, but no pneumonitis (Nyfors 1978). This figure is not significantly different from what we have found in patients with severe psoriasis, who did not receive MTX or other immunosuppressive agents systemically (Zachariae 1979).

Pulmonary fibrosis is rare as a consequence of MTX in psoriasis.

12.4.5 Neoplasias

Because MTX is immunosuppressive, the drug theoretically carries the risk of carcinogenesis, and cases have been reported of malignancies developing in patients treated with MTX, often in combination with other agents for psoriasis or cancer (International Agency for Research on Cancer, Working Group 1981). However, although among 6910 individuals discharged from Danish hospitals with a diagnosis of psoriasis there has been observed a 2.5-fold increased risk for non-melanoma skin cancer and also a significant increase in the incidence of non-cutaneous cancer (Olsen *et al.* 1992), no excess

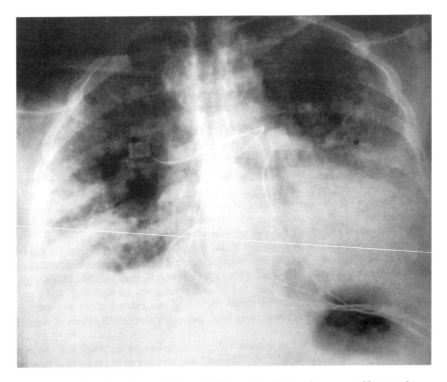

Fig. 12.3 Radiography showing bilateral, diffuse, interstitial pulmonary infiltrates of a methotrexate-induced pneumonitis. (From From 1975.)

of cancer was found in 248 Danish patients who received MTX for psoriasis (Nyfors 1978). Another study on MTX-treated psoriatic patients gave the same results (Bailin *et al.* 1975). These studies together with the analyses by Stern *et al.* (1982), in which 26 cases of non-cutaneous cancer and 80 cases of non-melanoma skin cancer and four times as many matched controls found relative risks for cancer of 0.96 for non-cutaneous and 1.2 for non-melanoma, indicate that MTX, as it is used in the treatment of severe psoriasis, does not significantly increase the risk of non-cutaneous or cutaneous malignancy.

12.4.6 Mutagenicity and teratogenicity

MTX gives negative results in the Ames test for mutagenicity (Benedict *et al.* 1977), and this has been confirmed in the white-ivory somatic mutation test (Clements *et al.* 1990), but MTX is teratogenic (Milunsky *et al.* 1968) and women should not become pregnant while taking the drug.

MTX is also still being used to terminate early pregnancies (Hausknecht 1995). The chromosomal studies have given variable results; whereas some authors have reported chromosome breaks in cultured lymphocytes from MTX-treated patients, others were unable to confirm this. Therefore, mutagenicity cannot be excluded with certainty.

We found greater differences in chromosomal studies (Nielsen & Zachariae 1973) between psoriatic patients and normal controls than between psoriatic patients receiving MTX and those not receiving systemic therapy. Oligospermi has been reported in MTX-treated psoriatic patients (Sussman & Leonard 1980), but El-Beheiry *et al.* (1979) found no deleterious effects of the drug in 26 male psoriatic patients, either in the semen, testicular histology or spermatogenic function as tested by radioactive phosphorus. Our group studied human semen in patients with psoriasis who were treated with topical steroids and in psoriatic patients who were on MTX (Grunnet *et al.* 1977). We also could not demonstrate any unfavourable effect on the semen quality during MTX therapy. In fact, the semen analyses were more frequently normal in the MTX-treated group.

So far, no malformations have been observed in the children of fathers receiving MTX near the time of the child's conception. This is in contrast to the children whose mothers were taking MTX during the first trimester of pregnancy (Briggs *et al.* 1994). Nonetheless, prudence dictates that MTX therapy without contraceptive measures should be avoided for both men and women planning to have children in the near future, and that these measures should be continued for 3 months after termination of therapy.

12.4.7 Renal complications

So far, with the dosages used in the treatment of psoriasis, renal impairment has not been reported. Kidney biopsies from 16 psoriatics treated for 1 month to 16 years with MTX (Zachariae *et al.* 1990) have been studied, using light and electron microscopy. Three of the patients were treated for more than 10 years. Fourteen of the 16 biopsies were normal, and the minor pathological changes in two biopsies were not considered to be MTX-related. Renal function has been studied earlier (Kennedy & Baker 1976), and shown to be normal.

12.4.8 Infections

In the Nijmegen study on the 113 patients treated at the department between 1970 and 1992 (van Dooren-Greebe *et al.* 1994) six patients had minor infections, and the infections were not more serious than those seen in normal subjects without immunosuppressive therapy. On the other hand, in contrast to MTX-treated psoriasis and psoriatic arthritis, opportunistic infections are increasingly reported in rheumatoid arthritis treated with low-dose MTX. This could be due to the patient group, as the infection rate during MTX treatment has been shown to be higher in severe rheumatoid arthritis than in patients with moderate disease (Boerbooms *et al.* 1995). At Aarhus we have not found infections to be a significant problem among the numerous psoriatic patients on MTX followed since 1970.

12.5 Methotrexate and the liver

Initial reports in 1955 (Colsky *et al.* 1955) on leukaemic patients were the first to indicate the hepatotoxicity of MTX. From 1968 there followed isolated cases of cirrhosis published on MTX-treated psoriatic patients (Coe & Bull 1969; Epstein & Craft 1969).

Later, cooperative (Weinstein *et al.* 1973) as well as single long-term studies (Rees *et al.* 1974; Zachariae *et al.* 1975; Nyfors 1978; Robinson *et al.* 1980; Zachariae & Søgaard 1987) confirmed that the drug may induce liver damage, which in some psoriatic patients will lead to fibrosis or cirrhosis. The biochemical basis for liver toxicity from MTX is unknown. An action on DNA is unlikely, and folate depletion has been suggested as an important factor. The changes in the livers of folate-deficient rats seem very similar to the MTX-induced liver changes of liver morphology of humans. Alcohol, an important cofactor for MTX-induced liver cirrhosis may add to the folate depletion of the liver. Polyglutamates of MTX within hepatocytes competing with hepatocyte folate polyglutamates may lead to chronic hepatocellular folate deficiency, which may be responsible for the toxicity (Barak *et al.* 1984).

12.5.1 Factors associated with methotrexate-induced liver damage

The first international study group evaluated 242 (Weinstein *et al.* 1973) and later more than 1000 (Roenigk *et al.* 1976) liver biopsy specimens. American centres continued their efforts in a prospective investigation (Roenigk *et al.* 1976) as did some European participants (Nyfors 1978; Zachariae & Søgaard 1987). The data from all these investigations indicated that increasing cumulative dosage, increased alcohol intake, the combination of diabetes and obesity, and increasing age were associated with liver damage in MTX-treated psoriatic patients. The minor abnormalities often found in pre-MTX biopsy specimens may also be a predisposing factor (Nyfors 1978; Zachariae 1991), as may a genetic factor (Olsen 1991). Previous intake of arsenic (Zachariae *et al.* 1975) and probably also long-term use of other hepatotoxic agents are similarly associated with liver damage. The general risk for increased toxicity to MTX in patients with a lowered renal function should not be forgotten (Olsen 1991). Table 12.4 shows data from eight patients from Aarhus (Zachariae *et al.* 1980), who developed liver cirrhosis before reaching a cumulative dose of 1600 mg MTX. The cumulative dose of approximately 1.5 g is an indication for performing a liver biopsy in patients without known risk factors (see later).

The international cooperative study (Weinstein *et al.* 1973) indicated that daily oral MTX therapy was associated with the highest degree of liver toxicity, but it is still unknown which of the other drug schedules is less damaging to the liver.

Table 12.4 Liver biopsy findings during methotrexate therapy in psoriasis and in control subjects.

Author	Year	n	Cumulative dose (g)	Fibrosis (%)	Cirrhoses (%)
Weinstein *et al.*	1973	200	0	22	1.5
Reese *et al.*	1974	35	0	3	0
Warin *et al.*	1975	68	0	6	1
Nyfors & Poulsen	1976	116	0	1	1
Roenigk *et al.*	1976	118	0	16	0
Zachariae *et al.*	1980	328	0	6	0.6
Ashton *et al.*	1982	38	0	0	0
Lanse *et al.**	1985	30	0	13	0
Weinstein †	1973	56799	0	–	3.05
Zachariae †	1975	60	0	7	3.3
Weinstein *et al.*	1973	372	1.8	34	3
Reese *et al.*	1974	35	2.1	31	3
Zachariae *et al.*	1975	96	1.164 ± 0.098	11	6
Nyfors & Poulsen	1976	88	0.175–4.590	6	7
Roenigk *et al.*	1977	51	Not stated	20	0
Nyfors	1977	92	0.050–5.075	7	1
Nyfors	1977	68	0.325–8.0	24	20
Robinson *et al.*	1980	43	0.35–3.56	26	0
Zachariae *et al.*	1980	183	2.2	Not stated	10
Zachariae *et al.*	1980	39	>4	Not stated	25
van de Kerkhof	1985	44	3.624 ± 2.929	16	4
Reynolds & Lee	1986	14	0.4–11	14	14
Zachariae	1986	390	2.9	Not stated	7.4
Themido *et al.*	1992	30	3.431	50	10
van Dooren-Greebe *et al.*	1994	50	4.803	13	4
Malatjalian *et al.*	1996	104	Not stated	23	3

* Included some patients with rheumatoid arthritis
† Autopsy material

In Danish long-term studies of serial biopsy specimens, 15 mg weekly by the divided intermittent oral dosage schedule (Zachariae and Søgaard 1987) seemed to give the same frequency of liver cirrhosis as a 25-mg weekly single oral dose schedule (Nyfors 1978) with approximately the same cumulative dosage. There is no difference between the two types of dosage schedules in relation to acute liver toxicity (Zachariae 1991).

12.5.2 Frequency of fibrosis and cirrhosis

There have been great variations in the reported frequencies of fibrosis and cirrhosis among the different studies on MTX-treated psoriatic patients (Table 12.4). From our own investigations (Zachariae 1991) it has appeared that with the exception of an increase in fatty infiltration all early data showed no significant differences between pre- and post-MTX biopsy specimens, and until 1975 cirrhosis was not found. At that time cirrhosis was detected in three patients (Zachariae *et al.* 1975), who had no signs of fibrosis in their pre-MTX biopsies. Our data published in 1987 (Zachariae and Søgaard), however, showed a frequency of 7.4% cirrhosis among 390 patients. The average cumulative dosage had risen from approximately 1 g to approximately 3 g.

It should be noted that among the 29 with MTX-induced liver cirrhosis, 20 were male and nine female; among all patients 195 were male and 195 female. Danish male psoriatic patients had at that time a higher alcohol consumption than female psoriatic patients (Grunnet 1974). Besides alcohol a high number of patients previously treated with arsenic and vitamin A (Zachariae 1991) could be a contributing factor to the relatively high frequency of cirrhosis in our group of patients.

Following the introduction of PIIINP in our control, and the decision to change to other therapies if a liver biopsy, taken subsequently to two increased PIIINP values, showed development of more than slight fibrosis, no new cases of MTX-induced liver cirrhosis have been found at our department.

12.5.3 Severity of methotrexate-induced liver cirrhosis

Data on serial liver biopsy specimens from 25 patients with MTX-induced liver cirrhosis were published by Zachariae and Søgaard in 1987. The patients were cirrhotic patients whose disease could not be controlled at the time of diagnosis by other means than MTX. They agreed to stop alcohol consumption or to limit their intake to an absolute minimum. Twenty-one received continued but reduced dosages prior to their latest biopsy. The cumulative dosages appear in Table 12.5. In 14 patients, an absence of cirrhosis was found in the latest biopsy specimen (Fig. 12.4), and in most patients there was a trend for later specimens to be of the same rather low grading as the original, or even lower, irrespective of continued treatment. This led us to conclude that the MTX-induced liver cirrhosis in general is not of an aggressive nature. This suggestion is supported by Baker (1982), who states that the patients he found to have cirrhosis have done well for years after MTX was stopped; and by Newman *et al.* (1989), who found meaningful improvement in histology in their patients with fibrosis and/or cirrhosis after MTX treatment had been withdrawn for 6 months or more.

In 1996 Zachariae *et al.* 1996 published a further 10-year follow-up on the same patients that were studied in 1985 and reported on in 1987 (Zachariae & Søgaard 1987).The investigations were carried out on 186 liver biopsies and five autopsies. Eleven of 12 surviving patients were also studied by PIIINP, which is in indicator of ongoing fibrogenesis. Two patients were still on MTX. Thirteen patients had died; one of these died of liver failure. Another patient died from an overdose due to misunderstanding of the prescribed dosage given elsewhere. The remaining deaths were non-MTX related, but all five autopsies showed some degree of cirrhosis. On the other hand, 13 had no histologically verified liver cirrhosis in their latest biopsy, and PIIINP was within normal range in all patients investigated, this in spite of total cumulative doses from 1 to 18.5 g (mean 7.2 g). We believe that the study confirmed that in most patients the MTX-induced liver cirrhosis is not aggressive. The lack of agreement between autopsies and the same patients' latest biopsies could partly be due to sampling error in a biopsy. However, continued low-dose MTX in an 84-year-old female led, in spite of normal liver tests, 8 years after the last biopsy to liver failure and death. PIIINP was unfortunately not available at that time, and we had decided to stop taking biopsies as her ordinary liver tests were all normal, and the dosages given varied between 2.5 and 7.5 mg weekly only.

12.5.4 Monitoring hepatic toxicity

This consists initially of a weekly, and later monthly, check-up of liver enzymes, with twice-yearly estimation of the alkaline phosphatases. Until recently, our department advocated serial liver biopsies at intervals of 1–1.5 years, depending on whether the patient belonged to a risk group or not, and on the findings of a preceding biopsy, when present. We also, as recommended in the guidelines (see p. 218) advised at least performing a first liver biopsy, when the cumulative dose of MTX reached 1.5 g.

Liver biopsies

The morbidity of liver biopsies were reported in the 1980s to range from 0.02 to 10% (Creswell & Burrows 1980; Sherlock *et al.* 1985; Piccinio *et al.* 1986) and the mortality to 0.01–0.1%. These figures are probably lower in psoriatic patients on MTX. In our hands we have had five cases of cholascus, of which two led to surgery, in more than 2000 liver biopsies, and no mortalities.

Haemorrhage, pneumothorax and sepsis were not recorded. On the other hand, besides obtaining a liver biopsy in eight cases, we also accidentally obtained a renal biopsy (Zachariae *et al.* 1976). We had until the introduction of the use of PIIINP found the risk of performing a biopsy outweighed by the risk of liver failure secondary to unmonitored MTX use.

Recommendations concerning the continuation or discontinuation of MTX are commonly based upon the following classification.

Grade I: Normal; mild fatty infiltration, nuclear variability and portal inflammation.

Table 12.5 Clinical, histological and serological information from 25 patients with methotrexate-induced liver cirrhosis. From Zachariae *et al.* 1996. Patient numbers are the same as in Zachariae *et al.* 1980 and Zachariae & Søgaard 1987, where the patients were studied at earlier stages. The age of the patients corresponds to the latest visit or age at death. There was no liver related death except for patient 18 (see p. 211). PIIINP normal range: 1.7–4.2 µg/L; 10 of these determinations were performed within a year of the study.

Pat. No	Sex/age	Cumulative MTX doses (mg)			Death	Cirrhosis in latest biopsy	No. of biopsies (total)	Observation after cirrhosis (years)	PIIINP µg/L.
		Before cirrhosis	At latest biopsy	In all					
1	M/78	810	5140	5980	-	-	15	23	2.7
2	M/70	1270	1775	1775	+	-	7	14	-
3	F/50	3250	5905	6325	+	-	10	10	-
4	M/81	3685	5930	6080	+	-	11	12	-
5	M/82	590	2780	2840	+	-	7	8	-
6	M/80	3080	10920	13 250*		-	11	16	4.1
7	F/44	3710	15790	17 470*		-	11	22	3.7
8	F/82	1465	2165	2165		+	8	19	3.4
9	M/72	8105	18645	18 645	+	+†	9	19	3.6
10	M/77	3290	5980	7660		+	11	12	2.3

No.	Sex/Age								
11	M/73	2145	3030	3450	+	++†	6	5	-
12	F/79	1720	4870	4870	+	-	5	10	-
13	M/86	1680	2030	2030		+	5	5	4.0
14	M/78	1000	1000	1000	+	+	5	11	-
15	M/56	1720	5080	5455		+	5	5	-
16	M/26	1025	4045	4295		-	7	18	4.2
17	M/79	1120	1120	1120		+	4	24	2.7
18	F/84	1680	2380	4060	++‡	++†	8	8	-
19	F/66	5600	7280	7280	+	++†	9	15	3.1
20	F/78	1900	2080	2080	+	-	5	3	-
21	M/66	6720	8400	8580	+	++†	8	6	2.7
22	F/70	3000	3910	3910		+	7	11	-
23	M/74	8000	8000	8000	+	-	3	10	-
24	F/64	9980	15180	17000		-	11	13	3.2
25	M/68	1745	1745	1745	+	-	3	4	-

*Still under MTX treatment at end of study.

†At autopsy.

‡Died in liver failure.

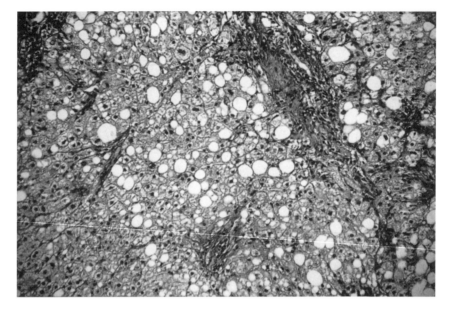

(a)

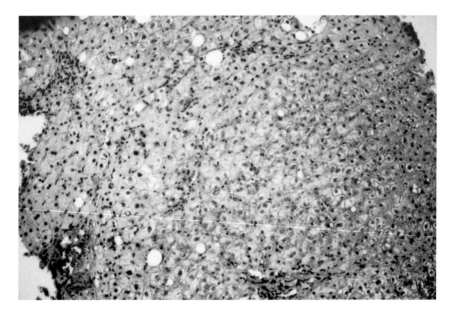

(b)

Fig. 12.4 (a) Liver biopsy specimen with active cirrhosis showing collagenous fibres, moderately destroyed liver cell parenchyma, and steatosis. (b) Liver biopsy specimen from the same patient as in (a) performed 6 years later and following treatment with further 5.5 g methotrexate and abstention from alcohol. The biopsy shows improvement with disappearing cirrhosis.

Grade II: Moderate to severe fatty infiltration, nuclear variability, portal tract expansion, portal tract inflammation and necrosis.

Grade III: (A) Mild fibrosis; (B) Moderate to severe fibrosis.

Grade IV: Cirrhosis.

The recommendations have been that patients with grade I and II may continue with MTX. Patients with grade IIIA may continue, but should have a new liver biopsy after approximately 6 months; and patients with grade IV should discontinue MTX, unless exceptional circumstances require further MTX therapy, and then this should be done with careful follow-up liver biopsies. We also still will advocate performing liver biopsies, but find that the number of necessary biopsies can be reduced significantly by the use of either one of two promising screening procedures: serum PIIINP measurement and dynamic hepatic scintigraphy. Several other attempts have been made earlier in the search for non-invasive screening; and the use of the galactose tolerance test, ultrasound, static scintigraphy of the liver, magnetic resonance imaging, and measurements of MTX and folate concentrations in erythrocytes have all previously been reviewed and reported as not sufficiently reliable (Zachariae 1991). The salivary antipyrine clearance was correlated with fatty changes in the liver but not with fibrosis (Paramsothy *et al.* 1988). Many rheumatologists who use MTX for rheumatoid arthritis have maintained that liver biopsies are unnecessary, and this assumption has also been the basis for the guidelines for the monitoring of patients with rheumatoid arthritis who are receiving MTX (Kremer *et al.* 1994).

A meta-analysis, however, of 636 rheumatoid patients showed, that 24% progressed to some fibrosis and 2.7% to cirrhosis (Whiting-O'Keefe *et al.* 1991). The lower frequency of cirrhosis in rheumatoid patients may be related to the higher number of women than men in rheumatoid arthritis studies, since women tend to consume less alcohol than men. Also, lower doses of MTX are usually used in rheumatoid arthritis than in psoriasis. Besides, there could also be a genetic factor, which together with the longer duration of the experience in psoriasis could be, in part, responsible for the differences.

Measurement of serum PIIINP

In collaboration with the researchers who developed a new rapid equilibrium type of radioimmunoassay for this purpose (Risteli *et al.* 1988), we have found good indications that analyses of PIIINP in serum, although the test is not organ specific, can be utilized as a valuable non-invasive marker of fibrogenesis in liver in MTX-treated psoriatic treatments. This had already been established in other chronic liver diseases (Frei *et al.* 1984). In hepatic fibrosis there is an increased synthesis and deposition of predominantly type III collagen. The assay measures the amino-terminal procollagen propeptides, which are cleaved off during collagen synthesis, and released into the circulation. In another study (Zachariae *et al.* 1988) 72 psoriatic patients were investigated by liver biopsy and PIIINP during MTX treatment, whereas 11 patients studied prior to treatment had no biopsy taken (Fig. 12.5). PIIINP from these two groups were compared with results from 127 healthy controls. Patients with fibrosis or cirrhosis in their liver had a mean PIIINP value of 5.2 ± 1.5 µg/L. This differed significantly from PIIINP in psoriasis without fibrosis, who had an average of 3.3 ± 0.6 µg/L, and from psoriasis investigated prior to MTX with an average of 3.4 ± 0.7 µg/L; these two groups had results similar to the healthy controls (Table 12.6).

In a further study in 170 patients with psoriasis including patients with psoriatic arthritis (Zachariae *et al.* 1991) these differences were confirmed; however, 38% of patients with arthritis had an increase in PIIINP in the absence of detectable liver fibrosis. Our conclusion was that in arthritic patients an increase in PIIINP may be related to the joint disease, and that for

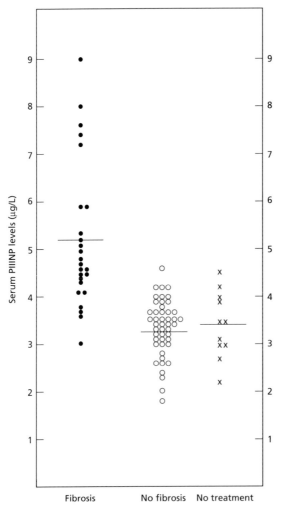

Fig. 12.5 Serum PIIINP levels in methotrexate-treated psoriatics fibrosis and/or cirrhosis in their liver biopsies, methotrexate-treated psoriatics without liver fibrosis, and psoriatics investigated prior to methotrexate. All values are in µg/L. (From Zachariae *et al.* 1988.)

Table 12.6 Exclusion criteria for methotrexate in psoriasis.

Pregnancy
Renal impairment
Recent hepatitis
Pre-methotrexate cirrhosis or pronounced liver fibrosis
Excessive alcohol intake
Patient unreliability
Unwillingness to adopt control measures
Unwillingness to use contraception
Active peptic ulcer
Severe infection
Pronounced anaemia
Leukopenia
Thrombocytopenia

these patients therefore the established guidelines should be followed for taking liver biopsies during MTX therapy of psoriasis (Roenigk *et al.* 1988). Two other groups have studied PIIINP as an indicator for development of liver fibrosis in MTX-treated psoriatic patients. Van Dooren-Greebe *et al.* (1996) from Nijmegen studied the value of dynamic hepatic scintigraphy together with PIIINP in 25 MTX patients. Their conclusion was that although a global relationship was demonstrated between PIIINP and hepatic damage, single measurements were not reliable. Mitchell *et al.* (1990) found similar results, when studying 51 patients. In 1996, however, the same group (Boffa *et al.* 1996) after studying patients for up to 6 years, and with a total of 87 patients, demonstrated that the patients with inflammation, fibrosis or cirrhosis had significantly higher levels than patients with normal histology or steatosis alone ($P < 0.0001$), and that among the patients with 3-monthly serum samples PIIINP was elevated at some time in all three patients who developed abnormal histology, but was consistently normal in eight of 11 patients whose histology remained or became normal. Their conclusion therefore was the same as ours (Zachariae *et al.* 1991), that as long as PIIINP remains normal in serial investigations, there seems to be no great risk of the development of a substantial liver fibrosis or cirrhosis, and that the number of liver biopsies in patients on MTX with continued normal PIIINP may be reduced to a minimum. We have not found any substantial fibrosis or cirrhosis developing among this category of patients since we began using PIIINP.

Dynamic hepatic scintigraphy

The study by van Dooren-Greebe *et al.* (1996) on dynamic hepatic scintigraphy in 22 patients showed that this new non-invasive technique can be valuable for sparing liver biopsies. The technique could not be used for the determination of severity of liver damage, but it showed that a demonstrated portal contribution of $> 52\%$ was associated with a $> 95\%$ chance of a liver biopsy classification grade I. With this cut-off value of 52%, it would have been possible to reduce the number of liver biopsies to at least 55% in the patients with a normal liver histology. Without doubt this promising new technique should be further explored.

12.6 Guidelines for methotrexate therapy

Indications and contraindications for the use of MTX in psoriasis as well as the way to monitor therapy has been presented in international guidelines (Roenigk *et al.* 1988; British Association of Dermatologists 1991). The guidelines presented below are apart from the already mentioned discrepancies concerning liver biopsies, and a few minor details in line with the international guidelines.

12.6.1 Indications

The decision to administer MTX should be individualized. Each patient should be evaluated with reference to disease severity, amount of discomfort, degree of incapacity and general medical and psychological conditions. The psoriasis should be severe and not adequately controlled by standard topical antipsoriatic therapy. In psoriatic arthritis it will be the first drug of choice for patients with active disease requiring disease-modifying agents.

12.6.2 Contraindications

Normal kidney, liver and bone-marrow functioning are prerequisites for MTX treatment. Pregnancy and alcohol abuse are absolute contraindications, as are active peptic ulcers or severe infections Exclusion criteria for MTX are given in Table 12.6. Circumstances may arise in which contraindications must be waived, such as when benefits can be expected to outweigh the risks of therapy in an individual patient, where another systemic treatment for one reason or the other cannot be used. Interfering mechanisms should be dealt with. Drug interactions are listed in Table 12.1. The most important are those with sulphonamides, especially if combined with trimethoprim, and salicylates. Concomitant medication with these two medications are absolutely contraindicated. The exception is low-dose aspirin therapy with 100–150 mg daily. Non-steroidal anti-inflammatory agents should be avoided on MTX-treatment days.

12.6.3 Premethotrexate screening

History

There should be a complete search for contraindications. It is the responsibility of the physician that MTX is not given to a pregnant woman, and it is recommended to perform a pregnancy test in any woman in the reproductive years, who is not using a safe method of contraception. Contraception is as already mentioned required during treatment and until 3 months following discontinuation of the drug. The history concerning risk factors for liver disease should include past and present intake of alcohol, past or present abnormal results of liver chemistry, history of any liver disease, previous or present use of known hepatotoxic drugs, and diabetes. Signs of obesity should be observed and registered.

It is of utmost importance that the patient is reliable and cooperative. Advice regarding alcohol intake, concomitant medication, contraception, precise MTX intake, and the importance of regular visits and laboratory control should be given, preferably in writing, and be taken seriously. Previous high intake of alcohol is not an absolute contraindication in a patient with normal liver function tests.

It is preferable that the patient abstains from alcohol intake during MTX therapy, but up to three units of alcohol per week can be allowed.

Laboratory investigations

Table 12.7 shows the laboratory examinations before and during the MTX

Table 12.7 Recommended laboratory examinations before and during methotrexate treatment of psoriasis.

Before therapy
      Haemoglobin, leucocyte and differential count, thrombocyte count
      Urine analyses, serum creatinine, creatinine clearance or preferable GFR
        (glomerular filtration rate)
      Liver transaminases, alkaline phosphatases, bilirubin
      PIIINP (if available)
      Serum albumin
      Chest radiography

During therapy
      Weekly to monthly
      Leucocyte and thrombocyte counts
      Liver transaminases

      Two to three times yearly
      Haemoglobin
      Alkaline phosphatases
      PIIINP (if available)
      Serum creatinine

      Yearly
      Creatinine clearance or preferable GFR
      Serum albumin
      Chest radiography

      At least after 1.5 g accumulated methotrexate
      Liver biopsy (see also p. 211)

---

treatment which we recommend. A creatinine clearance can with advantage be exchanged with glomerular filtration rate (GFR), i.e. by chromium EDTA clearance. We do not recommend pretreatment liver biopsies unless one is dealing with a high risk factor for liver disease. If available we recommend a baseline PIIINP.

Choice of dosage schedule and dose

The possible advantages of usage of one or the other of the two most common dosage schedules has already been discussed (see p. 200). Some authors (Roenigk *et al.* 1988) advise a test dose of 5–10 mg to avoid hypersensitivity reactions or rather any unusual sensitivity to toxic effects. Over the many years that we have used MTX, we have only done this in elderly patients, and have not encountered situations where we have regretted not having performed the test dose. With the divided oral dose schedule we would start with 5 mg at 12-h intervals for three doses each week to the average adult weighing approximately 70 kg, and reduce according to weight, with the lowest dose being 2.5 mg for each of the three doses. With the single weekly dose, we would normally not go above 25 mg per week. Occasional patients, however, will need a maximum of 37.5 mg/week. For parenteral treatment see p. 201.

12.6.4 Observations during therapy

Visits and laboratory investigations

A first visit 1–2 weeks after initiation of therapy is suitable. Further controls should be performed with 1–3-month intervals. The laboratory investigations required for control are shown in Table 12.8. We perform leucocyte and thrombocyte counts and liver transaminases initially weekly, later monthly. Every 3 months we include haemoglobin and alkaline phophatases. At least twice yearly we study PIIINP, and once yearly we study serum creatinine and preferably also GFR. Serum albumin is recommended yearly. Chest radiography should be undertaken yearly.

A liver biopsy is recommended after a cumulative dose of 1.5 g MTX. If increased PIIINP appears more than once during therapy, we recommend a liver biopsy be taken even if the 1.5-g level has not been reached. The guidelines (Roenigk *et al.* 1988) for patients having prolonged, significant abnormalities in liver chemistry values or one or more risk factors recommend an early liver biopsy and repeat liver biopsies at 1.0–1.5-g intervals of further cumulative MTX doses. They also advise repeat liver biopsies with the same intervals following the first 'normal biopsy'. We believe that with continuous normal PIIINP the number of repeat biopsies as a whole can be reduced to a minimum. Recently we decided to reduce them to be performed with a 5-

Table 12.8 Risks for increased toxicity potential in combination therapy with methotrexate.

Mechanism	Drugs
Additive immunosuppressive effects	Cyclosporin Corticosteroids
Additive antihaematopoietic effect	Azathioprine Hydroxycarbamide Other cytotoxic drugs
Additive carcinogenesis	Cyclosporin PUVA UVB
Enhanced MTX-toxicity due to decrease of MTX elimination	Cyclosporin
Increased hepatotoxicity	Retinoids (Cyclosporin?)
Increased phototoxicity	PUVA UVB

year interval. Probably they may be omitted in this group of patients. In all other cases we follow the guidelines.

Interpretation of laboratory studies

The clinical interpretation of liver biopsy results are shown on p. 211. A significant reduction in leucocyte and platelet counts necessitates reduction or temporary discontinuation of MTX therapy. It should be noted that the maximum depression usually occurs 7–10 days after a dose of MTX.

Leukopenia below 3.5×10^9/L continuing beyond 1 week needs special attention and in general discontinuation; the same applies to thrombocyte counts below 100×10^9/L. If the counts have returned to normal 2 weeks after discontinuation, MTX can be reinstituted with half dosage. Anaemia can be due to folate depletion, and in that case the depletion should be compensated.

Minor increases in liver enzymes can be tolerated, but persistent minor increases as well as major increases of 100% or more should lead to reduction in dose or temporary discontinuation. The patient's alcohol consumption should also be re-explored, and if necessary forbidden or adjusted. If a persistent abnormality lasts beyond 2 or 3 months a liver biopsy is recommended. Increases in PIIINP to pathological values more than once indicate liver biopsies to be performed according to the established guidelines (Roenigk *et al.* 1988).

Reductions in kidney function should, if they are mild, be compensated by reducing the dose. With a reduction in creatinine clearance to less than 50 mL/min MTX treatment should be stopped.

12.6.5 Dosage management during therapy

Dosage reductions according to laboratory findings have already been mentioned. They may also be necessary due to subjective side-effects, but in a number of cases the introduction of folic acid 5 mg twice weekly may be sufficient; other patients will benefit by methoclopramide for nausea. With an optimal doctor–patient relationship many minor complaints especially in anxious patients can be handled by counselling.

A 100% clearing should not be the aim of treatment. What can be expected is an improvement to approximately 75% clearing, and thereby a pronounced improvement in quality of life. The maximum effect will be found after a couple of months, this applies to both psoriasis and psoriatic arthritis. The goal of MTX in psoriatic arthritis is to arrest progression.

Most patients will experience reduction of pain and tenderness, less swelling, a decrease in morning stiffness and an improvement in grip strength if the hands are involved (see Table 12.1). Long-term treatment beyond the clearance phase of psoriasis and consolidation phase of arthritis will usually permit a gradual reduction in dose. Dosage reductions, unless for side-effects, should take place gradually over weeks and months in order to keep an optimal result.

If an overdose is given or taken by mistake or occurs in relation to interaction or decreased renal function, it should be countered within 12–24 h at the most by the antidote leucovorin, 6–12 mg i.m. every 6 h for four doses.

12.6.6 Concomitant therapy

The use of any drug in addition to MTX should be carefully evaluated. Interaction problems have already been discussed. The use of corticosteroids systemically together with MTX has been discouraged, and several authors claim a direct contraindication (Baker 1976; Roenigk *et al.* 1988). There are, however, situations where the combination can be justified for a short period, i.e. when introducing MTX in a patient already on systemic steroids for an erythroderma. It is also justified to give a patient with a severe and painful psoriatic arthritis non-steroidal anti-inflammatory agents together with MTX until the MTX effect appears, as long as the drug is not administered on MTX treatment days. MTX in combination therapy will be dealt with below. The combination with retinoids has already been mentioned in relation to interaction. The use of topical therapy with calcipotriol or topical steroids together with MTX should be encouraged in order to keep the long-term maintenance dose of MTX as low as possible.

12.7 Combination therapy

The degree of improvement following conventional systemic single-drug therapy may be impressive, but none of the drugs we use is curative, and every so often they do fail to clear the patient sufficiently within the dose range possible; therefore, combined approaches have been sought. These approaches are in accordance with experience gained in cancer chemotherapy and combined immunosuppressive therapy in organ transplantation, and suggest that it may be possible sometimes to increase efficacy while minimizing side-effects. In other instances, however, there may be risks of increased toxicity (Table 12.8). The following discussion will focus on some of the various possible treatment combinations that have included the use of MTX. The combinations have in general been found empirically because of lack of sufficient knowledge about combined pharmacodynamics and pharmacokinetics.

12.7.1 Methotrexate and topical therapy

Many patients on MTX are so well managed by the drug that they discontinue their topical therapy. Topical therapy, however, should generally be encouraged to help keep the MTX dose as low as possible. This is an assumption and is not based on controlled studies. It applies to the most common combination, MTX and topical steroids, as well as to the combinations MTX and dithranol, and MTX and tar preparations. At the department of dermatology of Marselisborg hospital in Aarhus, we have often added MTX to patients treated with tar on an inpatient basis to shorten their stay at the hospital, when hospitalization seemed likely to exceed a 4-week period. In these cases, the tar-resistant lesions cleared quickly, and the same applied to dithranol-based therapies.

Combined topical calcipotriene ointment 0.005% and various systemic therapies including MTX in treatment of plaque-type psoriasis was studied by a survey sent to academic and psoriasis treatment centre-based dermatologists who treat approximately 4000 psoriasis patients per month (Katz 1997). The survey requested that the dermatologists related their experience regarding the safety and efficacy of the combined treatment after 8 weeks of therapy. The conclusion was that the combination therapy with ointment and acitretin/etretinate, cyclosporin, MTX or phototherapy usually enhances efficacy, while improving the risk/benefit ratio by decreasing exposure to the systemic agent.

12.7.2 Methotrexate and cyclosporin

While this combination has been widely used by rheumatologists in rheumatoid arthritis as well as in psoriatic arthritis with favourable results (Mazzanti *et al.* 1994; Haagsma & van Riel 1997; Stein *et al.* 1997) and without serious problems, in dermatology it has been the advice that MTX and cyclosporin can be a dangerous combination (Korstanje *et al.* 1990), or that the drugs may be combined for short periods if one is converting a patient from MTX to cyclosporin or converting from cyclosporin to MTX (Roenigk 1994). Naturally one should be concerned about an abnormal renal function, which can occur from cyclosporin, and what effect this could have on MTX toxicity, and for this reason use a lower MTX dose, i.e. 2.5 mg three times with 12-h intervals once weekly. We have used the combination of MTX and cyclosporin in single patients for up to 1½ years without problems, when adhering to the guidelines for the two drugs. The indication was that it was not possible to control the patient's psoriasis with any of the two drugs within the recommended dose ranges or without unacceptable toxicity.

The mechanism of action of cyclosporin on T cells inhibiting IL-2, interferon-γ and IL-3, combined with an effect of MTX acting on IL-1 could suggest combined biological effects.

The effect could, however, also be due to cyclosporin-induced changes in MTX elimination (decreased GFR). An MTX–cyclosporin combination study group in a double-blind, cross-over study found MTX + cyclosporin superior to MTX + placebo in rheumatoid arthritis (Stein et al. 1997a). Similar controlled studies are lacking in psoriasis and/or psoriatic arthritis. The use of a combination of two drugs that may each result in liver toxicity raises the concern that additive hepatoxicity might occur with the combination therapy; however, the addition of cyclosporin to MTX in a 24-week trial in rheumatoid arthritis only resulted in a clinically unimportant increase in bilirubin and alkaline phosphatase concentrations, but did not affect livertransaminase concentrations (Stein et al. 1997b), thus suggesting that additive liver toxicity in the short term is unlikely. This fits with the assumption that the hepatotoxicity of the two drugs occurs through different mechanisms, for cyclosporin the most well known are through cholestasis and decreased biliary flow (Edwards et al. 1995). An increase in serum creatinine in patients on MTX + cyclosporin in comparison with MTX + placebo (Mazzanti et al. 1994; Stein et al. 1997) is only what can be expected, otherwise side-effects have not been substantially increased. It is too early to report if the combination will lead to a reduced frequency of morphological renal changes in these patients in relation to findings in psoriatic patients treated with cyclosporin alone (Zachariae et al. 1997). As well as renal and liver toxicity, the risk for malignancies should be considered in long-term follow-up.

12.7.3 Methotrexate and retinoids

Vanderveen et al. (1982) and Adams (1983) were the first to describe the benefits of this combination. Since the first reports a number of other patients have benefited from receiving MTX together with retinoids (Luderschmidt & Balda 1983; Rosenbaum & Roenigk 1984; Zachariae 1986), including patients with pustular psoriasis, Reiters's disease and pityriasis rubra pilaris. In our department, however, we have warned against the combination because two of 10 patients on the combination developed life-threaten-ing hepatitis, and in a pharmacological study Larsen *et al.* (1990) found that retinoids increase the maximum plasma concentration of MTX. If the combi-nation is to be tried, we recommend low acitretin or etretinate doses from 25 mg twice weekly to 25 mg daily and MTX not over 10–15 mg weekly by the divided intermittent oral dosage, and prolonged use of weekly laboratory controls, including liver enzymes, leucocytes and thrombocytes, even if the patient has been on MTX for long periods.

12.7.4 Methotrexate and PUVA or UVB

These treatments are certainly effective (Morison *et al.* 1982; Paul *et al.* 1982; Bronner & Morison 1986), and the combination of MTX and PUVA results in clearing at a considerably lower amount of UVA and psoralen than with PUVA alone (Morison *et al.* 1982). It should, however, be borne in mind that the possibility exists of a synergistic effect on tumour promotion (Fitzsimons *et al.* 1983), and that MTX may increase light sensitivity, which again may lead to phototoxic reactions (Plate 12.3, facing p. 180). Prolonged phototoxic re-actions have also been reported (Morison *et al.* 1982). When deciding to use MTX together with PUVA or switching from MTX to PUVA due to liver toxic-ity on MTX, it may be prudent to remember a case report with acute hepatic failure appearing during PUVA in a psoriatic patient with a prior MTX-in-duced cirrhosis (Markin *et al.* 1993). Submassive necrosis superimposed on cirrhosis appeared to produce the hepatic failure.

Patients have been treated with a 3-week course of MTX followed by a combination of UVB and MTX (Paul *et al.* 1982). MTX was stopped when the patient's skin was clear and maintenance was with UVB alone.

It must, however, be expected that if the patient has a severe psoriasis, it will often be necessary to restart MTX after reducing UVB. It was stated that no signs of the so-called recall of UV-induced erythema (Møller 1970) was seen in the study (Paul *et al.* 1982).

12.7.5 Methotrexate and other cytotoxic agents

Although combination treatment with several cytotoxic drugs is common in anticancer therapy, it has generally been recommended not to use such com-binations in psoriasis (van de Kerkhof 1986). Previously, when the available systemic therapies for psoriasis and psoriatic arthritis were limited, we found it justifiable to add azathioprine to MTX in cases of psoriatic arthritis, which did not respond sufficiently to MTX alone (Zachariae 1986), and have found benefit on the arthritis without any effect on psoriasis itself.

Hydroxycarbamide has also been used in combination with MTX. Sauer (1973) reported a satisfactory clinical response in 13 patients given the two drugs together in half their usual dosage, and also reported that no worsening

of laboratory results occurred in 11 patients. In this study, the MTX maintenance dose was close to that commonly used when MTX is given alone. With
hydroxycarbamide, as with azathioprine, the main risk of the combination
therapy is bone-marrow impairment. Levels of haemoglobin, white cells and
platelets may all be depressed, and anaemia is common during hydroxycarbamide therapy. Hepatotoxicity is not uncommon in treatment with azathioprine, but is not found following hydroxycarbamide.

12.7.6 Methotrexate and systemic corticosteroids

Corticosteroids administered systemically together with MTX should be
avoided where possible to prevent unintentionally induced immunosuppressive effects (van de Kerkhof 1986). However, there are situations where such
a combination may be considered. We have used the combination in patients
with a very severe, active and painful psoriatic arthritis, where other MTX
combination therapies for one or other reasons have not been available. The
combination was employed until the MTX effect on the arthritis appeared
after a couple of months. The steroid was then reduced gradually without
any problems, and especially without any rebound phenomenon. It should
be noted that dermatologists are accustomed to the use of combinations of
cytotoxic drugs and corticosteroids in a number of autoimmune diseases,
and often for much longer periods. It should also be noted that immunosuppression today is considered a part of the antipsoriatic effect of drugs, and
that we only advocate short-term use.

12.8 General considerations

The revised guidelines for MTX therapy in psoriasis (Roenigk *et al.* 1988; Edwards
et al. 1995) are recommendations that generally should be followed, although
as can be seen some suggestions for revision have been brought forward. It is
of the greatest importance that the patients are given clear and correct instruc-
tions. If these principles are adhered to, the risk for the patient is low. In almost
all of the few cases published (Baker 1976) that have had a fatal outcome, a
violation of the rules had occurred. MTX is, as already mentioned, the drug
used for systemic treatment of psoriasis that has by far the longest history.
When patients and physicians, often after much debate, have decided to use it,
there is a very high degree of compliance together with a high degree of efficacy. With the rising costs of medication both for the individual and for society
as a whole, it is worth comparing prices for the available systemic therapies for
psoriasis. Four years ago we found the monthly costs of MTX in US dollars to
be 75, against 170 for acitretin and 290 for cyclosporin (Zachariae 1993). Since
then, no greater changes in prices have appeared. If the rules for good control
are adhered to, the risk/benefit ratio for the drug is still very favourable, and
MTX should be considered one of the most valuable agents in psoriasis therapy.

References

Adams, J. (1983) Concurrent MTX and etretinate therapy for psoriasis. *Archives of Dermatology* **119**, 793.

Anderson, L., Collins, G., Ojima, Y. & Sullivan, R. (1970) A study of the distribution of methotrexate in human tissues and tumors. *Cancer Research* **30**, 1344–1348.

Ashton R., Millward-Sadler G. & White J. (1982) Complications in methotrexate treatment of psoriasis with particular reference to liver fibrosis. *Journal of Investigative Dermatology* **79**, 229–232.

Bailin, P., Tindall, J., Roenigk, H. & Hogan, M. (1975) Is methotrexate therapy for psoriasis carcinogenic? A modified retrospective-prospective analysis. *Journal of the American Medical Association* **232**, 359–362.

Baker, H. (1976) Methotrexate the conservative treatment for psoriasis. In: *Psoriasis: Proceedings of the Second International Symposium* (eds Farber, E. & Cox, A.), pp. 235–245. York Medical Books, New York.

Baker, H. (1982) Antimitotic drugs in psoriasis. In: *Psoriasis: Proceedings of the 3rd International Symposium* (eds Farber, E. & Cox, A.), pp. 119–126. Grune & Stratton, New York.

Barak, A., Tuma, D. & Beckenhauer, H. (1984) Methotrexate hepatotoxicity. *Journal of the American College of Nutrition* **3**, 93–96.

Benedict, W., Baker, L., Haroon, L., Choi, E. & Ames, B. (1977) Mutagenicity of cancer therapeutic agents in the salmonella/microsome test. *Cancer Research* **37**, 2209–2213.

Bjerring, P., Beck, H., Zachariae, H. & Søgaard, H. (1986) Topical treatment of psoriatic skin with methotrexate cream: a clinical, pharmacokinetic and histological study. *Acta Dermato-Venereologica* **66**, 515–519.

Black, R., Van O'Brien, W., Scott, E. *et al.* (1964) Methotrexate therapy in psoriatic arthritis. *Journal of the American Medical Association* **189**, 743–747.

Bleyer, W. (1978) The clinical pharmacology of methotrexate: New applications of an old drug. *Cancer* **41**, 35–51.

Boerbooms, A., van Kerstens, P., Loenhout, J., Mulder, J. & van de Putte, L. (1995) Infections during low-dose methotrexate treatment in rheumatoid arthritis. *Seminars in Arthritis and Rheumatism* **4**, 411–421.

Boffa, M., Smith, A., Chalmers, R. *et al.* (1996) Serum type III procollagen aminopeptide for assessing liver damage in methotrexate-treated psoriatic patients. *British Journal of Dermatology* **135**, 538–544.

Boomla, K., Aherne, G., Greaves, M. & Quinton, M. (1979) Radioimmunoassayable methotrexate concentrations in plasma and skin exudate of patients with psoriasis. *Clinical Experimental Dermatology* **4**, 457–463.

Briggs, G., Freeman, R. & Yaffe, S. (1994) *Drugs in Pregnancy and Lactation*, pp. 568–572. Williams & Wilkins, Baltimore.

British Association of Dermatologists (1991) Guidelines for management of patients with psoriasis. *British Medical Journal* **303**, 829–835.

Bronner, A. & Morison, W. (1986) Combination methotrexate, PUVA and UVB therapy in the treatment of psoriasis. *Photodermatology* **3**, 245–246.

Calabresi, P. & Parks, R. (1985) Antiproliferative agents and drugs used for immunosuppression. In: *The Pharmacological Basis of Therapeutics* (eds Gilman, A. & Goodman, L.), 7th edn, pp. 1263–1267. Macmillan, New York.

Chang, D., Baptiste, P. & Schur, P. (1990) The effect of antirheumatic drugs on interleukin 1 (IL-1) activity and IL-1 and IL-1 inhibitor production by human monocytes. *Journal of Rheumatology* **17**, 1148–1157.

Clements, J., Howe, D., Lowry, A. & Philips, M. (1990) The effects of a range of anticancer drugs in the white-ivory somatic mutation test in Drosophilia. *Mutation Research* **228**, 171–176.

Coe, R. & Bull, F. (1969) Cirrhosis associated with methotrexate treatment of psoriasis. *Journal of the American Medical Association* **1969** (206), 1515–1520.

Collins, P. & Rogers, S. (1992) The efficacy of methotrexate in psoriasis—a review of 40 cases. *Clinical Experimental Dermatology* **17**, 257–260.

Colsky, J., Greenspan, E. & Warren, T. (1955) Hepatic fibrosis in children with acute leukemia after therapy with folic acid antagonists. *Archives of Pathology* **59**, 198.

Comaish, S. & Juhlin, L. (1969) Site of action of methotrexate in psoriasis. *Archives of Dermatology* **100**, 99–105.

Cream, J. & Poll, D. (1980) The effect of methotrexate and hydroxyurea on neutrophil chemotaxis. *British Journal of Dermatology* **102**, 557–563.

Creswell, S. & Burrows, D. (1980) Liver biopsies in psoriatics—complications and evaluation. *International Journal of Dermatology* **19**, 217–219.

Cronstein, B. (1996) Molecular therapeutics. Methotrexate and its mechanisms of action. *Arthritis and Rheumatism* **39**, 1951–60.

Edmundson, W. & Guy, W. (1958) Treatment of psoriasis with folic acid antagonists. *Archives of Dermatology* **78**, 200–203.

Edwards, B., Bhatnagar, D., Mackness, M. *et al.* (1995) Effect of low-dose cyclosporine on plasma lipoproteins and markers of cholestasis in patients with psoriasis. *Quarterly Journal of Medicine* **88**, 109–113.

El-Beheiry, A., El-Mansy, E., Kamel, N. & Salama, N. (1979) Methotrexate and fertility in men. *Archives of Andrology* **3**, 177–179.

Epstein, E. & Craft, J. (1969) Cirrhosis following methotrexate administration for psoriasis. *Archives of Dermatology* **100**, 531.

Evans, W. & Christensen, M. (1985) Drug interactions with methotrexate. *Journal of Rheumatology* **12** (Suppl.), 15–20.

Fitzsimons, C., Long, J. & Mackie, R. (1983) Synergistic carcinogenic potential of methotrexate and PUVA in psoriasis. *Lancet* **i**, 235–236.

Frei, A., Zimmermann, A. & Weigand, K. (1984) The end-terminal propeptide of collagen type III in serum reflects activity and degree of fibrosis in patients with chronic liver disease. *Hepatology* **4**, 830–834.

From, E. (1975) Methotrexate pneumonitis in a psoriatic. *British Journal of Dermatology* **93**, 107–110.

Golden, M., Katz, R., Balk, R. & Golden, H. (1995) The relationship of pre-existing lung disease to the development of methotrexate pneumonitis in patients with rheumatoid arthritis. *Journal of Rheumatology* **22**, 1043–1047.

Grunnet, E. (1974) Alcohol consumption in psoriasis. *Dermatologica* **149**, 136–139.

Grunnet, E., Nyfors, A. & Hansen, K. (1977) Studies on human semen in topical corticosteroid-treated and in methotrexate-treated psoriatics. *Dermatologica* **154**, 78–84.

Gubner, R. (1951) Effects of aminopterin on epithelial tissues. *Archives of Dermatology and Syphilology* **64**, 688–699.

Haagsma, C. & van Riel, P. (1997) Combination of second-line antirheumatic drugs. *Annals of Medicine* **29**, 169–173

Hausknecht, R. (1995) Methotrexate and misoprostol to terminate early pregnancy. *New England Journal of Medicine* **333**, 537–540.

Hendel, L., Hendel, J., Johnsen, A. & Gudmand-Høyer, E. (1982) Intestinal function and methotrexate absorption in psoriasis patients. *Clinical and Experimental Dermatology* **7**, 491–498.

Hendel, J. & Nyfors, A. (1984) Nonlinear renal elimination kinetics due to saturation of renal tubular reabsorption. *European Journal of Clinical Pharmacology* **26**, 121–124.

Hills, R. & Ive, F. (1992) Folinic acid rescue used routinely in psoriasis with known methotrexate sensitivity. *Acta Dermato-Venereologica* **72**, 438–440.

International Agency for Research on Cancer, Working Group (1981) Methotrexate. *IARC Monographs on the Evaluation of the Carcinogenic Risk of Chemicals to Humans* **26**, 267–292.

Jeffes, E., McCullough, J. & Pittelkow, M. (1995) Methotrexate therapy of psoriasis: differential sensitivity of proliferating lymphoid and epithelial cells to the cytotoxic and growth-inhibitory effects of methotrexate. *Journal of Investigative Dermatology* **104**, 183–188.

Katz, H. (1997) Combined topical calcipotriene ointment 0.005% and various systemic therapies in the treatment of plaque-type psoriasis vulgaris: review of the literature and results of a survey sent to 100 dermatologists. *Journal of the American Academy of Dermatology* **37**, S62–S68.

Kennedy, C. & Baker, H. (1976) Renal function in methotrexate treated psoriatics. *British Journal of Dermatology* **94**, 702–703.

Korstanje, M., van Breda Vriesman, C. & van de Staak, W. (1990) Cyclosporine and methotrexate: a dangerous combination. *Journal of the American Academy of Dermatology* **23**, 320–321.

Kragballe, K., Zachariae, E. & Zachariae, H. (1982) Methotrexate in psoriatic arthritis: a retrospective study. *Acta Dermato-Venereologica* **63**, 165–167.

Kremer, J. (1996) Methotrexate update. *Scandinavian Journal of Rheumatology* **25**, 341–344.

Kremer, J., Alarcón, G., Lightfoot, R. *et al.* (1994) Methotrexate for rheumatoid arthritis: suggested guidelines for monitoring liver toxicity. *Arthritis and Rheumatism* **37**, 316–328.

Lammers, A. & van de Kerkhof, P.C.M. (1987) Reduction of leukotriene B4-induced intraepidermal accumulation of polymorphonuclear leukocytes by methotrexate in psoriasis. *British Journal of Dermatology* **116**, 667–671.

Lanse S., Arnold G., Gowans J. & Kaplan M. (1985) Low incidence of hepatotoxicity associated with long-term, low-dose oral methotrexate in treatment of refractory psoriasis, psoriatic arthritis, and rheumatoid arthritis. An acceptable risk/benefit ratio. *Digestive Diseases and Sciences* **30**, 104–109.

Larsen, F., Nielsen-Kudsk, F., Jacobsen, P., Schrøder, H. & Kragballe, K. (1990) Interaction of etretinate with methotrexate pharmacokinetics in psoriatic patients. *Journal of Clinical Pharmacology* **30**, 802–807.

Luderschmidt, C. & Balda, B.-R. (1983) Reiter's disease, effective combination drug therapy with methotrexate, etretinate and prednisolone. *Münchener Medizinische Wochenschrift* **76**, 936–940.

Malatjalian D., Ross J., Colwell S. & Eastwood B. (1996) Methotrexate hepatotoxicity in psoriasis: report of 104 patients from Nova Scotia, with analysis of risk from obesity, diabetes and alcohol consumption during long term follow-up. *Canadian Journal of Gastroenterology* **10**, 369–375.

Markin, R., Donovan, J., Shaw, B. & Zetterman, R. (1993) Fulminant hepatic failure after methotrexate and PUVA therapy for psoriasis. *Journal of Clinical Gastroenterology* **17**, 311–313.

Mazzanti, G., Coloni, L., De Sabbata, G. & Paladini, G. (1994) Methotrexate and cyclosporin combined therapy in severe psoriatic arthritis. A pilot study. *Acta Dermato-Venereologica* **186** (Suppl.), 116–117.

Milunsky, A., Graef, J. & Gaynor, M. (1968) Methotrexate-induced congenital malformations. *Journal of Pediatrics* **72**, 790–795.

Mitchell, D., Smith, A., Rowan, B. *et al.* (1990) Serum type III procollagen peptide, dynamic liver function tests and hepatic fibrosis in psoriatic patients receiving methotrexate. *British Journal of Dermatology* **122**, 1–7.

Møller, H. (1970) Methotrexate and the ultraviolet light inflammation in the guinea pig. *Dermatologica* **140**, 225–230.

Morison, W., Momtaz, K., Parrish, J. & Fitzpatrick, T. (1982) Combined methotrexate-PUVA therapy in the treatment of psoriasis. *Journal of the American Academy of Dermatology* **1982** (6), 46–51.

Moscow, J., Gong, M., Rui, H. *et al.* (1995) Isolation of a gene encoding a human reduced folate carrier (RFC1) and analyses of its expression in transport-deficient, methotrexate-resistant human breast cancer cells. *Cancer Research* **55**, 3790–3794.

Newman, M., Auerbach, R., Feine, R.H. *et al.* (1989) The role of liver biopsies in psoriatic patients receiving long-term methotrexate treatment. Improvement in liver abnormalities after cessation of treatment. *Archives of Dermatology* **125**, 1218–1224.

Nielsen, J. & Zachariae, H. (1973) Chromosome aberrations in severe psoriasis. *Acta Dermato-Venereologica* **53**, 192–194.

Nyfors A. (1977) Liver biopsies from psoriatics related to methotrexate therapy. *Acta Pathologica et Microbiologica Scandinavica* **85**, 511–518.

Nyfors, A. (1978) Benefits and adverse drug experiences during long-term methotrexate treatment of 248 psoriatics. *Danish Medicine Bulletin* **25**, 208–211.

Nyfors A. & Poulsen H. (1976) Liver biopsies from psoriatics related to methotrexate therapy. *Acta Pathologica et Microbiologica Scandinavica* **84**, 262–270.

Olsen, E. (1991) The pharmacology of methotrexate. *Journal of the American Academy of Dermatology* **25**, 306–318.

Olsen, J., Møller, H. & Frentz, G. (1992) Malignant tumors in patients with psoriasis. *Journal of the American Academy of Dermatology* **27**, 716–722.

Paramsothy, J., Strange, R., Sharif, H. *et al.* (1988) The use of antipyrine clearance to measure liver damage in psoriatic patients receiving methotrexate. *British Journal of Dermatology* **119**, 761–765.

Paul, B., Momtaz, K., Stern, R., Arndt, K. & Parrish, J. (1982) Combined methotrexate-ultraviolet B therapy in the treatment of psoriasis. *Journal of the American Academy of Dermatology* **7**, 758–762.

Piccinio, F., Sagnelli, E., Pasquale, G. & Giusti, G. (1986) Complications following percutaneous liver biopsy: a multicenter retrospective study on 68,276 biopsies. *Journal of Hepatology* **2**, 166–173.

Rees, R., Bennet, J. & Bostick, W. (1955) Aminopterin for psoriasis. *Archives of Dermatology* **72**, 133–143.

Rees, L., Grisham, J., Aach, R. & Eisen, A. (1974) Effects of methotrexate on the liver in psoriasis. *Journal of Investigative Dermatology* **62**, 597–602.

Reynolds F. & Lee W. (1986) Hepatotoxicity after long-term methotrexate therapy. *Southern Medical Journal* **79**, 536–539.

Risteli, J., Søgaard, H., Oikarinen, A. *et al.* (1988) Aminoterminal propeptide of type III procollagen in methotrexate-induced liver fibrosis and cirrhosis. *British Journal of Dermatology* **119**, 321–325.

Robinson, J., Baughman, R., Auerbach, R. & Cimis, R. (1980) Methotrexate hepatotoxicity in psoriasis. *Archives of Dermatology* **110**, 413–415.

Roenigk, H. (1994) Methotrexate. In: *Psoriasis* (ed. Dubertret, L.), pp. 162–173. ISED, Brescia.

Roenigk, H., Auerbach, R., Bergfeld, W. *et al.* (1976) Cooperative, prospective study of the effects of chemotherapy of psoriasis on liver biopsies. In: *Psoriasis: Proceedings of the Second International Symposium* (eds Farber, E. & Cox, A.), pp. 243–248. Yorke Medical Books, New York.

Roenigk, H., Auerbach, R., Maibach, H. & Weinstein, G. (1988) Methotrexate in psoriasis: revised guidelines. *Journal of the American Academy of Dermatology* **19**, 145–156.

Roenigk, H., Fowler-Bergfeld, W. & Curtis, G. (1969) Methotrexate for psoriasis in weekly oral doses. *Archives of Dermatology* **99**, 86–93.

Rosenbaum, M. & Roenigk, H. (1984) Treatment of generalised pustular psoriasis with etretinate (RO 10–0359) and methotrexate. *Journal of the American Academy of Dermatology* **10**, 357–361.

Rothenberg, R., Graziano, F., Grandone, J. *et al.* (1988) The use of methotrexate in steroid-resistant lupus erythematosus. *Arthritis and Rheumatism* **5**, 612–615.

Said, S., Jeffes, E. & Weinstein, G. (1997) Systemic treatment; methotrexate. *Clinics in Dermatology* **15**, 781–797.

Sauer, G. (1973) Combined methotrexate and hydroxyurea therapy for psoriasis. *Archives of Dermatology* **107**, 369–370.

Schwartz, P., Barnett, S. & Milstone, L. (1995) Keratinocytes differentiate in response to inhibitors of deoxyribonucleotide synthesis. *Journal of Dermatological Science* **9**, 129–135.

Segal, R., Dayan, M., Zinger, H. & Mozes, E. (1995) Methotrexate in murine experimental systemic lupus erythematosus (SLE): Clinical benefits associated with cytokine manipulation. *Clinical and Experimental Immunology* **101**, 66–72.

Sherlock, S., Dick, R. & van Leeuwen, D. (1985) Liver biopsy today. The Royal Free Hospital experience. *Journal of Hepatology* **1**, 75–85.

Stein, C., Brooks, R. & Pincus, T. (1997a) Effect of combination therapy with cyclosporine and methotrexate on liver function test results in rheumatoid arthritis. *Arthritis and Rheumatism* **40**, 1721–1723.

Stein, C., Pincus, T., Yocum, D. *et al.* (1997b) Combination treatment of severe rheumatoid arthritis with cyclosporine and methotrexate for forty-eight weeks: an open-label extension study. The methotrexate-cyclosporine combination study group. *Arthritis and Rheumatism* **40**, 1843–1851.

Stern, R., Zierler, S. & Parrish, J. (1982) Methotrexate used for psoriasis and the risk of noncutaneous or cutaneous malignancy. *Cancer* **50**, 869–872.

Straub, R., Müller-Ladner, U., Lichtinger, T. *et al.* (1997) Decrease of interleukin 6 during the first 12 months is a prognostic marker for clinical outcome during 36 months treatment with disease-modifying anti-rheumatic drugs. *British Journal of Rheumatology* **36**, 1298–1303.

Sussman, A. & Leonard, J. (1980) Psoriasis, methotrexate, and oligospermia. *Archives of Dermatology* **116**, 215–217.

Ternowitz, T., Bjerring, P., Andersen, P., Schröder, J. & Kragballe, K. (1987) Methotrexate inhibits the human C5a-induced skin response in patients with psoriasis. *Journal of Investigative Dermatology* **89**, 192–196.

Themido R., Loureiro M., Pecegueiro M., Brandao M. & Canpos M. (1992) Methotrexate hepatoxicity in psoriatic patients submitted to long-term therapy. *Acta Dermato-Venereologica (Stockh)* **72**, 361–364.

van de Kerkhof, P.C.M. (1986) Methotrexate. In: *Textbook of Psoriasis* (eds Mier, P. & van de Kerkhof, P.C.M.), pp. 231–251. Churchill-Livingstone, Edinburgh.

van de Kerkhof, P.C.M. & Mali, J. (1982) Methotrexate maintenance following Ingram therapy in difficult psoriasis. *British Journal of Dermatology* **106**, 623–627.

van de Kerkhof P.C.M., Hoefnagels W., van Haelst U. & Mali J. (1985) Methotrexate maintenance therapy and liver damage in psoriasis. *Clinical and Experimental Dermatology* **10**, 194–200.

van den Hoogen, F., Boerbooms, A., Swaak, A. *et al.* (1996) Comparison of methotrexate with placebo in the treatment of systemic sclerosis; a 24 week randomized double-blind trial, followed by a 24 week observational trial. *British Journal of Rheumatology* **35**, 364–372.

van Dooren-Greebe, R., Kuijpers, A., Buijs, W. *et al.* (1996) The value of dynamic hepatic scintigraphy and serum aminoterminal propeptide of type III procollagen for early detection of methotrexate-induced hepatic damage in psoriasis patients. *British*

Journal of Dermatology **134**, 481–487.

van Dooren-Greebe, R., Kuijpers, A., Mulder, J., De Boo, T. & van de Kerkhof, P. (1994) Methotrexate revisited: effects of long-term treatment in psoriasis. *British Journal of Dermatology* **130**, 204–210.

Vanderveen, E., Ellis, C., Campbell, J., Case, P. & Voorhees, J. (1982) Methotrexate and etretinate as concurrent therapies in severe psoriasis. *Archives of Dermatology* **118**, 660–662.

Warin A., Landells J., Levene G. & Baker H. (1975) A prospective study of the effects of weekly oral methotrexate on liver biopsy. *British Journal of Dermatology* **93**, 321–327.

Weinstein, G. & Frost, P. (1971) Methotrexate for psoriasis: a new therapeutic schedule. *Archives of Dermatology* **103**, 33–38.

Weinstein, G., Roenigk, H., Maibach, H. *et al.* (1973). Methotrexate therapy for psoriasis – revision of guidelines. *Archives of Dermatology* **108**, 36–42.

Whiting-O'Keefe, Q., Fye, K. & Sach, K. (1991) Methotrexate and histologic hepatic abnormalities: a metaanalysis. *American Journal of Medicine* **90**, 711–716.

Zachariae, H. (1979) Pathological findings in internal organs of patients with severe psoriasis. *Acta Dermato-Venereologica* **87** (Suppl.), 87–89.

Zachariae, H. (1986) Combination cytotoxic therapy. In: *Psoriasis: Proceedings of the 4th International Symposium* (eds Farber, E. & Cox, A.J.), pp. 240–247. Elsevier Scientific Publishing, New York.

Zachariae H. (1986) Liver biopsy findings during methotrexate therapy. In: *Psoriasis* (ed. Dubertret L.), p. 168. ISED, Brescia.

Zachariae, H. (1991) Psoriasis and the liver. In: *Psoriasis* (eds Roenigk, H. & Maibach, H.), 2nd edn, pp. 59–82. Marcel Dekker, New York.

Zachariae, H. (1993) Methotrexate therapy. Risk assessment for patient and dermatologist. *Fitzpatrick's Journal of Clinical Dermatology* **1**, 14–20.

Zachariae, H. (1996) Methotrexate—past, present and future. *Life Chemistry Reports* **14**, 187–191.

Zachariae, H. & Søgaard, H. (1987) Methotrexate-induced liver cirrhosis. A follow-up. *Dermatologica* **75**, 178–182.

Zachariae, E. & Zachariae, H. (1987) Methotrexate treatment of psoriatic arthritis. *Acta Dermato-Venereologica* **67**, 270–273.

Zachariae, H., Aslam, H., Bjerring, P. *et al.* (1991) Serum aminoterminal propeptide of type III procollagen in psoriasis and psoriatic arthritis: Relation to liver fibrosis and arthritis. *Journal of the American Academy of Dermatology* **25**, 50–53.

Zachariae, H., Grunnet, E. & Søgaard, H. (1975) Liver biopsy in methotrexate-treated patients—a re-evaluation. *Acta Dermato-Venereologica* **55**, 291–296.

Zachariae, H., Grunnet, E. & Søgaard, H. (1976) Accidental kidney biopsies in psoriasis. *British Journal of Dermatology* **94**, 655–661.

Zachariae, H., Hansen, H., Søgaard, H. & Olsen, T. (1990) Kidney biopsies in methotrexate-treated psoriatics. *Dermatologica* **181**, 273–276.

Zachariae, H., Kragballe, K., Hansen, H., Marcussen, N. & Olsen, S. (1997) Renal biopsy findings in long-term cyclosporin treatment of psoriasis. *British Journal of Dermatology* **136**, 531–535.

Zachariae, H., Kragballe, K. & Søgaard, H. (1980) Methotrexate induced liver cirrhosis. *British Journal of Dermatology* **102**, 407–412.

Zachariae, H., Søgaard, H. & Heickendorff, L. (1988) Serum aminoterminal propeptide of type III procollagen—A non-invasive test for liver fibrogenesis in methotrexate-treated psoriatics. *Acta Dermato-Venereologica* **69**, 241–243.

Zachariae, H., Søgaard, H. & Heickendorff, L. (1996) Methotrexate-induced liver cirrhosis, clinical, histological and serological studies—A further 10-year follow-up. *Dermatology* **192**, 343–346.

Chapter 13: Topical and Systemic Retinoids

H.P.M. Gollnick and B. Bonnekoh

During the last 2 decades retinoids as important representatives in dermato-logical therapy have mainly been used via the systemic route. However, very recently an effective topical retinoid has also been introduced to the market. It is now possible to use a topical retinoid in minor forms of psoriasis and systemic retinoids in major forms (Gollnick and Orfanos 1986; Orfanos *et al.* 1987; Gollnick 1996).

The topical therapeutics in psoriasis such as tazarotene and in particular vitamin D_3 derivatives on the one hand are limited in the expression of their efficacy in widespread psoriasis due to a limited surface area for application and on the other hand the benefit/risk ratio and the cost-efficacy ratio are low in chronic plaques when psoriatic area and severity (PASI) scores exceed 10–15.

Therefore, systemic treatment with cyclosporin A, fumaric esters, meth-otrexate and, in particular, systemic retinoids is indicated (Gollnick & Kirsten 1996; Gollnick & Dümmler 1997).

This chapter will discuss the use of topical and systemic retinoids in monotherapy and in particular the various possibilities for combining the systemic retinoids with other topical agents and UV light.

13.1 Historical background

Despite the detection of a possible role of retinol around the turn of this century its biological significance was first described in depth by Wolbach and Howe (1925) demonstrating tissue changes following deprivation of fat-soluble retinol.

Phrynoderma as a characteristic skin hyperkeratosis with excessive follicular keratinization was discovered in the 1930 to be a deficiency of reti-nol. Consequently vitamin A was used to treat follicular hyperkeratosis in dermatology, but soon it was found to lead to severe hypervitaminosis A syndrome particularly in high-dose treatment regimens. When in 1962 Stüttgen and later Baer discovered the use of retinol acid for topical treat-ment an important breakthrough was achieved in particular for the treat-ment of acne (Stüttgen 1962). However, the low therapeutic index (ratio of required efficacy to toxicity) after oral application of the natural retinol and of oral retinol acid has led to the development of synthetic retinoids. Neither topical isotretinoin nor the new adapalene have a considerable antipsoriatic profile. Tazarotene is an novel third-generation acetylenic retinoid and represents the first efficacious antipsoriatic topical retinoid (Weinstein & Grenn 1994; Krueger *et al.* 1998).

Pharmacological development of retinol molecules and derivatives began when continuous pharmaceutical research started in 1968 (Bollag 1985). The retinol molecule was in particular changed at the polar marginal group, the polyen chain or the cyclic end-group. This search has led to the derivatives such as all-trans retinoic acid (ATRA/tretinoin) and 13-*cis*-retinoic-acid (isotretinoin) (Fig. 13.1). The latter was a major breakthrough for the treatment of conglobate acne (Ward *et al.* 1984). Isotretinoin has in addition a role in the treatment of severe pustular psoriasis, in particular in combination with psoralen and UVA (PUVA).

Monoaromatic retinoids such as etretinate and its first metabolite acitretin were discovered, and named second-generation retinoids. Both led to a revolution in the systemic treatment of psoriasis. Today, acitretin as the first metabolite of etretinate is in use worldwide not only for psoriasis but for ichthyoses, palmoplantar keratoses, Darier's disease, pityriasis rubra pilaris, hyperkeratotic hand eczema, keratosis lichenoides chronica and lichen ruber.

Due to the immunomodulating and cell-differentiating properties not only of keratinocytes, but also of lymphocytes and neutrophils or fibroblasts dermatological diseases such as bullous diseases, lichen sclerosus et atrophicus and cutaneous lupus erythematosus are additional indications. Moreover, during the last decade systemic retinoids have been shown to be very effective not only in the prevention but also in the therapy of skin cancer either

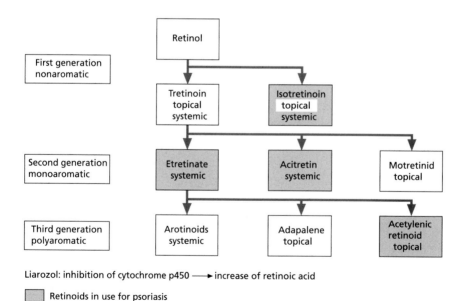

Liarozol: inhibition of cytochrome p450 ⟶ increase of retinoic acid

Retinoids in use for psoriasis

Fig. 13.1 Retinoid generations.

alone or in combination with other agents or modalities such as PUVA or interferon-α (Tsambaos & Orfanos 1981; Mahrle 1985; Gollnick & Orfanos 1991).

During the early 1980s the third-generation retinoids were developed; however, the efficacy/toxicity ratio was quite difficult to estimate because of serum level monitoring, in particular with regard to the teratogenic potential of retinoids and the use in females of childbearing age.

Finally, a topical aromatic retinoid, motretinid (Tasmaderm) has been registered in Switzerland for the treatment of hyperkeratotic disorders.

A new way of using endogenous tretinoin was tried by introducing an imidazol derivative, liarozole, an inhibitor of cytochrome P-450 inhibiting the 4-hydroxylation of retinoic acid which consequently increases concentration of retinoic acid within the cell (van Wauwe 1990; Dockx et al. 1995).

Kuijpers et al. (1998) recently performed a study comparing liarozole and acitretin in 20 patients with severe plaque-type psoriasis during a 24-week course. As evaluated by the PASI score both were equally effective by working with different modes of action.

13.2 Mechanisms of action

During the last decade, development of novel research methods on the molecular level brought new fundamental insights into the mechanisms of action of different retinoids. With these sensitive methods, it has become possible to elucidate where retinoids induce their effects on the cellular and nuclear level.

The term 'retinoids' is applied to a family of substances that comprises retinol, retinal and its isoforms, including retinylester, ATRA, 13-*cis*-retinoic acid and 9-*cis*-retinoic acid. In addition, newly developed substances, such as 3,4-di-dehydroretinoic acid and 14-hydroxy-retro-retinol or so-called selective retinoid receptor agonists have been studied.

13.2.1 Retinoid receptors

Biological effects of retinoids, mainly of the natural stereoisomers ATRA and 9-*cis*-retinoic acid, are transmitted through cytoplasmic retinoid binding proteins and nuclear retinoid receptors. At present, we know at least two kinds of retinoid receptors, both in a variety of isoforms: the RARs and the RXRs.

Although each cell possesses only about 1000–1500 receptor molecules, binding of a ligand causes a cascade of substantial effects through transcriptional activation. (Brand et al. 1988; Gollnick & Kirsten 1996) Nuclear retinoid receptors are members of the steroid–thyroid receptor superfamily. The ability to form heterodimers divides this superfamily into two classes: the first class has retinoid receptors, thyroid-hormone receptors and vitamin D receptors; the other has glucocorticoid receptors, the oestrogen-hormone receptor, androgen- and mineralocorticoid hormone receptors, acting only as homodimers.

13.2.2 Regulation on the protein level

The search for more effective retinoids is focusing on the new agonists and antagonists of which a binding to the known retinoid receptors is expected (RAR-α, -β, -γ and RXR-α, -β, -γ). The retinoid receptors RARs and RXRs are nuclear receptors, acting as ligand (retinoid-homone)-activated transcription factors. Through activation of alternative promoters and post-transcriptional splicing, each of these subclasses possess a variety of isoforms. As with the other members of the closely related steroid–thyroid receptor superfamily, sequence comparisons between the RARs and RXRs revealed six functional domains, designated A–F.

Three functional domains are assigned to the sections B,C and E. The first domain is a multifunctional domain at the carboxy-terminal end of the receptor, with sections for ligand binding (LBD), ligand-dependent transactivation function, hetero- or rather homodimerization, nuclear trans-location, and interactions with heat-shock proteins.

The second domain is flexibly connected with LBD. It is a central DNA-binding and dimerization domain (DBD), which is characterized in this receptor family by two highly conserved zinc-finger sections. The third domain is associated with an amino-terminus that constitutes an acting domain of transactivation (AF-1).

Binding of retinoid receptors to different retinoids or their metabolites, rather than association with different DNA sections and the further DNA context, influences the activation or inhibition of transcription by changing protein conformation or binding to other associated proteins (Chen & Privalsky 1995; Hackney 1995).

13.2.3 Effects on the cellular level

Investigations of embryonic and adult tissue, including skin, show distinct as well as overlapping expression of different isoforms of RARs and RXRs. Cell-specific expression of the receptor could explain the pleotropic effects. Cell-specific expression is also important in differentiation of basal keratinocytes and in the formation of other epidermal cell layers as well as in dedifferentia-tion and tumour progression. For example RAR-γ1 is detected only in adult skin, whereas RAR-α1 is ubiquitous in adult tissue.

Knock-out experiments of individual RARs do not show as a rule morphologic or functional alterations of the epithelium as a consequence. This leads to the assumption of functional redundancy of individual receptors.

RXR-α is the dominant RXR transcript in the skin; in fact, RXR concentration is fivefold higher than RAR concentration. RXR-α/RAR-γ heterodimers are postulated to be the main regulating protein complex of retinoid-sensitive target genes in adult human skin (Fisher *et al.* 1994; Xiao *et al.* 1995).

The cellular retinoic acid binding protein (CRABP) and the cellular retinol binding protein (CRBP) were proposed to serve as specific transport proteins of retinoic acid, or retinol, to the nucleus (Takase *et al.* 1986). In contrast to etretinate, acitretin competes with retinoic acid for binding at the CRABP (Saurat *et al.* 1987). High concentrations of CRABP are found in epidermal tissue, even in lamellar ichthyosis, Darier's disease, pityriasis rubra pilaris and keratosis pilaris. All these diseases show good clinical response to the treatment with retinoids. In the past, CRABP and CRBP were proposed to serve as receptors for retinoids; however, the cellular binding proteins are not present in all retinoid-responsive cell lines. For example, the human promyelocytic cell line HL-60, a model for studying retinoid-induced differentiation, does not express these binding proteins. Further evidence for a receptor distinct from CRBP and CRABP was presented by the findings that etretinate and also the new adapalene did not bind to these receptors, although it exhibited all the typical retinoid effects. In 1987, the first evidence for transmission of the specific retinoid effect through a nuclear retinoid receptor was reported (Petkovich *et al.* 1987; Benbrook *et al.* 1988). Acitretin has low affinity to RARs, but it activates receptors; therefore, one can deduce that a metabolite binds to the receptor (Fig. 13.2).

13.2.4 Effects in psoriatic skin

Through their influence on proliferation, keratinization and differentiation of epithelial cells, and through additional effects on cellular and humoral

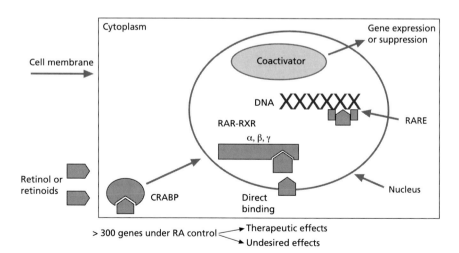

Fig. 13.2 Retinoid action at the cellular level. CRABP, cellular retinoic acid-binding protein; RA, retinoic acid; RAR/RXR, retinoic acid receptors; RARE, retinoic acid response elements.

immune response and their anti-inflammatory abilities, such as influence on the arachidonic acid cascade and on the migration of polymorphonuclear leucocytes (PMNs), acitretin and etretinate are highly effective drugs in the treatment of psoriasis.

Acitretin has been shown to moderate cell proliferation in a number of *in vitro* investigations on animal and human cell lines. The results in cultured cells do not always provide confirmation; on the one hand, they give evidence for inhibition of cell proliferation, and other studies have shown increased growth of cells in culture under retinoid influence (Priestley 1987; Harper 1988; Imcke *et al.* 1991).

Both acitretin and etretinate possess immunosuppressive and immunostimulating abilities. In fact, the exact and predominating operation and mechanisms in the treatment of the different types and phases of psoriasis still remain speculative to a certain degree. Effects through influence on the T-cell system have been discussed recently. Both metabolites show significant anti-inflammatory effects in the delayed murine hypersensitivity inhibitory test and in the animal model of arthritic rats. Acitretin has been shown to modulate the reaction of peripheral blood lymphocytes to different stimuli (Bauer & Orfanos 1984). It has been demonstrated in several studies that acitretin inhibits the release of reactive oxygen species from PMNs (Struy *et al.* 1996). Together with a decrease in keratinocytes production of interleukin 8 (IL-8) this combinatory effects weakens important steps in the pathogenesis of psoriasis. In addition, acitretin decreases the ability of antigen presentation of phytohaemagglutinin-stimulated lymphocytes (Dupuy *et al.* 1989).

Further evidence of immunostimulating properties is the inhibition of tumour growth in the animal model, increased numbers of Langerhans cells in normal and psoriatic skin after acitretin treatment, and immunostimulation of natural killer (NK) lymphocytes (Fig. 13.3 and Table 13.1).

Polyamine levels as markers of growth and differentiation of epidermal keratinocytes, which are increased in psoriatic skin, decrease significantly under treatment with retinoids.

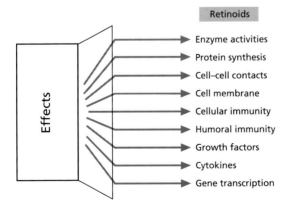

Fig. 13.3 Effects of retinoids.

Table 13.1 Immunomodulatory properties of etretinate/acitretin.

Evidence for immunosuppression	Evidence for immunostimulation
Murine delayed hypersensitivity: inhibitory effects	Tumour growth inhibition test: inhibitory in animal models
In vitro depression of T-cell blast transformation	Increased numbers of Langerhans cells in normal and psoriatic skin
	Type IV reaction increased in humans
PMN migration inhibition	Immunostimulation of NK cells

PMN, polymorphonuclear leucocytes; NK, natural killer cells.

Transduction of cyclic nucleotides regulates differentiation and growth of keratinocytes, as well as anti-inflammatory reactions.

Recently a group of investigators reported that alterations of cyclic adenosine monophosphate (cAMP) content in psoriatic skin could be normalized by retinoid treatment (Raynaud *et al.* 1994).

Migration inhibitory factor-related protein (MRP-8), a marker of hyperproliferative as well as abnormal keratinocyte differentiation, is strongly expressed in the epidermis of psoriatic lesions but not in normal skin. DiSepio *et al.* demonstrated that retinoids inhibit the expression of MRP-8 by a direct action at the promoter level. The MRP-8 promoter is activated by the nuclear factor of IL-6 (NF-IL6) and retinoids inhibit MRP-8 expression by antagonizing this activity of NF-IL6. It has been reported that interferon-γ (a key cytokine in the psoriatic process), induces MRP-8 expression. Using a chloramphenicol acetyl transferase (CAT) reporter assay incorporating the MRP-8 promoter, the authors demonstrated that the induction of MRP-8 by interfon-γ is inhibited by retinoid receptors in a ligand-dependent manner (DiSepio *et al.* 1997).

13.2.5 Retinoid resistance, receptor mutation and relevance for neoplasia

Certain mutants of retinoid receptors show decreased affinity to retinoids, but they maintain their DNA-binding capacity. This is called a dominant negative activity of the retinoid receptor. The result is competition at the DNS-binding domain, but binding on DNS segments is not always followed by transcriptional activity. The phenomenon of dominant negative activity is proposed to be an important factor in the development of neoplasia. In acute promyelocytic leukaemia (APL), a large amount of promyelocyte (PML)-RAR fusion protein is produced in the cells; this is caused by chromosomal translocation of the PML gene next to the RAR gene. Inhibition of differentiation of the PMLs in an early stage of development by this fusion protein is postulated.

The exact mechanism by which ATRA could induce complete remission in patients with acute promyelocytic leukaemia is still not clearly understood (Parkinson & Smith 1992; Weis *et al.* 1994).

13.3 Pharmacokinetics

After oral intake, acitretin is resorbed in the bowel, and in the mucosal bowel epithelium acitretin is metabolized to 13-*cis*-acitretin (Cotler *et al.* 1992; Pilkington & Brogden 1992). Monitoring plasma concentrations of oral retinoids and their metabolites under short- or long-term treatment permits early identification and a better understanding of the so-called 'non-responders', either due to a disturbed metabolism of retinoids or to non-compliance. Monitoring of 13-*cis*-acitretin in plasma after cessation of treatment with etretinate or acitretin in women of childbearing age seems to be more sensitive than measurement of plasma levels of etretinate or acitretin. These measurements are helpful for defining the strategy of oral retinoid therapy and for reliable information for women who wish to become pregnant after cessation of drug therapy (Gollnick *et al.* 1990). Because of the lack of clinical investigations, it still remains unclear, whether the metabolite 13-*cis*-acitretin itself has antipsoriatic effects (Geiger & Brindley 1988).

Absolute maximal plasma concentrations (C_{max}) after oral treatment with acitretin and etretinate are similar. Resorption of acitretin is faster than that of etretinate, and the time to reach its maximal plasma concentration (P_{max}) is shorter (Wiegand & Chou 1998). Bioavailability of both substances increases with food ingestion.

Absolute bioavailability of acitretin and etretinate are rather low, 59% and 40%, respectively; both show high variations of resorption after oral administration. In most subjects mean maximum plasma concentrations (C_{max}) vary between 400 and 500 ng/mL 2 h after single dosing.

Because of long-term storage of etretinate in deeper compartments, particularly in the subcutaneous adipose tissue, acitretin, at first glance, seems to be the more advantageous drug in clinical treatment, although both show similar efficacy (Gollnick & Orfanos 1986). After oral absorption, etretinate is metabolized to acitretin (Fig. 13.4). In animal experiments, it was shown that the carboxylic acid of etretinate, acitretin, is not stored in adipose tissue. There is evidence that these results are not at all transferable to the metabolism in humans (Wiegand & Chou 1998).

Acitretin is isomerized to 13-*cis*-acitretin, and this is a reversal reaction; however, there are no hard data about the equilibrium of this reaction. Mean elimination half-life of acitretin is about 2 days, whereas etretinate has a half-life time of about 120 days. This was thought to be the most important advantage of acitretin, because of the teratogenicity of oral retinoid treatment. Etretinate is detectable in the subcutis for about 18 months after drug cessation (Rollman & Vahlquist 1983). In the treatment of women of childbearing age with acitretin,

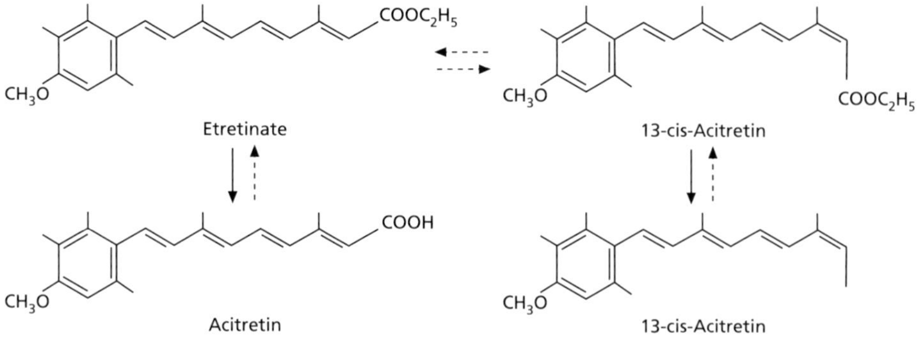

Fig. 13.4 Chemical formula of acitretin and etretinate and their main metabolites.

post-therapeutic contraception for about 2 months was considered sufficient in the early phases of drug development in clinical trials; however, in monitoring the plasma levels of acitretin-treated patients, etretinate was detected, and, as a consequence, contraception after drug treatment had to be continued for a period of 2 years or more, depending on local regulations. Obviously there is a metabolism of re-esterification from acitretin to etretinate.

The results of animal experiments and clinical investigations indicate that one of the most important cofactors of re-esterification seems to be ethanol (Almond-Roesler & Orfanos 1996). Table 13.2 lists the pharmacokinetic properties of etretinate and acitretin.

13.4 Clinical use

13.4.1 Clinical efficacy of topical application of retinoids

Topical retinoids

Usually the management of mild to moderate psoriasis involves topical treatment with tar preparations, anthralin, supporting agents such as salicylic acid and urea, and the new developments such as calcipotriol, tacalcitol and tazarotene. Corticosteroids are used in different classes of potency depending on

Table 13.2 Pharmacokinetics of etretinate and acitretin.

	Acitretin	Etretinate
Half-life period	≈ 50 h	80–100 days
Protein binding	Albumin	Lipoproteins
Lipid solubility		50-fold higher than acetrin
Elimination rate	50-fold faster than etretinate	
Bioavailability	59% (35–90)	40%

the type of psoriasis, local differences in the health systems and different characters of a more inpatient- or outpatient-based dermatology. The topical retinoid tazarotene has been investigated as a topical treatment for psoriasis for about 5 years (Weinstein & Grenn 1994; Krueger *et al.* 1998).

The first two initial dose-ranging studies were performed to evaluate the efficacy in mild to moderate plaque psoriasis. The first study involved 45 psoriatic patients treated either with tazarotene 0.01% gel, 0.05% gel or ve-hicle gel. In this 6-week study the 0.05% tazarotene gel was significantly more effective than 0.01% gel or vehicle gel, concerning the reduction of plaque elevation and scaling of lesions. The success rate with 0.05% gel when compared to the vehicle gel was already significant after the second week of treatment. The overall success rate was 45% for tazarotene gel 0.05%, 31% for the 0.1% formulation and 13% for the vehicle gel.

In the second study, also a dose-ranging study with 0.1% and 0.05% tazarotene, 105 patients were included. By the end of the treatment the suc-cess rate ranged from approximately 50–60% in both groups. The 8-week post-treatment phase showed that the success rates were generally main-tained (40–58%).

In another study tazarotene 0.1% and 0.05% applied once daily were compared to fluocinonide 0.05% cream applied twice daily. The treatment lasted for 12 weeks followed by a 12-week post-treatment evaluation. The high-potency corticosteroid produced a significantly higher reduction in ery-thema throughout the treatment period. During the 12-week treatment both concentrations of tazarotene were associated with significant reductions from baseline levels in lesion severity scores. After week 4 of the treatment phase, the overall success was similar for fluocinonide and the two tazarotene con-centrations (tazarotene 0.1% gel, 65%; 0.05% gel, 52%; and fluocinonide, 66%). During the post-treatment phase both tazarotene gel concentrations showed significantly better reductions in plaque elevation severity on the knees and elbows than the corticosteroid. Fluocinonide produced a signifi-cantly greater reduction in scaling during the early treatment phase, but dur-ing week 4 of the post-treatment phase the tazarotene concentrations were superior to fluocinonide in reducing scaling of knee/elbow lesions.

Typically, after the discontinuation of treatment, during the follow-up phase, those patients who received fluocinonide declined in their treatment success rate more rapidly than those who had been treated with tazarotene. So, patients with treatment successes at end of week 12 of treatment and after 12 weeks of therapy were: tazarotene (0.1%) 59%, tazarotene (0.05%) 58% and fluocinonide 40%. It is important to note that no rebound phe-nomena occurred with the topical retinoid as can usually be seen in treat-ment with topical corticosteroids.

All clinical trials so far demonstrate that tazarotene is generally well tol-erated. Because of its very low absorption rate the adverse effects were only of a local nature as expected, which are mild to moderate erythema, pruritus and burning or stinging. The local adverse effects were greater with the higher concentration of 0.1% compared to 0.05%.

Very recently two clinical trials using tazarotene gel in combination with low-, medium-, and high-potency corticosteroids in a daily or in an alternate-day regimen were performed. The results of the first study, in which 300 patients had been included, demonstrated that the additive combination of the treatment using tazarotene once daily in the evening plus a low-, mid- or high-potency corticosteroid once daily in the morning significantly increased the percentage of plaques achieving treatment success at the end of the treatment period, compared with tazarotene plus placebo (91% and 95% versus 80% respectively). In addition, tazarotene combined with a mid- or high-potency topical steroid reduced the incidence of patients withdrawing from the trial when compared to those who had been treated with tazarotene plus placebo only or low-potency corticosteroids.

The results of the second study, which involved 398 patients, clearly showed that a combination regimen which alternates daily between tazarotene gel and a high-potency topical corticosteroid treatment significantly increased the treatment success rate compared with regimens using tazarotene alternating with a mid-potency corticosteroid or placebo (75% versus 55% and 54%, respectively at the end of the treatment period). Furthermore, there was a trend towards a lower incidence of local side-effects with the stronger corticosteroid.

In those countries currently not favouring the use of topical corticosteroids to treat chronic plaque psoriasis, the results of these two studies are likely to lead to a revival in the use of corticosteroids and thus a change in the therapeutic armanentarium. It seems logical to treat chronic plaque-like psoriasis with two agents with additive or synergistic effects. In the consensus paper of the *European Advisory Panel Meeting for Tazarotene* (May 1998) it is recommended that, in certain cases, the most effective therapy available appears to be the combination of tazarotene plus corticosteroid instead of tazarotene monotherapy. If tazarotene monotherapy is not sufficient, or if a local irritation becomes a problem, the topical corticosteroid should be added to the therapy as early as possible. This combination therapy regimen may either be tazarotene and corticosteroid on alternate days, or one agent in the morning and the other in the evening. Although this combination therapy is highly effective, patients should discontinue the corticosteroid application after 4 weeks of treatment to minimize the risk of side effects developing from long-term corticosteroid exposure.

The combination of tazarotene with phototherapy has recently been evaluated in a multicentre study. Fifty-four patients received tazarotene gel, vehicle gel or no treatment 3 times a week for 2 weeks before starting UVB-therapy. The patients were exposed to UVB 3 times per week for 10 weeks. Tazarotene gel was applied after each UVB-session, or the vehicle gel or no topical treatment was given. The results clearly demonstrated that the patients treated with UVB plus tazarotene experienced more rapid clearance of their plaques than those treated with UVB and vehicle gel or UVB therapy alone. The study also demonstrated that patients treated with the combination therapy needed less cumulative UV-light to achieve a similar treatment success compared with those receiving UVB alone. Therefore, the risk of skin cancer is reduced by this combination treatment. When vitamin D_3 derivatives are compared with tazarotene, the available data that support tazarotene's lack of phototoxicity makes it a more favourable option.

Considering the clinical data currently available, the Advisory Panel recommends that tazarotene be used for the treatment of chronic, stable, plaque-type psoriasis on the trunk or limbs, covering up to 20% of the body area.

Efficacy was generally apparent by 4 weeks, at the latest, of start-up of the treatment, after which continuing improvement tended to plateau at around 8–12 weeks. Improvement was maintained for up to 12 weeks after stopping application of tazarotene. Concerning the use of tazarotene, the rule is to apply the product on the plaque lesion, avoiding normal skin in order to reduce local irritation.

With regard to possible troublesome local irritations with tazarotene, the advisory panel in the consensus paper recommended the following:
1   reducing the concentration to 0.05%;
2   reducing the frequency of application to every other day;
3   add a topical corticosteroid to therapy; and
in rare cases where severe irritation persists the patient should stop tazarotene treatment.

The combination treatment with systemic retinoids has so far not been evaluated. With regard to an additive risk of retinoid dermatitis, careful observation during clinical management of severe cases should be performed.

13.4.2 Clinical efficacy of oral application of retinoids

Monotherapy

During the last decade, treatment of moderate to severe psoriasis was dominated by the use of systemic application of retinoids such as etretinate in the past and acitretin today (Gollnick 1996). It is an essential outcome of nearly 20 years of experimental and clinical experience with these drugs in psoriasis treatment that in the chronic plaque-like type acitretin, and where etretinate is still available, both are a domain for combination therapy with topical antipsoriatic agents such as dithranol, vitamin D_3 derivatives (calcipotriol/tacalcitol) and UVA/B with or without tar. However, in the erythrodermic variants of psoriasis or in severe pustular psoriasis, including acrodermatitis continua suppurativa (Hallopeau's disease), oral monotherapy with retinoids still represents the therapy of choice; in addition, etretinate and acitretin show good efficacy as maintenance drugs for chronic plaque psoriasis after clinical remission (Gollnick *et al.* 1993).

Standard dosage of acitretin is about 0.25–0.6 mg/kg daily, but it has to be adapted in terms of indication and individual response (Table 13.3). Absence of severe diseases of the liver and kidney or other metabolic diseases, including severe diabetes and impairment of lipid metabolism, are preconditions for the oral treatment with retinoids. The dynamics of the clinical response is dependant on the clinical types of psoriasis to be treated: relatively slowly occurring in chronic stable thick plaque type, but dramatically fast in the pustular and even the erythrodermic variant. Maximal therapeutic efficiency can be achieved with about 0.5 mg/kg daily after 2–3 months of treatment.

For further stabilization after clearing the acute disease, a constant maintenance dose of 0.2–0.4 mg/kg daily is advisable for about 3–6 months. During the entire period of treatment, adjuvant topical skin care is useful.

Administration of oral retinoids significantly decreases the number of inpatients and the duration of residential treatment required (Gollnick & Orfanos 1985; Ellis *et al.* 1987). Thanks to its non-immunosuppressive but immunomodulating properties, oral application of acitretin is an adequate regimen also in the treatment of the severe plaque-like types of psoriasis in immunosuppressed and human immunodeficiency virus (HIV)-positive patients.

Palmoplantar psoriasis. In the hyperkeratotic type of palmoplantar psoriasis it is advisable in our experience to treat the patient initially for 10–14 days with a retinoid pulse dose of 1.0–1.5 mg/kg. Thereafter the dose is tapered down to 0.25 mg/kg for another 2 weeks. Usually, a desquamation of the hyperkeratotic plaques occurs after 12–18 days. A maintenance dose of twice-weekly 20 mg/day is only necessary to stabilize the disease combined with a urea or salicylic acid containing emollient.

Nail involvement in psoriasis. It is well-known from clinical observations that during etretinate/acitretin treatment, the nail plate becomes thinner, and even brittleness can occur; however, in thick hyperkeratotic psoriatic nails or in those cases in which only nails are affected, this otherwise adverse drug effect is rather desirable. Therefore, one should use low-dose acitretin

Table 13.3 Dosing of acitretin.

Manifestation	Initial dose (mg/kg/day)	Maintenance dose (mg/kg/day)
Chronic plaque psoriasis (in combinations)	0.25–0.5	0.125–0.5
Erythrodermic psoriasis	0.25–0.4	0.125–0.5 change to combined therapy
Pustular localized or generalized psoriasis	0.75–1.0	0.125–0.5

1×10 mg/day over a 6-month period, which is recommended to improve >75–90% of the psoriatic nail involvement. Side-effects such as paronychia will not occur, if manipulation of the nail fold is avoided.

Scalp psoriasis. Retinoid treatment is known to affect scalp psoriasis only relatively moderately. A complete remission does not usually occur; however, reduction of a scalp PASI score of 30–50% can be achieved after 4–6 weeks. Therefore, combination treatment of a retinoid with a keratolytic agent, corticoid lotion and a UV combination is necessary. Note: split acitretin dose to twice daily not exceeding 2×10 mg/day to avoid a retinoid telogen effluvium! Not much is known yet about the combination with a calcipotriol lotion, but this also seems promising. The treatment of severe scalp psoriasis with an oral retinoid alone is not advisable. Hair loss as a possible adverse event of the retinoid or originally caused by the psoriatic inflammation, mechanical irritation and the patient's manipulation or all together is not easy to discriminate from each other, but more importantly it may not be easy to explain to the patient. The efficacy of the combination of low-dose acitretin with topical tazarotene has to be proven by a clinical trial.

Childhood psoriasis. The indication for retinoids in childhood psoriasis should be considered carefully. In those cases which are very severe, frequently relapsing, and of the plaque-like type, acitretin may be indicated; but it should be combined with dithranol, balneophototherapy, or short-term UV irradiations except PUVA. The adverse effects of acitretin in children are similar to the spectrum in adults; although, in general, less severe: careful observation of symptoms of diffuse ideopathic skeletal hyperostosis (DISH) is obligatory.

Psoriatic arthropathy. A study comparing ibuprofen and etretinate in psoriatic arthropathy demonstrated advantage of the retinoid (Hopkins *et al.* 1985). In general, in mild cases a trial of at least 4–8 weeks with acitretin is justified. Sometimes, comedication with non-steroidal anti-inflammatory drugs (NSAIDs) can be reduced or even stopped. Compared with methotrexate (MTX) or cyclosporin A (CyA), the position of acitretin is lower with regard to this indication. When acitretin is combined with bath-PUVA, significant improvement can be achieved, and it is well accepted by the patients.

Combination therapy

With the exception of the erythrodermic and pustular forms of psoriasis, oral application of retinoids should always be combined with adjuvant topical antipsoriatic substances (Fig. 13.5).

Oral retinoid treatment in combination with topical agents shows long-term clinical success particularly in refractory and exanthematic courses of chronic plaques types. Combination is possible with local applications of tar,

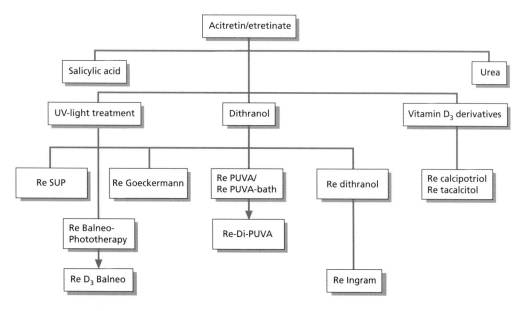

Fig. 13.5 Options to combine acitretin or etretinate with topical regimens in chronic plaque-type psoriasis.

dithranol and calcipotriol/tacalcitol; in addition, UV treatments with selective UV phototherapy (SUP), narrow-band UVB, PUVA, bath-PUVA or balneophototherapy are very effective (Tables 13.4 and 13.5). Balneophototherapy and the development of the topical vitamin D$_3$ derivatives calcipotriol and tacalcitol have especially widened the spectrum of combination therapies during recent years. The configuration of individual combination therapy for the out- and the inpatient has to be designed carefully in terms of the patient's mobility, amount of time available for residential treatment, and therapeutic response.

Combination with topical antipsoriatic drugs. Combination of retinoids with topical treatment, such as dithranol and the new vitamin D$_3$ analogues represents a very effective therapeutic procedure. In general, one would prefer a regimen with dithranol during an inpatient treatment, whereas calcipotriol and tacalcitol are easier to apply at home; however, the improvement of the galenic formulations dithranol, such as the development of a washable dithranol paste or the introduction of dithranol microencapsulated by crystalline monoglycerides (Biogram) makes ambulatory treatment with dithranol increasingly attractive (Christensen *et al.* 1989; De Jong & van de Kerkhof 1992). In addition, short-contact treatment with dithranol was introduced as an attractive alternative for outpatient treatment during recent years (Schaefer *et al.* 1980; de Mare *et al.* 1989).

The therapeutic response of acitretin in combination with topical antipsoriatic treatment is not well documented so far, even though it is used

Table 13.4 Combinations of PUVA – bath with retinoids.

	Topical	Systemic
RePUVA		
Initial: acitretin 0.5–0.75 mg/kg/day for 10 days		
Morning	Shower or bath Moisturizer UVA: 0.5–5 J/cm^2 30 min–2 h Enhance dosage	Acitretin 10–20 mg 5-MOP 8-MOP $\Big\}$ 0.3–0.6 mg/kg/day TMP
Evening	Moisturizer	Acitretin 10 (–20) mg
Caution: patient has to wear UV-sunglasses: sun protection!		
RePUVA-bath		
Initial: acitretin 0.5–0.75 mg/kg/day for 10 days		
Morning	Psoralen bath ↓ UVA Shower Moisturizer	Acitretin 10 (–20) mg
Evening	Moisturizer	Acitretin 10 (–20) mg

TMP, tri-methony psoralen

in most dermatological departments by experience without any doubts. Recently, topical application of calcipotriol or either vehicle in addition to oral acitretin treatment was investigated in 135 patients with extensive psoriasis vulgaris. Combination of calcipotriol ointment with oral acitretin produced a significantly better treatment response achieved with a lower cumulative acitretin dose in patients with severe psoriasis vulgaris (van de Kerkhof *et al.* 1996). In earlier studies it was determined that the addition of topical dithranol to systemic etretinate application increased the antipsoriatic effects of both (Orfanos & Goerz 1978). Addition of dithranol ointment to the retinoid showed better clinical response in psoriatic patients than oral etretinate alone. A similar study has not been performed for acitretin; however, a similar situation with this metabolite has to be expected. For the combination treatment of acitretin and dithranol the following interference is important to know: usually the dithranol concentration is increased stepwise (0.01/0.02/0.1 ... 2%) every 3–5 days twice daily (inpatient regimen) or dose and application time are variably augmented (outpatient regimen). After 10–12 days the irritative potential of both can cumulate, in particular at the margin and within the centre of the plaque. Therefore, in this combination regimen the dithranol

Table 13.5 Good working UV – combinations with acitretin.

	Topical	Oral
Goeckermann*		
Morning	Tar bath followed by selective UV bands and moisturizer	Acitretin 10–15 mg
Evening	Urea plus emollient	Acitretin 10–15 mg
Ingram*		
Morning	Tar bath followed by selective UV bands and classical or short-contact dithranol plus emollient	Acitretin 10–15 mg
Evening	Classical or short-contact dithranol plus emollient	Acitretin 10 (–20) mg
Balneophototherapy		
Morning	15% saltwater (sole) bath followed by selective UV bands plus emollient	Acitretin 10–15 mg
Evening	Urea plus emollient	Acitretin 10–15 mg

*Modified regimen.

dose has to be increased more slowly due to additive clinical and irritative effects of both. The time needed for clearance is shorter than with either monotherapies.

Combination with UV irradiation. Etretinate and acitretin have shown enhanced clinical response in combination therapy with SUP or PUVA (Tables 13.4 and 13.5) (Ruzicka *et al.* 1990; Meigel 1991; Tanew *et al.* 1991). The combination of retinoids with UV irradiation and balneophototherapy is more favourable in comparison with other systemic antipsoriatic drugs such as MTX, CyA or fumaric acid because of a better benefit/risk ratio.

One of the most effective antipsoriatic regimens available is the combination of retinoids and PUVA (RePUVA). This type of therapy allows significant reduction of the cumulative UVA dose. The oral retinoid most probably also reduces the risk of initiation and promotion of skin cancer by UV. In addition, enhanced duration of remission is achieved when therapy is stopped (Grupper & Berretti 1981). If possible, oral retinoid application should commence 10 days before UV treatment. Compared with acitretin monotherapy, the acitretin dose is lower at about 2×10 mg/day. After clinical clearance, dosage should be reduced, maintenance administration is advised for another 3 months. After 6 weeks of treatment with RePUVA in a dosage of about 10–15 mg acitretin twice daily and a total dose of 30–60 J/cm² UVA, significant clinical response of >90% can be expected in about 90–95% of patients. RePUVA or RePUVA-bath are both equally successful in severe psoriasis. Today we prefer RePUVA-bath in a day-care setting. Moreover, even in cases with moderate to severe primary or reactive secondary arthropathy, this treatment procedure is well accepted by the patients, who shortly experience marked improvement of clinical symptoms.

The practice of RePUVA-bath is convenient for the patient and produces fewer side-effects.

During RePUVA-bath, the patient takes a psoralen-containing bath, for example methoxsalen (8-MOP), bergapten (5-MOP) or trioxsalen, for a period of about 15 min before exposure to UVA light. A reduced risk of developing skin cancer after treatment with PUVA-bath in a trioxsalen solution compared to PUVA therapy with oral application of 8-MOP is reported (Lindelöf et al. 1992). The greatest advantage is achieved by starting acitretin supplementation 10–14 days before PUVA-bath is commenced. It is possible to select from among the variations of a whole-body bath, partial bath or foil-bath; thus, one can choose an individual therapy for each patient, and the consumption of 5- or 8-MOP/trioxsalen can be reduced. Patients with severe pustular palmoplantar psoriasis show good clinical response of hands and feet after the treatment with local PUVA-bath. RePUVA-bath is a particularly acceptable alternative for patients who suffer from gastrointestinal discomfort after ingestion of oral psoralen. As there is nearly no systemic resorption of psoralen through the skin, side-effects are reduced; and under these conditions it is not necessary to wear UVA sunglasses after PUVA-bath treatment. In addition, RePUVA-bath treatment is a practicable regimen for patients who tend to develop cataracts. The use of retinoid-balneo-phototherapy (15 min of 10–20% sole bath, followed by SUP) provides special comfort for the patient, but it shows a lower efficiency rate as compared to RePUVA-bath. It is the therapy of choice in moderate courses of psoriasis, or it has to be combined with additional topical ointment such as dithranol or calcipotriol.

The combination regimen is less limited in terms of the side-effects of the retinoid due to lower dosage, but there are contraindications of UVA exposure. Patients with light-sensitive skin, chronic UV damage and a history of dysplastic nevus cell nevus syndrome, multiple pigment naevi, pre-existing basal cell carcinoma, arsenic exposure, actinic keratosis, squamous cell carcinoma, or melanoma should not be treated either with PUVA or RePUVA.

Combination therapy: the retinoid plus topical treatment and UV irradiation. There has been good experience in the modification of well-established combination regimens such as Goeckermann's or Ingram with acitretin. The severity grade (PASI >12) of the disease and the individual patient's response and pretreatment history determine the choice of those modifications. An important consideration is whether the patient has to be treated as an inpatient or outpatient. Additional combination schemes of acitretin with calcipotriol or dithranol together with balneophototherapy, or acitretin with dithranol and PUVA/PUVA-bath are possible (Fig. 13.5).

Contraindicated combination therapies. Even if there is an immense spectrum of possible combination therapies with retinoids, we emphasize that some substances are not useful for combination. On the one hand, they may produce additional side-effects, on the other, they may interact in their pharmacological metabolism. For example, combinations of acitretin with MTX, CyA or fumaric acid have to be avoided because of their metabolism and/or interactions. Mainly the increase of hepatotoxicity limits the application of at least two of these drugs. Hepatotoxicity of CyA is less pronounced compared with MTX, but additional side-effects, for example on the kidney, leads to an incalculable short- and long-term risk. Retinoids can inhibit the metabolism of CyA, and thereby increase CyA plasma levels (Webber & Black 1993). However, a short period of days to a few weeks of overlap can be accepted. For example, CyA or MTX are first given as a crisis intervention modification, then the dose is weaned and the retinoid is introduced, and, finally the CyA or MTX tapered down to zero.

13.5 Side-effects and interactions

Acitretin has a characteristic spectrum of side-effects similar to chronic hypervitaminosis A syndrome (Table 13.6). Retinoid-induced cheilitis is unavoidable and occurs more or less rapidly, depending on the dosage administered. At the same time, it is also a parameter for the drug's absorption and patients's compliance. Particularly under isotretinoin, dryness of the nasal mucosa can sometimes lead to epistaxis at dosages of 0.8–1.0 (or more) mg/kg per day. Dryness of the mouth associated with thirst is observed, and rhagades may occasionally appear. Increased keratolysis may also appear as an undesired side-effect in those patients having no palmoplantar involvement of psoriasis, in others the palmoplantar desquamation is desirable. In addition, skin xerosis, pruritus, and the feeling of a burning, or rather sticky skin may result as a common side-effect. Hair loss and brittle nails are observed more or less frequently, depending on the dose. All these effects are reversible after cessation of acitretin treatment, but in some cases they can be the reason for interruption of administration. In multicentre investigations with comparison of etretinate and acitretin, acitretin shows a slightly higher amount of mucocutaneous side-effects, especially in a dosage of about 50 mg daily (Kragballe *et al.* 1989; Gollnick *et al.* 1993).

   Increase of serum triglycerides is a common side-effect under retinoid treatment; increased serum cholesterol and liver enzymes are observed less frequently. In most cases the changes in laboratory parameters are transient (Vahlquist *et al.* 1987). The increase of serum lipids can be prevented by a fat-

Table 13.6 Most important adverse drug effects of systemic retinoid treatment

Affected area	Effect
Skin and mucous membranes	Cheilitis, dryness of eyes, nasal and oral mucosa (100%) Epistaxis (10%) Xerosis, pruritus (100%) Brittle nails (20%) Hair loss (20–50%) Feeling of burning or sticky skin (20%)
Muscle and skeletal system	Ossification of ligaments, such as longitudinal ligament of the spine Degenerative spondylosis, osteoporosis
Liver	Elevation of liver enzymes (20%) Severe liver damage (<1%)
Lipid metabolism	Increase of serum triglycerides and cholesterol Decrease of HDL cholesterol (isotretinoin)
Teratogenicity	Malformation of the craniofacial (such as, cleft palate), thymic, cardiac, skeletal, and central nervous system
Various	Fatigue, headache, nausea

and carbohydrate-reduced diet. Less frequently combinations with serum lipid-reducing drugs are necessary. Rarely, inflammation of the liver has been observed (Berbis *et al.* 1989; Gupta *et al.* 1989). Only in one case was severe hepatotoxic reaction with progression to cirrhosis of the liver reported (van Ditzhuijsen *et al.* 1990).

In some patients, especially in chronic and frequently relapsing courses of pustular psoriasis, retinoid therapy may become long standing, even for years. In these cases it becomes particularly important to pay attention to the problem of retinoid-induced harmful effects on the bones. It is advisable to take an X-ray of the spine before starting the therapy and to document carefully skeletal pains and mobility restriction. If there is any clinical doubt, radiographic control of symptomatic parts of the skeleton is necessary. After long-term acitretin application, diffuse ideopathic skeletal hyperostosis (DISH syndrome), degenerative spondylosis, arthritis of the vertebral articulations, and development of syndesmophytes at the vertebral spine have been observed. In addition, the development of bone spurs and chondrosis of the ligamentum longitudinale, the premature epiphyseal closure, and osteoporosis have been reported (Di Giovanna *et al.* 1995). In a clinical study with 135 long-term acitretin-treated patients, the development of DISH was examined through X-rays of the spine. In this investigation DISH syndrome shows no correlation with the duration of treatment but instead with the age of patients (van Dooren-Greebe *et al.* 1996).

Regarding the results of *in vitro* investigations, which provided evidence that acitretin inhibits collagen synthesis in murine cranial bones, we have to consider potentially severe bone disorders occurring as a rare result of long-term acitretin treatment; and as a consequence careful observation is reasonable.

Teratogenicity of retinoids is generally an unsolved problem. Even if the plasma half-life of acitretin is only about 50–60 h, re-esterification of acitretin to etretinate requires very safe contraceptive measures during acitretin treatment for women of childbearing age. Contraception should be started about 1 month before application and continued at least for 2 years after cessation of the therapy depending on local regulations (Table 13.7).

13.6 Interactions

Interactions are possible with tetracyclines, phenytoin, barbiturates, NSAIDs, ketoconazol, and CyA. Combination therapy with MTX is contraindicated because of additional hepatotoxic side-effects. Recent investigations have provided evidence that retinoids inhibit the CyA metabolism and lead to increased drug plasma levels.

13.7 Contraindications

The contraindications are listed below, where A = absolute and R = relative.
1   Pregnancy, or planning for pregnancy < 2 years, nursing (A).
2   Severe hepatic dysfunction (A).
3   Insufficient patient compliance (A).
4   Moderate hepatic disturbances (R).
5   Severe renal impairment (R).

Table 13.7 Guidelines for treatment with acitretin.

Pretreatment laboratory and clinical monitoring
    Exclude severe disease of liver, kidney, and metabolism, such as diabetes, hyperlipidemia
    Exclude concomitant treatment with interacting drugs or abuse of alcohol
    Ask for skeletal pains and mobility restriction on a regular basis; radiographic control of symptomatic areas; spinal X-ray

In female patients
    Pregnancy test, oral and written information concerning clinical effectiveness, side effects
    Need for adequate contraception from at least one month prior to treatment until two years post-treatment in fertile female patients
    During therapy
    Control serum lipids, liver enzymes and serum creatinine; initially every two weeks, later every 6–12 weeks
    Control contraception

---

6 Strongly elevated serum levels of cholesterol/triglycerides (R).
7 Concomitant treatment with tetracyclines (risk factor for intracranial hypertension), or phenytoin (competition of plasma-protein binding) (R).
8 Concomitant use of hepatotoxic drugs, for example MTX (R).

13.8 Future perspectives

Introduction of retinoids has led to a revolution in the treatment of psoriasis and other dermatological diseases. In fact, they have become indispensable in mono- and combination therapy during recent years. The newly developed topical antipsoriatic retinoid tazarotene, and the systemic cytochrome P-450 inhibitor liarozole, which enhance retinoic acid cytoplasma levels, show promising prospects for the future. Clinical introduction will determine if these drugs are able to reduce significantly the dissociation between therapeutic efficacy and side-effects. It would be a great advantage to develop oral retinoid derivatives that lack their most unacceptable side-effect: teratogenicity.

Receptor-specific drug targeting or the specific block (knock-out) of receptors by receptor antagonists are future prospects.

References

Almond-Roesler, B. & Orfanos, C.E. (1996) Trans-Acitretin wird in Etretinat rück-metabolisiert. *Hautarzt* **47**, 173–177.

Apfel, C., Crettaz, M., Siegentaler, G. *et al.* (1991) Synthetic retinoids: binding to retinoic acid receptors. In: *Retinoids 10 Years On* (ed. Saurat, H.-J.), pp. 110–121. Karger, Basel.

Bauer, R. & Orfanos, C.E. (1984) Effects of synthetic retinoids on human peripheral blood lymphocytes and polymorphonuclears *in vitro*. In: *Retinoid Therapy: A review of Clinical and Laboratory Research* (ed. Cunliffe, W.J.), pp. 101–118. MTP Press, Boston.

Benbrook, D., Lernhardt, E. & Pfahl, M. (1988) A new retinoic acid receptor identified from hepatocellular carcinoma. *Nature* **333**, 669–672.

Berbis, P., Geiger, J.M., Vaisse, C. *et al.* (1989) Benefit of progressively increasing doses during the initial treatment with acitretin in psoriasis. *Dermatologica* **178**, 88–92.

Bollag, W. (1985) New retinoids with potential use in homans. In: *Retinoids: New Trends in Research and Therapy* (ed. Saurat, J.H.), pp. 274–288. Karger, Basel.

Brand, N., Petkovitch, M., Krust, A. *et al.* (1988) Identification of a second human retinoid acid receptor. *Nature* **332**, 850–853.

Chen, H. & Privalsky, L. (1995) Cooperative formation of high-order oligomers by retinoid X receptors: an unexpected mode of DNA recognition. *Proceedings of the National Academy of Science of the USA.* **92**, 422–426.

Christensen, O.B., Holst, R., Hradil, E. *et al.* (1989) Clinical response and side effects in the treatment of psoriasis with UVB and a novel dithranol formulation. *Acta Dermato-Venereologica* **146** (Suppl.), 96–101.

Cotler, S., Chang, D., Henderson, L. *et al.* (1992) The metabolism of acitretin and isoacitretin in the in situ isolated perfused rat liver. *Xenobiotica* **22**, 1229–1237.

De Jong, E.M.G.J. & van de Kerkhof, P.C.M. (1992) Short contact dithranol treatment of psoriasis, using a novel emulsifying ointment (Hermal-AWR): Changes in clinical scores and in parameters for inflammation, proliferation and keratinization. *British*

Journal of Dermatology **2**, 552–558.

Di Giovanna, J.J., Sollitto, R.B., Abangan, D.L. *et al.* (1995) Osteoporosis is a toxic effect in a long-term etretinate therapy. *Archives of Dermatology* **131**, 1321–1322.

DiSepio, D., Malhotra, M., Chandraratna, A.S. & Nagpal, S. (1997) Retinoic acid receptor-nuclear factor-interleukin 6 antagonism. *Journal of Biological Chemistry* **41**, 25555–25559.

Dockx, P., Decree, J. & Degreef, H. (1995) Inhibition of the metabolism of endogenous retinoic acid as treatment for severe psoriasis: an open study with oral liarozole. *British Journal of Dermatology* **133**, 426–432.

Dupuy, P., Bagot, M., Heslan, M. *et al.* (1989) Synthetic retinoids inhibit the antigen presenting properties of epidermal cells in vitro. *Journal of Investigative Dermatology* **93**, 455–459.

Ellis, C.N., Hermann, R.C., Gorsulowsky, D.C. *et al.* (1987) Etretinate therapy reduces inpatient treatment of psoriasis. *Journal of the American Academy of Dermatology* **17**, 787–791.

Fisher, G.J., Talwar, H.S., Xiao, J.H. *et al.* (1994) Immunological identification and functional quantitation of retinoic acid and retinoid X receptor protein in human skin. *Journal of Biological Chemistry* **269**, 20629–20635.

Geiger, J.M. & Brindley, C.J. (1988) Cis-trans-interconversion of acitretin in man. *Skin Pharmacology.* **1**, 230–236.

Gollnick, H. (1996) Oral retinoids-efficacy and toxicity in psoriasis. *British Journal of Dermatology* **135**, 6–17.

Gollnick, H. (1998) Psoriasis: treatment and patient. *Journal of Dermatology Treatment*

Gollnick, H. & Dümmler, U. (1997) Retinoids. *Clinics in Dermatology* **15**, 799–810.

Gollnick, H. & Kirsten, S. (1996) Retinoide-Wo stehen wir heute? Ein Überblick zu den Wirkmechanismen und Hauptindikationen. *Y X. Hautkrankheiten.* **71**, 442–452.

Gollnick, H. & Menter, A. (in press) Tazarotene in combination treatment with corticoids. *British Journal of Dermatology*

Gollnick, H. & Orfanos, C.E. (1985) Etretinat Pro und Contra. Nutzen-Risiko-Abwägung der systemischen Retinoidtherapie bei Psoriasis und neue Entwicklungen. Freie aromatische Säure Arotinoide. *Hautarzt* **36**, 2–9.

Gollnick, H. & Orfanos, C.E. (1986) Retinoids. In: *Textbook of Psoriasis* (ed. Mier, P.D. & van de Kerkhof, P.C.M.), pp. 252–267. Churchill Livingstone, Edinburgh.

Gollnick, H. & Orfanos, C.E. (1991) Theoretical aspects of the use of retinoids as anticancer agents. In: *Retinoids in Cutaneous Malignancy* (ed. Marks, R.), pp. 41–65. Blackwell Science, Oxford.

Gollnick, H., Bauer, R., Brindley, C. *et al.* (1988) Acitretin versus etretinate in psoriasis. Clinical and pharmacokinetic results of a German multicenter study. *Journal of the American Academy of Dermatology* **19**, 458–469.

Gollnick, H., Rinck, G., Bitterling, T. *et al.* (1990) Pharmakokinetik von Etretinat, Acitretin und 13-cis-Acitretin: neue Ergebnisse und Nutzen der Blutspiegel-orientierten klinischen Anwendung. *Y X. Hautkrankheiten.* **65**, 40–50.

Gollnick, H., Zaun, H., Ruzicka, T. *et al.* (1993) Relapse rate of severe generalised psoriasis after treatment with acitretin or etretinate. Results of the first randomised double-blind multicenter half-year follow up study. *European Journal of Dermatology* **3**, 442–446.

Grupper, C. & Berretti, B. (1981) Treatments of psoriasis by oral PUVA therapy combined with aromatic retinoid (Ro 10–9359; Tigason®). *Dermatologica* **162**, 440–413.

Gupta, A.K., Goldfarb, M.T., Ellis, C.N. *et al.* (1989) Side effect profile of acitretin therapy in psoriasis. *Journal of the American Academy of Dermatology*, 1088–1093.

Hackney, D.D. (1995) Polarity-specific activities of retinoic acid receptors determined by a co-repressor. *Nature* **377**, 451–454.

Harper, R.A. (1988) Specificity in the synergism between retinoic acid and EGF on the growth of adult human skin fibroblasts. *Experimental Cell Research* **178**, 254–263.

Hopkins, R., Brid, H.A., Jones, H. *et al.* (1985) A double-blind controlled trial of etretinate (Tigason®) and ibuprofen in psoriatic arthritis. *Annals of Rheumatic Disease* **44**, 189–193.

Imcke, E., Ruszczak, Z.B., Mayer-da-Silva, A. *et al.* (1991) Cultivation of human dermal microvascular endothelial cells in vitro: Immunocytochemical and ultrastructural characterization and effect of treatment with three synthetic retinoids. *Archives of Dermatological Research* **283**, 149–157.

Kragballe, K., Jansen, C.T., Geiger, J.-M. *et al.* (1989) A double-blind comparison of acitretin and etretinate in the treatment of severe psoriasis. *Acta Dermato-Venereologica* **69**, 35–40.

Krueger, G.G., Drake, L.A., Elias, P.M. *et al.* (1998) The safety and efficacy of tazarotene gel, a topical acetylenic retinoid, in the treatment of psoriasis. *Archives of Dermatology* **134**, 57–60.

Kuijpers, A.L.A., van Pelt, H.P.A., Bergers, M. *et al.* (1998) Effects of oral liarozole on epidermal proliferation and differentiation in severe plaque psoriasis: a double-blind comparative study with acitretin. *Journal of Investigative Dermatology* **110** (4), 553.

Lindelöf, B., Sigurgeirson, B., Tegner, E. *et al.* (1992) Comparison of the carcinogenic potential of trioxalen bath PUVA and oral methoxsalen PUVA. *Archives of Dermatology* **128**, 1341–1344.

Mahrle, G. (1985) Retinoids in oncology. *Current Problems in Dermatology* **13**, 128–163.

de Mare, S., Calis, N., den Hartog, G. *et al.* (1989) Out patient treatment with short contact dithranol. The impact of frequent concentration adjustments. *Acta Dermato-Venereologica* **69**, 449–451.

Meigel, W. (1991) Acitretin and PUVA or UVB. In: *Retinoids: 10 Years On. Retinoid Symposium Geneva, 1990* (ed. Saurat,. J.H.), pp. 214–227. Karger, Basel.

Orfanos, C.E. & Goerz, G. (1978) Orale Psoriasis-Therapie mit einem neuen aromatischen Retinoid. *Deutsche Medizinische Wochenschrift.* **103**, 195–199.

Orfanos, C.E., Ehlert, R. & Gollnick, H. (1987) The retinoids. A review of their clinical pharmacology and therapeutic use. *Drugs* **34**, 459–503.

Parkinson, D.R. & Smith, M.A. (1992) Retinoid therapy for acute promyeloic leukemia: a coming of age for the differentiation therapy of malignancy. *Annals of Internal Medicine* **117**, 338–339.

Petkovich, M., Brand, N.J., Krust, A. *et al.* (1987) A human retinoic acid receptor which belongs to the family of nuclear receptors. *Nature* **330**, 444–450.

Pilkington, T. & Brogden, R.N. (1992) Acitretin: a review of its pharmacology and therapeutic use. *Drugs* **43**, 597–627.

Priestley, G.C. (1987) Proliferation and glycosaminoglycans secretion in fibroblasts psoriatic skin: differential responses to retinoids. *British Journal of Dermatology* **117**, 575–583.

Raynaud, F., Gerbaud, P. & Evian-Brion, D. (1994) Benefical effect of a combination of retinoids and long-acting theophylline in treatment of psoriasis vulgaris. *British Journal of Dermatology* **31**, 740–742.

Rollmann, O. & Vahlquist, A. (1983) Retinoid concentrations in skin, serum and adipose tissue of patients treated with etretinate. *British Journal of Dermatology* **109**, 439–447.

Ruzicka, T., Sommerburg, C., Braun-Falco, O. *et al.* (1990) Efficiency of acitretin in combination with UV-B in the treatment of severe psoriasis. *Archives of Dermatology* **126**, 482–486.

Saurat, J.-H., Hirschel-Scholz, S., Salomon, D. *et al.* (1987) Human skin retinoid-binding proteins and therapy with synthetic retinoids: a still unexplained link. *Dermatologica* **175** (Suppl. 1), 13–19.

Schaefer, H., Faber, E.M., Goldberg, L. *et al.* (1980) Limited application period for dithranol in psoriasis. *British Journal of Dermatology* **102**, 571–573.

Struy, H., Bohne, M., Morenz, J. *et al.* (1996) Effects of retinoids on human neutrophil-derived free radicals (Abstract). *European Journal of Haematology* **59** (Suppl. 57), 52.

Stüttgen, G. (1962) Zur Lokalbehandlung von Keratosen mit Vitamin A-Säure. *Dermatologica* **124**, 65–80.

Takase, S., Ong, D.E. & Chytil, F. (1986) Transfer of retinoic acid from ist complex with cellular retinoic acid-binding protein to the nucleus. *Archives of Biochemistry and. Biophysics* **247**, 328–334.

Tanew, A., Guggenbichler, A., Hönigsmann, H. *et al.* (1991) Photochemotherapy for severe psoriasis without or in combination with acitretin: a randomized double-blind comparisation study. *Journal of the American Academy of Dermatology* **25**, 682–684.

Tsambaos, D. & Orfanos, C.E. (1981) Chemotherapy of psoriasis and other skin disorders with oral retinoids. *Pharmacological Therapy* **14**, 355–374.

Vahlquist, C., Lithell, H., Michaelsson, G. *et al.* (1987) Plasma fat elimination, tissue lipoprotein lipase activity and plasma fatty acid composition during sequential treatment with atretinate and isotretinoin. *Acta Dermato-Venereologica* **67**, 139–144.

van de Kerkhof, P.C.M., Hutchinson, P.E. & the Calcipotriol Study Group (1996) Topical use of calcipotriol improves outcome in acitretin treated patients with severe psoriasis vulgaris. *British Journal of Dermatology* **135** (Suppl. 47), 30 (Abstract).

van Ditzhuijsen, T.J., van Haelst, U.J., van Dooren-Greebe, R.J., van de Kerkhof, P.C. & Yap, S.H. (1990) Severe hepatotoxic reaction with progression to cirrhosis after use of a novel retinoid (acitretin). *Journal of Hepatology* **11**, 185–188.

van Dooren-Greebe, R.J., Lemmens, J.A., de Boo, T. *et al.* (1996) Prolonged treatment with oral retinoids in adults: no influence on the prevalence, incidence and severity of spinal abnormalities. *British Journal of Dermatology* **134**, 71–76.

van Wauwe, J.P. (1990) Liarozol an inhibitor of retinoic acid metabolism of all trans retinoic acid in rats. *Journal of. Pharmacology and Experimental Therapeutics* **252**, 365–369.

Ward, A., Brogden, R.N., Heel, R.C. *et al.* (1984) Isotretinoin. A review of ist pharmacological properties and therapeutic efficacy in acne and other skin disorders. *Drugs* **28**, 6–37.

Webber, I.R. & Black, D.J. (1993) Effect of etretinate on cyclosporin metabolism *in vitro*. *British Journal of Dermatology* **128**, 42–44.

Weinstein, G.D. & Grenn, L. (1994). New topical retinoid gel for therapy of psoriasis: dose ranging study of AGN 190168. Abstract. *Sixth International Psoriasis Symposium*, July 20–24, Chicago.

Weis, K., Pambaud, S., Lavau, C. *et al.* (1994) Retinoic acid regulates aberrant nuclear localization of PML-RARa in acute promyelotic leukemia cells. *Cell* **76**, 345–356.

Wiegand, U.W. & Chou, R.C. (1998) Pharmacokinetics of oral isotretinoin. *Journal of the American Academy of Dermatology* **39** (2), 8–12.

Wolbach, S.B. & Howe, P.R. (1925) Tissue changes following deprivation of fat-soluble A-vitamin. *Journal of Experimental Medicine* **42**, 753–778.

Xiao, J.H., Durand, B., Chambon, P. *et al.* (1995) Endogenous retinoic acid receptor (RAR)–retinoid X-receptor (RXR) heterodimers are the major functional forms in adult human keratinocytes. *Journal of Biological Chemistry* **270**, 2001–2011.

Chapter 14: Cyclosporin and Immunotherapy

M.A. de Rie and J.D. Bos

14.1 Introduction

Although the pathogenesis of psoriasis is controversial, it is generally accepted that T lymphocytes play a pivotal role in this skin disease. This concept that psoriasis is an immunodermatosis first emerged from the histopathological demonstration that T cells are abundantly present in lesional skin of psoriasis patients. Later it was found that these T cells are activated as indicated by their HLA DR and interleukin 2 receptor (IL-2R) expression. In addition, systemic administration of the T-cell growth factor IL-2 exacerbates psoriasis. The effectiveness of cyclosporin has further supported the view that T-cell-mediated immunomodulation is implicated in the pathogenesis of psoriasis (Bos 1988).

During the last decade much effort has been directed at the development of T-cell-specific immunomodulating agents for the treatment of psoriasis. Cyclosporin A, the prototype T-cell-selective agent, served as the pioneer drug in this field. The group of cyclic immunosuppressants, which includes cyclosporin A, comprises several interesting molecules that are now studied for psoriasis treatment (Table 14.1).

Although cyclosporin A and S are cyclic peptides and the others belong to the group of macrolides, they all have almost indistinguishable cellular effects. Tacrolimus, which is the best known macrolide from this group, and the undecapeptide cyclosporin A both inhibit certain calcium-dependent cellular processes including transcriptional activation of lymphokine genes such as that of IL-2 in helper T cells following the T-cell-receptor-mediated signal transduction (Fig. 14.1). Cyclosporin A and the major representatives from this group of cyclic immunosuppressive peptides including ascomycin will be discussed in further detail.

Table 14.1 Cyclic immunosuppressive agents.

Peptides	Macrolides
Cyclosporin A	Tacrolimus (FK506)
Cyclosporin S (SDZ IMM 125)	Ascomycin (SDZ 281-240 and SDZ ASM 981)
	Sirolimus (rapamycin)
	Didemnin B
	Tetranactin

T-cell directed immunosuppressive agents at work

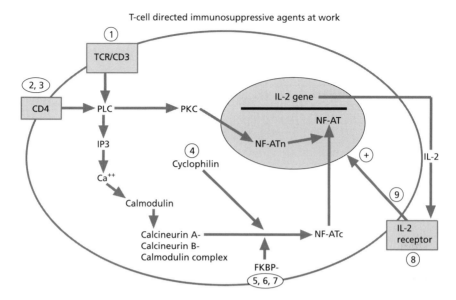

Fig. 14.1 T-cell-directed immunosuppressive agents at work. Schematic representation of the T-cell activation pathway that leads to transcription of the IL-2 gene and subsequent IL-2 production. T-cell activation can be blocked by anti-CD3 monoclonal antibodies (1), anti-CD4 monoclonal antibodies (2) and peptide T (3) that bind to the TCR/CD3 complex and the CD4 molecule, respectively. Alternatively, T-cell activation can be blocked by cyclosporins (4) that bind to cyclophilins and thereby inhibit the formation of the NF-ATc complex. Tacrolimus (= FK-506) (5) and the ascomycins SDZ 281–240 (6) and SDZ-ASM-981 (7) bind to FKBP and consequently inhibit T-cell activation. The interleukin 2 (IL-2) receptor can be blocked by the lymphocyte-selective toxin DAB$_{389}$IL-2 (8). Sirolimus (9) also binds to a FK binding protein but does not inhibit IL-2 production but a later stage of the cell cycle. TCR, T-cell receptor; PLC, phospholipase C; PKC, protein kinase C; IP$_3$, inositol-triphosphate; FKBP, FK-506 binding protein; NF-ATn,c, nuclear factor of activated cells *n*ucleus, *c*ytosol. Redrawn from de Rie & Bos (1997) with permission from Elsevier Science.

Monoclonal antibodies (Mab) against T-cell membrane molecules (CD3 and CD4) have been used in a limited series of patients with sometimes dramatic remission of their psoriasis. Since antimonoclonal sensitization (anti-idiotypic and anti-isotypic) is a major problem in this field, recombinant chimeric Mab are now under research. A summary of the state of the art in relation to treatment of psoriasis will be given.

As well as the T-cell-selective agents mentioned above, various chemical compounds that modulate the immune system have been developed. Cytokines including tumour necrosis factor-α (TNF-α), the lymphocyte-selective diphtheria toxin DAB$_{389}$IL-2 and antireceptor peptides, have been tested in several trials. Although it is premature to interpret these data, since they are derived from uncontrolled trials in a limited number of patients, they are promising not only for therapeutic reasons but also to improve our understanding of the pathogenesis of psoriasis. These new therapeutic strategies will be discussed below.

14.2 Cyclic immunosuppressive drugs

14.2.1 Cyclosporin A and S

History and mode of actions

Cyclosporin A is a neutral lipophilic cyclic polypeptide consisting of an 11-amino-acid sequence. It was isolated from a sample of the fungus *Tolypocladium inflatum Gams*, which was first found during 1969 in a soil sample from the Hardanger Vidda in Norway. At first cyclosporin A was screened for antibiotic properties. The immunosuppressive properties of cyclosporin A were later discovered by Borel in 1972. The early reports of cyclosporin A in psoriasis were serendipitous case stories that reported clearing of psoriasis in patients suffering from psoriatic arthritis (Müller & Herrmann 1979).

Since then, multiple open and controlled studies with systemically administered cyclosporin A have been reported (review in de Rie & Bos 1997).

Recently, cyclosporin S (SDZ IMM 125), a new derivative of the cyclosporin family, was developed. Cyclosporin S is the hydroxyethyl derivative of D-serine-cyclosporin. In experimental studies, the immunosuppressive activity of this compound was at least equivalent to that of cyclosporin A. Cyclosporin S has a dose-related beneficial effect on psoriasis. However, the occurrence of abnormal liver function tests and the effect of long-term cyclosporin S on renal function require further evaluation (Witkamp *et al.* 1995).

To date, no effective topical cyclosporin A formulations have yet been developed for psoriasis (de Rie *et al.* 1991). Since cyclosporin A has a molecular weight of 1202.6 Da, it is unlikely that topically applied cyclosporin A will penetrate the skin barrier. Intralesional injections of cyclosporin A have a beneficial effect on psoriasis.

The biologic activity of cyclosporin A is attributed to the amino acid at position 1, *N*-methyl-L-threonine, in conjunction with the amino acids γ-aminobutyric acid at position 2 and *N*-methyl-L-valine at position 11 (Fig. 14.2).

10 MeLeu	11 MeVal	1 MeBmt	2 Abu	3 Ser
9 MeLeu				
D-Ala 8	Ala 7	MeLeu 6	Val 5	MeLeu 4

Fig. 14.2 Molecular structure of the undecapeptide cyclosporin A. Biological activity is mediated by the amino acids at position 1: *N*-methyl-L-threonine (MeBmt), position 2: γ-aminobutyric acid (Abu) and position 11: *N*-methyl-L-valine (MeVal). Other abbreviations: Ser, serine; MeLeu, *N*-methyl-leucine; Val, valine; Ala, alanine.

Cyclosporin A engages the active site of cyclophilin, a family of isomerases found in almost all mammalian cells. Cyclosporin A complexed with cyclophilin is the active drug and mediator of the immunosuppressive effects. This complex inhibits the enzyme calcineurin, which is a key enzyme in calcium-dependent signalling processes. Calcineurin is essential for signal transduction from the T-cell receptor to the cytokine promoters, triggering the transcription of many cytokines including the T-cell growth factors IL-2 and IL-4 (see Fig. 14.1) (Wong *et al.* 1993). Cyclosporin A nephrotoxicity may also be mediated via the cyclophilin–calcineurin pathway similar to its immunosuppressive effects.

The action of tacrolimus (FK-506) is similar to that of cyclosporin A, although tacrolimus binds to an FK binding protein (FKBP), which is another member of the family of isomerases. FKBP and cyclophilin together are called immunophilins. The FKBP–FK-506 complex also inhibits calcineurin and has therefore similar inhibitory effects on cytokine production by T cells (Schreiber & Crabtree 1992).

Immunosuppression induced by both cyclosporin A and tacrolimus is not restricted to T cells alone, since the secretion of T-cell cytokines important in the immunological functions of keratinocytes, antigen-presenting cells and polymorphonuclear leucocytes, are also inhibited. Moreover, cyclosporin A and possibly also tacrolimus may have direct downregulating immunomodulatory effects on keratinocytes and antigen-presenting cells (Wong *et al.* 1993).

Pharmacokinetics

The first market form of cyclosporin A (Sandimmun) achieved a bioavailability of 30% and an incomplete and highly variable systemic absorption. The latter was mainly due to a non-negligible presystemic first-pass metabolism and poor cyclosporin A permeability of the intestinal mucosa. Therefore a new galenical principle, namely microemulsion technology, was used. The present formulation, now registered as Neoral, is in fact a microemulsion preconcentrate based on a mixture of a hydrophillic solvent, a lipophilic solvent, a surfactant and cyclosporin A. With Neoral absorption of cyclosporin A is more complete and rapid, and results in a single narrow peak concentration and a consistent blood-concentration profile. Data from transplant- and non-transplant patients indicate that more rapid beneficial treatment effects can be reached with Neoral compared with Sandimmun.

By switching from Sandimmun to Neoral an increased exposure to cyclosporin A (area under the curve, C_{max}) could be anticipated. Large-scale studies have found that there is no increased risk for unwanted side-effects, provided that appropriate dose reductions are made on the basis of trough blood cyclosporin A concentration measurement (Erkko *et al.* 1997).

Indications and contraindications

Cyclosporin A is indicated in patients with severe psoriasis, in whom conventional therapy is ineffective (topical treatments, UVB phototherapy, psoralen and UVA (PUVA), methotrexate and etretinate) or inappropriate (Bos *et al.* 1989). Before the start of cyclosporin A therapy a detailed history must be taken (kidney disease, hypertension, malignancy, medication). Other treatments for psoriasis such as arsenic compounds and photo(chemo)therapy, which may increase the risk of cutaneous malignancy, should be taken into account.

Major exclusion criteria for cyclosporin A treatment are impaired kidney function, uncontrolled hypertension, past or present malignancy, infection, pregnancy and lactation, concomitant immunosuppressive therapy, primary or secondary immunodeficiency, severe chronic organ dysfunction and hypersensitivity.

Minor exclusion criteria are drug or alcohol abuse, malabsorption, noncompliance, recent and/or excessive photo(chemo)therapy, and concomitant treatment with drugs that affect cyclosporin A pharmacokinetics (Table 14.2).

Onset of action

Results from several double-blind, placebo-controlled trials showed that after 4 weeks of treatment with cyclosporin A in patients with chronic plaque-type psoriasis, a PASI (psoriasis area and severity index) reduction of 60–70%, can be achieved (Zachariae & Steen Olsen 1995).

Table 14.2 Drug interactions with cyclosporin A.

Increased serum [cyclosporin A]	Decreased serum [cyclosporin A]	Increased risk of nephrotoxicity
Diltiazem	Barbiturates	Aminoglycosides (i.v./i.m.)
Doxycycline	Carbamazepine	Amphotericin B
Ketoconazol	Metamizol	Ciprofloxacine
Macrolide antibiotics (e.g. erythromycin)	Nafcilline	Melphalan
Methylprednisolone	Phenytoin	NSAIDS
Nicardipin	Rifampicin	Trimethoprim
Oral contraceptives	Sulfadimidine with trimethoprim (i.v.)	
Propafenon		
Verapamil		

Induction of remission

The effectiveness of cyclosporin A has been established in a programme of large-scale studies, which have shown a clear dose–response relationship, with regard to both the number of patients who respond and the time to response. The five European multicentre dose-finding studies analysed and published by Timonen are typical examples showing the efficacy and dose-dependent PASI reduction of cyclosporin A in psoriasis patients (Timonen *et al.* 1990). In this report 457 adult patients suffering from severe psoriasis (PASI ≥ 18) were treated with 1.25, 2.5–3 and 5 mg cyclosporin A/kg/day. After 3 months of treatment, the reduction of PASI was 35% with 1.25 mg/kg/day, 57% with 2.5–3 mg/kg/day and 86% with 5 mg/kg/day. The rates of success, defined by a PASI ≥ 75%, or a score ≤ 8, were 24%, 52% and 88%, respectively. Several other groups of investigators have confirmed these findings (Zachariae & Steen Olsen 1995).

Based on these studies it is now recommended to start with an initial daily oral dose of 3 mg cyclosporin A/kg, in two divided doses, increased every 2 weeks if needed to a maximum daily dose of 5 mg cyclosporin A/kg, or decreased depending on the clinical response. Complete remission should not be the objective; a few lesions are allowed to be sure that the patient is not overdosed.

Maintenance of remission

Patients may be maintained in remission for long periods with cyclosporin A: a group of 44 patients is reported to have been treated for up to 50 months (mean 17 months) at a mean dose of 3.3 mg cyclosporin A/kg/day. Although 5 mg/kg/day of cyclosporin A is significantly more effective than 2.5 mg/kg/day in the treatment of chronic plaque-type psoriasis, remission (PASI reduction of ≥ 75%) can be maintained in most patients on a daily dose of 3 mg cyclosporin A/kg (Ellis *et al.* 1995; Shupack *et al.* 1997). When the dosage of cyclosporin A is reduced for maintenance therapy, there is a trend for laboratory values affected by cyclosporin A during induction to return towards pretherapy levels. However, even at low dosages, cyclosporin treatment for psoriasis generally should be limited to a course of less than 1 year since long-term treatment with cyclosporin A is not only dose-related but also time-related to nephrotoxicity and hypertension (Grossman *et al.* 1996).

Relapse characteristics

The elimination of cyclosporin A is mainly via bile and related to the age of the patient, with a dose-dependent half-life varying from 8.1 h (350 mg oral Sandimmun) to 14.4 h (1400 mg oral Sandimmun). It is therefore not surprising that the effects of cyclosporin A are rapidly reversible after treatment is stopped.

Relapse is often defined as PASI increasing again to more than 50% of baseline value. After cyclosporin A treatment is abruptly stopped relapse occurred within 2 months (Ellis *et al.* 1995). Substantial variability occurred in the rate of recurrence of psoriasis; some patients had relapses in as little as 2 weeks, and some had not relapsed after 4 months. Cyclosporin A does not lead to severe deterioration of the disease ('rebound') after drug withdrawal (Mrowietz *et al.* 1995).

A number of different approaches to stopping cyclosporin A therapy have been evaluated. It was found that even when cyclosporin A was tapered off over 9 weeks, relapse occurred during this tapering phase. There are no substantial data available to advocate a particular tapering off protocol for cyclosporin A.

Response in subforms of psoriasis

Most published studies are concerned with treatment of patients with chronic plaque-type psoriasis, but cyclosporin A has also proven to be effective in other subforms of psoriasis as well. It should be noted, however, that some studies showing efficacy of cyclosporin A in these subforms are uncontrolled studies with a limited number of patients. A summary of these studies is given in Table 14.3.

Table 14.3 Efficacy of cyclosporin A in subforms of psoriasis.

Subform of psoriasis	Dosage (mg/kg/day)	Reference
Erythrodermic psoriasis	≤ 5	Reitamo & Mustakallio (1989)
	≤ 5	Cimitan *et al.* (1989)
	≤ 5	Bonifati *et al.* (1989)
Generalised pustular psoriasis	< 7.5	Fradin *et al.* (1990)
	8	Korstanje *et al.* (1989)
	≤ 12	Meinardi *et al.* (1987)
Palmo-plantar pustulosis	1–6	Meinardi *et al.* (1990)
	1.25–2.5	Reitamo *et al.* (1993)
	2.5–5	Peter *et al.* (1994)
Psoriatic arthritis	≤ 6	Gupta *et al.* (1989)
	2.7	Mahrle *et al.* (1996)
	≤ 6	Olivieri *et al.* (1997)
	2.5–5	Mahrle *et al.* (1995)
	3–5	Riccieri *et al.* (1994)
	2.5	Schopf *et al.* (1994)
Nail psoriasis	2.5–5	Mahrle *et al.* (1995)

Safety and tolerability

Cyclosporin A is effective in the treatment of plaque-type and other subforms of psoriasis. However, cyclosporin A is potentially toxic. Since psoriasis is not a life-threatening disease and life-long therapy can be foreseen, side-effects (e.g. nephrotoxicity) are relatively more important than in clinical transplantation patients. As well as renal side-effects, hypertension, malignancies and infections, other side-effects may occur during treatment with cyclosporin A.

The renal effects of cyclosporin A can be separated into functional and structural changes involving tubules and blood vessels. Functional changes have no morphological substrate and are due to vasoconstriction of the afferent arteriole of the glomerulus. Hence the glomerular filtration rate is lowered and serum urea and creatinine levels are increased.

The increase of serum creatinine is dose dependent and related to the duration of cyclosporin A treatment (de Rie *et al.* 1990). Functional changes are relatively common, can also occur at low doses and are fully reversible. Structural changes are less common than functional changes. In general, structural changes can be divided into two groups: tubulopathy (damage of the proximal tubule) and vasculopathy of the afferent arteriole. Tubulopathy is reversible, vasculopathy is not. For classification of kidney biopsies, a panel of expert pathologists has been formed. This classification can serve as guidance for the definition of cyclosporin toxicity in patients with autoimmune diseases including psoriasis (Mihatsch *et al.* 1994). Age at biopsy and increase of creatinine over baseline were found to be most important risk factors for development of morphological changes. Detailed analysis of psoriatic patients showed that patients without a creatinine increase over 30% had no nephropathy (Feutren *et al.* 1990).

Hypertension, defined according to WHO criteria, may occur in 10% of patients who were normotensive at baseline, during long-term treatment with cyclosporin A. Multivariate analysis of 122 patients on long-term treatment showed that a diastolic blood pressure of more than 75 mmHg before starting was the only risk factor for development of hypertension. We have previously shown that the risk of hypertension is not only dose related but also time dependent. In most series, hypertension resolves after discontinuation of treatment. For antihypertensive treatment during cyclosporin A use, calcium-entry inhibitors are generally recommended (Mihatsch & Wolff 1992).

Any immunosuppressive drug carries the risk of increased incidence of tumours. An increased incidence of lymphoma and squamous cell carcinoma has been shown in transplant patients receiving cyclosporin A. In psoriasis patients only an increased risk of cutaneous squamous cell carcinoma has been reported. This increased risk can be attributed to previous treatments with photo(chemo)therapy and arsenic compounds. Cyclosporin A has no mutagenic effects (Grossman *et al.* 1996).

The incidence of serious infections in patients treated with cyclosporin A does not differ from patients treated with placebo or etretinate. At present it seems more likely that long-term treatment with immunosuppressive drugs such as cyclosporin A increases the incidence of human papillomavirus infection and thereby facilitates the development of malignant neoplasms (e.g. squamous cell carcinomas of the cervix) (Penn 1995).

Other side-effects include gastrointestinal disorders (nausea, vomiting, diarrhoea), hypertrichosis, paraesthesia, gingival hyperplasia, headache, vertigo, muscle cramps and tremor. Clinical experience has shown that these side-effects are manageable by dose reduction or direct treatment. Discontinuation of treatment because of persistence of these side-effects is sometimes required.

Guidelines

Guidelines have previously been published (Bos *et al.* 1989; Mihatsch & Wolff 1992). In summary, cyclosporin is indicated in patients with severe psoriasis who do not have major contraindications (see above). The minimum effective dose should be used and this should not exceed 5 mg cyclosporin A/kg/day. Serum creatinine and blood pressure should be monitored frequently (once every 2–3 weeks during the first 3 months; after that once every 4–6 weeks). Patients older than 50 years need more careful monitoring of creatinine, and lower doses of cyclosporin A are preferable. In cases of creatinine increase of ≥30% over baseline the following strategy is recommended: reduce the cyclosporin A dose for 1 month by 0.5–1 mg/kg/day; if there is no significant improvement in the creatinine values (creatinine increase remains ≥10% over baseline) cyclosporin A therapy should be stopped.

Sustained hypertension should be controlled with calcium-entry blocking drugs. In cases of uncontrolled hypertension cyclosporin A therapy should be stopped. Co-medication with drugs known to interfere with the pharmacokinetics (bioavailability) of cyclosporin A must be avoided (see above). Cyclosporin A monotherapy should not be given for more than 1 year. A scheme for changing the therapeutic regimens before toxicity becomes evident has recently been proposed and should be considered ('rotational therapy') (Weinstein & White 1993).

Combination with other psoriasis treatments

Since particularly the renal side-effects of cyclosporin A therapy are dose related, low-dose treatment regimens are advisable. In order to increase the efficacy of low-dose cyclosporin A treatment, topical steroids and calcipotriol can be used. The combination with potential mutagenic modalities such as photo(chemo)therapy and other immunosuppressive drugs is not recommended because of the increased risk of (skin) malignancies and excessive immuno-suppression. Combination therapies are discussed in Chapter 15.

14.2.2 Tacrolimus (FK-506)

Tacrolimus (FK-506) is a macrolide antibiotic of molecular weight 822 Da, first isolated in 1984 from the soil fungus *Streptomyces tsukubaensis* by Fujisawa (Osaka). The immunosuppressive potency of tacrolimus *in vitro* is 10–100 times greater than that of cyclosporin. Tacrolimus interferes with IgE receptor-mediated processes (skin mast cells and basophils), prostaglandin D_2 synthesis (skin mast cells), leukotriene C_4 secretion (basophils) and T-cell activation (MacLoad & Thompson 1991). Like cyclosporin, tacrolimus binds to an intracellular protein, which is termed FKBP. This complex binds to the enzyme calcineurin, which is pivotal in calcium-dependent intracellular T-cell activation pathways.

Consequently, both cyclosporin A and tacrolimus inhibit IL-2 production and other T-cell-derived growth-promoting cytokines (see Section 2.1 and Fig. 14.1).

Tacrolimus has been intensely studied in the prevention of cardiac, liver and kidney allograft rejection. The customary dose varies between 0.1 and 1 mg/kg/day. Adverse effects include nephrotoxicity and hypertension, among others, most being similar to those in cyclosporin A.

Recently a multicentre, double-blind, placebo-controlled study was presented showing that tacrolimus is effective in psoriasis at a dose of 0.05–0.15 mg/kg/day (European FK-506 Multicentre Study Group 1996). Most of the adverse events (especially renal dysfunction and hypertension) were mild to moderate in severity and resolved completely.

To avoid the occurrence of nephrotoxicity and other side-effects observed with systemic tacrolimus in transplantation and psoriasis, topical formulations have now been developed (Meingassner & Stütz 1992). Since tacrolimus has a lower molecular weight (822 Da) than cyclosporin A (1202 Da), a higher efficacy was anticipated. Indeed initial studies with topical tacrolimus (0.1–1%) have shown promising results in patients suffering from atopic dermatitis (Ruzicka *et al.* 1997). Studies employing topical tacrolimus formulations in psoriasis patients are now being conducted, but initial findings are negative.

14.2.3 Ascomycin

Ascomycin is another representative of the family of immunosuppressive macrolides. Recently SDZ 281–240, an ascomycin derivative, was developed. SDZ 281–240 has strong anti-inflammatory actions similar to tacrolimus.

SDZ 281–240 also binds *in vitro* to the macrophilin-binding protein FKBP-12 thereby inhibiting the phosphatase activity of calcineurin and preventing the assembly and activation of transcription factors NF-AT and NF-κB (see Fig. 14.1) (Meingassner & Stütz 1992). Consequently, activated T cells are downregulated and cytokine-mediated proliferation of keratinocytes is decreased.

Topical application of SDZ 281–240 has recently been studied in a randomized, double-blind, placebo-controlled trial in psoriasis patients. After 10 days a dramatic improvement of plaque-type lesions was seen using two concentrations (0.1% and 1%) in a Finn chamber assay (Rappersberger *et al.* 1996).

Studies have now been performed with a new ascomycin derivative SDZ-ASM-981 (molecular weight 810 Da) (Meingassner *et al.* 1997). SDZ-ASM-981 probably does not pass the normal skin barrier and is therefore only effective in patients with a defective skin barrier. Indeed, topical 1% SDZ-ASM-981 cream is effective in atopic dermatitis patients (van Leent *et al.* 1998).

14.2.4 Sirolimus (rapamycin)

Similar to cyclosporin A, sirolimus (molecular weight 914 Da) was originally isolated in a discovery programme for novel antifungal agents. Sirolimus is a macrocytic triene antibiotic produced by *Streptomyces hygroscopicus*, an actinomycete that was isolated from a soil sample collected from Rapa Nui (Easter Island). Although sirolimus has a similar structure to tacrolimus, its mechanism of action as an immunosuppressive agent is different. Rapamycin forms complexes with the macrophilin-binding protein FKBP and thereby inhibits activation of a family of calcium-independent kinases (P70 S6), that are responsible for the phosphorylation of S6 ribosomal subunits.

In contrast to tacrolimus and cyclosporin A, sirolimus does not inhibit the production of the T-cell growth factors IL-2 and IL-4, but acts on a later stage of the T-cell activation pathway (see Fig. 14.1). The net result is that T-cell proliferation is blocked in the G1 phase (Javier *et al.* 1997). *In vitro* and *in vivo* studies have demonstrated the synergistic effect of sirolimus and cyclosporin A. It has been shown that sirolimus produced a more than 25-fold greater immunosuppressive effect when combined with cyclosporin A.

In patients with recalcitrant psoriasis, both single and multiple (given over 14 days) oral doses have been well tolerated, up to a maximum dose of 1.0 mg/m²/day (unpublished observations). From studies in humans for treatment of allograft rejection it is known that sirolimus administration can cause hypertriglyceridemia, thrombocytopenia and elevations in liver enzymes. Drug interaction studies have not yet been conducted. Because of its toxicity in immunosuppressive doses it is likely that further efforts will be directed at combination treatment with cyclosporin A, thereby decreasing the side-effects of both drugs. A pilot, phase II study of sirolimus and cyclosporin A combination treatment of severe psoriasis, is ongoing. Since tacrolimus and şirolimus have a common intracellular binding protein (FKBP) they are considered to be their respective antagonists and therefore tacrolimus is not suitable for fruitful combination therapy with sirolimus.

At present no studies have been performed with topical sirolimus. As sirolimus is structurally related to tacrolimus, topical formulations may be considered for development although its molecular weight would perhaps be to high for penetration of the human skin.

14.3 Monoclonal antibodies

Therapeutic Mab have been investigated in a wide spectrum of clinical settings including immunosuppression. Anti-CD3 Mab is the most extensively studied specificity since OKT3 was the first marketed Mab.

Other specificities that have been investigated as immunosuppressive tools are anti-CD4, anti-IL-2 receptor (= CD25), antileucocyte function antigen 1 (LFA-1) and anti-intercellular adhesion molecule 1 (ICAM-1) Mab (Bach *et al.* 1993).

Treatment of patients suffering from psoriasis has been limited to anti-CD3 and anti-CD4 Mab therapies. Although the exact mechanism is unknown, it is generally believed that administration of anti-CD3 and anti-CD4 Mab leads to depletion of T cells and T-helper cells, respectively. Controlled studies with anti-CD3 and anti-CD4 Mab have not been published yet.

Since patients treated with these Mab became sensitized against murine Mab and developed antimurine antibodies, recombinant chimeric Mab were constructed. Cm-T412 is a chimeric CD4 Mab that is constructed of the antigen-binding variable region of the murine CD4 Mab M-T412, and the constant regions of a human IgG, κ-immunoglobulin. Treatment with this chimeric Mab induced long-lasting decrease of disease activity in not only psoriasis patients but also in patients suffering from cutaneous lupus erythematosus and rheumatoid arthritis (Prinz *et al.* 1996). Independently, another group of investigators found, using a novel humanized anti-CD4 Mab, clinical improvement in only three out of eight patients suffering from chronic plaque-type psoriasis (Isaacs *et al.* 1997). So far, Mab treatment has not led to a status of general immunosuppression or other irreversible serious side-effects.

Since clinical experience with Mab treatments in psoriasis patients is very limited, more studies are needed to estimate the future of this potent immunosuppressive therapy. It can be anticipated that Mab treatment will be restricted to patients with extensive chronic recalcitrant psoriasis and psoriatic arthritis.

14.4 Cytokines

Cytokines regulate immune reactivity and direct the maturation, activation and migration of inflammatory cells. Cytokines can be grouped in several networks that affect haemapoiesis (e.g. granulocyte/macrophage colony-stimulating factor (GM-CSF)), lymphopoiesis (e.g. IL-2), pro-inflammatory cytokines (e.g. TNF-α), cytokine networks that affect T-helper cell differentiation (e.g. IL-12) and chemokines. Cytokine networks can be manipulated via cytokine administration, by Mab that bind to specific cytokines, by cytokine-receptor antagonists (e.g. anti-IL-2R Mab), or by administration of soluble cytokine receptors. Clinical experience with cytokine therapy has been limited to case reports in which the pro-inflammatory cytokine TNF-α was given to patients with severe plaque-type psoriasis. Although it has been suggested that TNF-α has a role in the pathogenesis of psoriasis, the rationale for giving TNF-α to psoriasis patients is lacking.

Together with our understanding of the role of chemokines such as IL-8, growth-related oncogene α (GRO-α; is not an oncogene) and interferon-inducible protein 10 (IP-10) in the pathophysiology of psoriasis, evidence is growing that neutralization of chemokine activity may have therapeutic value. However, these studies have not been presented yet.

14.5 Fusion proteins

Since activated T cells in psoriatic lesions express IL-2 receptors, Gottlieb and coworkers used an IL-2 bearing toxin for the selective destruction of these IL-2 receptor-bearing lymphocytes (Gottlieb *et al.* 1995). This lymphocyte-selective toxin ($DAB_{389}IL-2$) is a fusion protein in which the receptor-binding domain of diphtheria toxin is replaced by human IL-2 and the membrane-translocating and cytotoxic domains have been retained.

Ten patients were treated systemically with low doses of this fusion protein (100–200 kU/kg) in comparison with those in trials in T-cell lymphomas (≥ 1000 kU/kg). Four patients showed striking clinical improvement and four moderate improvement after two cycles of this IL-2 toxin. No serious toxicity was encountered. Interestingly, a marked reduction of intraepidermal CD3 and CD8 positive cells was noticed, again pointing at the pivotal role of T cells in the pathogenesis of psoriasis.

Recently, the fusion protein LFA3TIP was developed. LFA3TIP is a protein comprised of the first LFA-3 extracellular domain fused to the hinge, C_H2 and C_H3 regions of a human IgG1. LFA3TIP binds to CD2 thus leading to inhibition of proliferation of human T cells *in vitro* (Majeau *et al.* 1994). Study results in psoriasis have not been published yet.

14.6 Peptide T

Peptide T is a synthetic octapeptide designed to bind to the HIV-1 binding site on the CD4 molecule. This octapeptide is termed peptide T because of its high threonine content. The concomitant improvement of psoriatic lesions in an HIV-1-positive patient treated with peptide T encouraged further clinical investigations in psoriasis patients. At present only a limited number of studies have been published using low-dose peptide T in psoriasis treatment (Marcusson *et al.* 1991). Clinical responses to this new treatment have been promising and most interestingly a majority of patients enjoyed an improvement of their skin disease for more than 1 year after treatment was stopped.

14.7 Miscellaneous

Several antimetabolites frequently used for treatment of autoimmune diseases and malignant haematologic conditions have been used in psoriasis treatment. Notably, azothioprine and 6-thioguanine have been employed successfully in psoriasis patients who failed to respond to conventional systemic agents. Next to general antimetabolic effects on proliferating cells, these drugs show evidence for selective immunosuppression.

Azathioprine is a purine antagonist that not only inhibits mitosis via inhibition of DNA and RNA synthesis, but also affects monocyte and polymorphonuclear functions. In addition, it inhibits B-cell proliferation, diminishes T-cell-mediated responses and suppresses antibody production. Azathioprine has proved to be an effective immunosuppressive drug commonly used for treatment of autoimmune diseases. In dermatology, azathioprine has a well-established place in management of potentially fatal blistering diseases, atopic dermatitis and actinic reticuloid. In 1974, the largest study to date, Du Vivier reported that azathioprine benefited 19 of 29 patients suffering from severe psoriasis. An initial dose of 100 mg/day was increased to 200 mg/day after 2 weeks. A few patients needed 300 mg/day for up to 6 months. No serious side-effects occurred. The recommended dosage for azathioprine in psoriasis is 150 mg/day or less. Azathioprine can be considered as an effective and relatively safe drug as long as the duration of treatment does not exceed 3–4 years, because of possible development of hepatotoxicity or myelodepression (Younger *et al.* 1991).

6-Thioguanine is a purine analogue structurally related to azathioprine that has been in clinical use since the 1950s. The mechanism of action of this drug is similar to that of azathioprine. Zackheim studied 81 patients who were treated with a variety of dosages of 6-thioguanine (40–160 mg/day) (Zackheim *et al.* 1994).

Thirty-nine per cent of patients with plaque-type psoriasis were effectively maintained with 6-thioguanine for a median of 33 months. Four of five patients with palmoplantar pustular psoriasis experienced substantial benefit. The most common side-effect was myelosuppression; it is therefore not recommended as a first-line treatment. 6-Thioguanine has not been approved for treatment of psoriasis by the Food and Drug Administration.

Extracorporeal photochemotherapy (EPCT) is a promising and safe alternative treatment of some diseases of suspected autoimmune pathogenesis and psoriatic arthritis. The principle of treatment of EPCT is identical to PUVA therapy; the difference lies in the UVA exposure of the lymphocytes concentrated in the leukapheresed blood fraction in EPCT. Although the mechanism of action of EPCT is not fully understood, photodamage and modulation of the immune system has been reported. Evidence has been presented indicating that EPCT modifies cytokine release by lymphocytes and suppresses immunity. Although psoriasis skin lesions did not respond to EPCT, some measurable effect in improving psoriatic arthropathy has been documented in patients with long-standing arthropathy resistant to conventional therapy (de Misa *et al.* 1994). Since EPCT is an expensive and invasive treatment which is not widely available, it should be restricted to patients with severe joint complaints and limited skin lesions, unresponsive to regular treatments.

14.8 Conclusions

The introduction of cyclosporin A in dermatology, especially in treatment of psoriasis patients, has led to the discovery of a new field of highly potent cyclic immunosuppressive drugs. Although the major representatives of these compounds have proven to be effective in systemic treatment of psoriasis, their use has been limited by their side-effects. For the near future topical application of cyclic immunosuppressive drugs seemed to be promising. Unfortunately, these molecules are too large to cross the skin barrier in psoriatic lesions. It is therefore crucial that new immunomodulating agents are developed. Fusion proteins may well emerge as a new field of immunomodulating drugs for the systemic treatment of severe psoriasis.

References

Bach, J.-F., Fracchia, G.N. & Chatenoud, L. (1993) Safety and efficacy of therapeutic monoclonal antibodies in clinical therapy. *Immunology Today* **14**, 421–425.

Bonifati, C., Clerico, R., Potenza, C.M. & Carlesimo, M. (1989) Cyclosporin A, preliminary results in the treatment of psoriasis. *Acta Dermato-Venereologica (Stockh)* Suppl **146**, 151–154.

Bos, J.D. (1988) The pathomechanisms of psoriasis; the skin immune system and cyclosporine. *British Journal of Dermatology* **118**, 141–155.

Bos, J.D., Van Meinardi, M.M.H.M., Joost, Th. *et al.* (1989) Use of cyclosporin in psoriasis. *Lancet* **30**, 1500–1502.

Cimitan, A., Fantini, F. & Gianetti, A. (1989) Clinical trial with cyclosporin A. *Acta Dermato-Venereologica (Stockh)* Suppl **146**, 159–163.

de Misa, R.F., Azana, J.M., Harto, A. *et al.* (1994) Psoriatic arthritis: one year of treatment with extracorporeal photochemotherapy. *Journal of the American Academy of Dermatology* **30**, 1037–1038.

de Rie, M.A. & Bos, J.D. (1997) Cyclosporine immunotherapy. *Clinics in Dermatology* **15**, 811–821.

de Rie, M.A., Meinardi, M.M.H.M. & Bos, J.D. (1990) Analysis of side-effects of medium- and low-dose cyclosporin maintenance therapy in psoriasis. *British Journal of Dermatology* **123**, 347–353.

de Rie, M.A., Meinardi, M.M.H.M. & Bos, J.D. (1991) Lack of efficacy of topical cyclosporin A in atopic dermatitis and allergic contact dermatitis. *Acta Dermato-Venereologica* **71**, 452–454.

Ellis, C.N., Fradin, M.S., Hamilton, T.A. & Voorhees, J.J. (1995) Duration of remission during maintenance cyclosporin therapy for psoriasis: relationship to maintenance dose and degree of improvement during initial therapy. *Archives of Dermatology* **131**, 791–795.

Erkko, P., Granlund, H., Nuutinen, M. & Reitamo, S. (1997). Comparison of cyclosporin A pharmacokinetics of a new microemulsion formulation and standard oral preparation in patients with psoriasis. *British Journal of Dermatology* **136**, 82–88.

European FK-506 Multicentre Study Group. (1996) Systemic tacrolimus FK (506) is effective for the treatment of psoriasis in a double-blind placebo-controlled study. *Archives of Dermatology* **132**, 419–423.

Feutren, G., Abeywickrama, K., von Friend, D. & Graffenried, B. (1990) Renal function and blood pressure in psoriatic patients treated with cyclosporin A. *British Journal of Dermatology* **122** (Suppl. 36), 57–69.

Fradin, M.S., Ellis, C.N. & Voorhees, J.J. (1990) Efficacy of cyclosporin A in psoriasis: a summary of the United States' experience. *British Journal of Dermatology* **122** (Suppl 36), 21–25.

Gottlieb, S.L., Gilleaudeau, P., Johnson, R. *et al.* (1995) Response of psoriasis to a lymphocyte-selective toxin (DAB$_{389}$IL-2) suggests a primary immune, but not keratinocyte, pathogenic basis. *Nature Medicine* **1**, 442–447.

Grossman, R.M., Chevret, S., Abi-Rached, J., Blanchet, F. & Dubertret, L. (1996) Long-term safety of cyclosporine in the treatment of psoriasis. *Archives of Dermatology* **132**, 623–629.

Gupta, A.K., Matterson, E.L., Ellis, C.N. *et al.* (1989) Cyclosporin in the treatment of psoriatic arthritis. *Annals of the Rheumatic Diseases* **125**, 507–510.

Isaacs, J.D., Burrows, N., Wing, M. *et al.* (1997) Humanized anti-CD4 monoclonal antibody therapy of autoimmune and inflammatory disease. *Clinical Experimental Immunology* **110**, 158–166.

Javier, A.F., Bata-Csorgo, Z., Ellis, C.N. *et al.* (1997) Rapamycin (sirolimus) inhibits proliferating cell nuclear antigen expression and clocks cell cycle in the G1 phase in human keratinocyte stem cells. *Journal of Clinical Investigations* **99**, 2094–2099.

Korstanje, M.J., Bessems, P.J.M.J., Hulsmans, R.F.H.J. & Van de Staak W.J. (1989) Pustular psoriasis and acrodermatitis continua (Hallopeau) need high doses of systemic cyclosporin A [Letter]. *Dermatologica* **179**, 90–91.

MacLoad, A.M. & Thompson, A.W. (1991) FK506: an immunosuppressant for the 1990s? *Lancet* **337**, 25–27.

Mahrle, G., Schulze, H.J., Färber, L.,Weidinger, G. & Steigleder G.K. (1995) Low-dose short-term cyclosporin versus etretinate in psoriasis: improvement of skin, nail, and joint involvement. *Journal of the American Academy of Dermatology* **32**, 78–88.

Mahrle, G., Schulze, H.J., Brautigam, M. *et al.* (1996) Anti-inflammatory efficacy of low-dose cyclosporin A in psoriatic arthritis. A prospective multicentre study. *British Journal of Dermatology* **135**, 752–757.

Majeau, G.R., Meier, W., Jimmo, B., Kioussis, D. & Hochman, P.S. (1994) Mechanism of Lymphocyte Function-Associated molecule 3-Ig fusion proteins inhibition of T cell responses. *Journal of Immunology* **152**, 2753–2767.

Marcusson, J.A., Talme, T., Wetterberg, L. & Johansson, O. (1991) Peptide T a new treatment for psoriasis? A study of nine patients. *Acta Dermato-Venereologica* **71**, 479–483.

Meinardi, M.M.H.M., Westerhof, W. & Bos, J.D. (1987) Generalized pustular psoriasis (von Zumbusch) responding to cyclosporin A. *British Journal of Dermatology* **116**, 269–270.

Meinardi, M.M.H.M., De Rie, M.A. & Bos, J.D. (1990) Oral cyclosporin A is effective in clearing persistent pustulosis palmaris et plantaris. *Acta Dermato-Venereologica (Stockh)* **70**, 77–79.

Meingassner, J.G. & Stütz, A. (1992) Immunosuppressive macrolides of the type FK 506: a novel class of topical agents for treatment of skin diseases? *Journal of Investigative Dermatology* **98**, 851–855.

Meingassner, J.G., Grassberger, M., Fahrngruber, H. *et al.* (1997) A novel anti-inflammatory drug, SDZ ASM 981, for the topical and oral treatment of skin diseases: *in vivo* pharmacology. *British Journal of Dermatology* **137**, 568–576.

Mihatsch, M.J. & Wolff, K. (1992) Consensus conference on cyclosporin for psoriasis. *British Journal of Dermatology* **126**, 621–623.

Mihatsch, M.J., Antonovych, T., Bohman, S.-O. *et al.* (1994) Cyclosporin A nephropathy: standardization of the evaluation of kidney biopsies. *Clinical Nephrology* **41**, 23–32.

Mrowietz, U., Färber, L., von Henneicke-Zepelin, H.-H. *et al.* (1995) Long-term maintenance therapy with cyclosporine and posttreatment survey in severe psoriasis: results of a multicenter study. *Journal of the American Academy of Dermatology* **33**, 470–475.

Müller, W. & Herrmann, B. (1979) Cyclosporin A for psoriasis [correspondence]. *New England Journal of Medicine* **301**, 555.

Olivieri, I., Salvarani, C., Cantini, F. *et al.* (1997) Therapy with cyclosporin in psoriatic arthritis. *Seminars in Arthritis and Rheumatism* **27**, 36–43.

Penn, I. (1995) Malignancy after immunosuppressive therapy. *Clinical Immunotherapy* **4**, 207–218.

Peter, R.U., Färber, L., Weiss, J. *et al.* (1994) Low-dose cyclosporin A in palmoplantar psoriasis: evaluation of efficacy and safety. *Journal of the European Academy of Dermatology and Venereology* **3**, 518–524.

Prinz, J.C., Meurer, M., Reiter, C. *et al.* (1996) Treatment of severe cutaneous lupus erythematosus with a chimeric CD4 monoclonal antibody, cM-T412. *Journal of the American Academy of Dermatology* **34**, 244–252.

Rappersberger, K., Meingasser, J.G., Fialla, R. *et al.* (1996) Clearing of psoriasis by a novel immunosuppressive macrolide. *Journal of Investigative Dermatology* **106**, 701–710.

Reitamo, S. & Mustakallio, K.K. (1989) Cyclosporin in erythrodermic psoriasis. *Acta Dermato-Venereologica (Stockh)* Suppl **146**, 140–141.

Reitamo, S., Erkko, P., Remitz, A., Lauerma, A.I., Montonen, O. & Harjula K. (1993) Cyclosporin in the treatment of palmoplantar pustulosis. *Archives of Dermatology* **129**, 1273–1279.

Riccieri, V., Sili-Scavalli, A., Spadaro, A., Bracci, M., Taccari, E. & Zoppini, A. (1994) Short-term 'Cyclosporin A' therapy for psoriatic arthritis. *Acta Dermato-Venereologica (Stockh)* Suppl **186**, 94–95.

Ruzicka, T., Bieber, T., Schöpf, E. *et al.* (1997) A short-term trial of tacrolimus ointment for atopic dermatitis. *New England Journal of Medicine* **337**, 816–821.

Schopf, R.E., Bräutigam, M., Morsches, B. (1994) Cyclosporin A benefits both skin and joint diseases in psoriatic arthritis. *Journal of Investigative Dermatology* **102**, 616.

Schreiber, S.L. & Crabtree, G.R. (1992) The mechanism of action of cyclosporin A and FK506. *Immunology Today* **13**, 136–142.

Shupack, J., Abel, E., Bauer, E. *et al.* (1997) Cyclosporine as maintenance therapy in patients with severe psoriasis. *Journal of the American Academy of Dermatology* **36**, 423–432.

Timonen, P., Friend, D., Abeywickrama, K. *et al.* (1990) Efficacy of low-dose cyclosporin A in psoriasis: results of dose-finding studies. *British Journal of Dermatology* **122** (Suppl.) (36), 33–40.

Van Leent, E.J., Gräber, M., Thurston, M., Wagenaar, A., Spuls, P.I. & Bos, J.D. (1998) Effectiveness of the ascomycin macrolactam SDZ ASM 981 in the topical treatment of atopic dermatitis. *Archives of Dermatology* **134**, 805–809.

Weinstein, G.D. & White, G.M. (1993) An approach to the treatment of moderate to severe psoriasis with rotational therapy. *Journal of the American Academy of Dermatology* **28**, 454–459.

Witkamp, L., Zonneveld, I.M., Jung, E.G. *et al.* (1995) Efficacy and tolerability of multiple-dose SDZ IMM 125 in patients with severe psoriasis. *British Journal of Dermatology* **133**, 95–103.

Wong, R.L., Winslow, C.M. & Cooper, K.D. (1993) The mechanisms of action of cyclosporin A in the treatment of psoriasis. *Immunology Today* **14**, 69–73.

Younger, I.R., Harris, D.W.S. & Colver, G.B. (1991) Azathioprine in dermatology. *Journal of the American Academy of Dermatology* **25**, 281–286.

Zachariae, H. & Steen Olsen, T. (1995) Efficacy of cyclosporin A (CyA) in psoriasis: an overview of dose/response, indications, contraindications and side-effects. *Clinical Nephrology* **43**, 154–158.

Zackheim, H.S., Glogau, R.G., Fisher, D.A. & Maibach, M.I. (1994) 6-Thioguanine treatment of psoriasis: experience in 81 patients. *Journal of the American Academy of Dermatology* **30**, 452–458.

Chapter 15: Comparisons and Combinations

P.C.M. van de Kerkhof

This chapter provides an overall comparison between various treatments, and a summary on combination treatments will be given. In the chapters of Part 3 on therapy, comparisons and combination treatment have been highlighted by the individual authors. The aim of this chapter is to provide an overall *'Gestalt'* on comparisons and combinations in the treatment of psoriasis.

Based on comparative studies, guidelines may be constructed for the therapeutic management of psoriasis. However, individualization of treatments is crucial for an optimal therapeutic result. Not only the expression of psoriasis but also its significance in the psychosocial context of each patient has to be reconciled.

15.1 Comparisons

Comparisons between treatments have to be evaluated in controlled trials. In the chapters of Part 3 comparisons have been made based on comparative studies. However, comparisons between treatments may be difficult since sometimes treatments are preferentially indicated in widespread and or recalcitrant psoriasis; whereas other treatments are indicated in minor manifestations of psoriasis. In most studies the psoriasis area and severity index (PASI) has been used as the primary efficacy marker. The validity of this marker has been debated in view of the large interobserver variability and the inconvenience that erythema, induration and scaling are listed as one single value which also includes the extent of the lesions. For example, a patient with dithranol irritation might still have a considerable PASI.

The therapeutic result can be measured in various ways. Clearing time is of importance if a 'quick fix' is the intention. Clearing capacity is of importance to adjust the treatment strength; some patients urge their dermatologist for 100% clearing, whereas other patients are satisfied with a considerable reduction of the expression of psoriasis. Maintenance capacity is another criterion of importance for the long-term management. Most patients prefer long-term control and use a treatment for more than a few weeks. Table 15.1 provides a comparative analysis of efficacy data, clearing time, clearing capacity and maintenance capacity (Young 1970; Weinstein & Frost 1971; Baker 1976; Nyfors 1978; Boer *et al.* 1980; Levine & Parrish 1980; Henseler *et al.* 1981; Wolff & Hönigsmann 1982; Katz *et al.* 1987; Gollnick *et al.* 1988; Bos *et*

Table 15.1 Clearance and maintenance of different monotherapies in psoriasis.

Therapy	Clearing time (weeks)	Clearing capacity	Maintenance capacity	Chapter	References
Calcipotriol	8	++/+++	++	8	Dubertret et al. (1992); Kragballe et al. (1991)
Potent topical corticosteroids	2–4	+++	–	9	Katz et al. (1987)
Dithranol					
Home treatment	8–16	+	–	10	van de Kerkhof (1991)
Daycare	3–10	++	–	10	van de Kerkhof (1991)
Inpatient	3–6	+++	–	10	van de Kerkhof (1991)
Tar	?	++	+		Young (1970)
UVB	8–10	+++	–	11	Levine & Parish (1980); Boer et al. (1980)
PUVA	4–8	+++	–	11	Henseler et al. (1981); Wolff & Hönigsmann (1982)
Methotrexate	8–16	+++	+++	12	Weinstein & Frost (1971); Nyfors 1978; Baker (1976)
Acitretin	8–12	+	+++	13	Gollnick et al. (1988)
Cyclosporin	4–8	+++	–	14	Bos et al. (1989); Labarte et al. (1994)

–, not recommended; +, poor; ++, moderate; +++, excellent

al. 1989; Kragballe *et al.* 1991; van de Kerkhof 1991; Dubertret *et al.* 1992; Labarte *et al.* 1994).

A particularly pronounced clearing capacity has been well established for potent topical corticosteroids, inpatient treatment with dithranol, photo-therapy (UVB) and photochemotherapy (PUVA), methotrexate and cyclo-sporin. The efficacy of calcipotriol is comparable to a medium-strength corticosteroid and is superior to outpatient treatment with dithranol; how-ever, comparison with dithranol inpatient treatment revealed that calcipotriol might approach the efficacy of potent topical corticosteroids and dithranol inpatient treatment (Ortonne 1994; Bruse *et al.* 1994; van der Vleuten *et al.* 1995; Lebwohl *et al.* 1996). A low efficacy has been reported for home treat-ment with dithranol in cream bases and for acitretin; however, both treat-ments can be valuable in combination with other treatments.

With respect to patient acceptability and side-effects treatments differ considerably (Table 15.2). Tar and dithranol are time-honoured principles and safe treatments. However, both treatments are more demanding as home treatments for reason of staining and irritation of the skin. Particularly at day-care centres and inpatient departments these treatments are a mainstay. Topical corticosteroids and topical vitamin D_3 analogues are cosmetically ac-ceptable approaches. However, if these treatments are applied on large body surface areas, systemic absorption may be a serious hazard. Atrophy of the skin is a side-effect of topical corticosteroids and irritation is a drawback of vitamin D_3 treatment.

With respect to systemic treatments, phototherapy and photochemo-therapy, the need for an efficacious treatment should be balanced against possible side-effects. In particular the long-term toxicity of these treatments should be taken into account if maintenance treatment is initiated. The deci-sion to provide maintenance therapy or to restrict the goal only to clearance is not easy. Most treatments have a cumulative toxicity potential; on the other hand prolonged remissions permit the patient to escape from his or her social isolation. In view of the cumulative toxicity potential it is advised that corticosteroids, photo(chemo)therapy and cyclosporin should be avoided as maintenance treatments. Treatments that are useful for maintenance are calcipotriol, methotrexate, acitretin and tar.

The treatment result is highly dependent upon the manifestation of pso-riasis. Guttate psoriasis has the most favourable spontaneous course; there-fore major therapies should be avoided. In palmoplantar pustulosis and acrodermatitis continua Hallopeau, topical treatments are not sufficient and systemic treatments are required for a substantial therapeutic effect. The same holds true for generalized pustular psoriasis and erythrodermic psoriasis where systemic treatments are indicated. In patients with chronic plaque psoriasis of limited extent, topical treatments are indicated; however, photo(chemo)-therapy is indicated in the more extensive manifestations. In recalcitrant forms of psoriasis, systemic treatments are indicated.

Table 15.2 Main side effects of treatments.

Treatment	Side effect
Topical vitamin D$_3$ (Chapter 8)	Irritation of the skin Hypercalcemia
Topical corticosteroids (Chapter 9)	Athrophy of the skin Precipitation of psoriasis after withdrawal Dermatitis perioralis Increased hair growth Adrenal gland suppression
Dithranol (Chapter 10)	Staining Burning Precipitation of new lesions
Tar (Chapter 14)	Staining Folliculitis Irritation of the skin
Phototherapy (Chapter 11)	Burning Erythema Ageing of the skin Cutaneous cancer
Photochemotherapy (PUVA) (Chapter 11)	Erythema Pigment disturbances Nausea Pruritus Deep burning Cutaneous cancers
Methotrexate (Chapter 12)	Liver impairment Subjective complaints Hematopoietic suppression Skin and mucosal membrane pathology Mutagenicity Immunosuppression
Retinoids (Chapter 13)	Skin and mucosal membrane disturbances Elevation of triglycerides and cholesterol Subjective complaints Liver impairment Diffuse hair loss Teratogenicity
Cyclosporin (Chapter 14)	Renal impairment Hypertension Cutaneous cancers Gastrointestinal discomfort Hypertrichosis Gingival hyperplasia Headache Vertigo Muscle cramps Tremor

15.2 Combinations

The combination of different treatments is used by the majority of patients. In a recent survey of patients in the Dutch Psoriasis Association, 68% of the patients were shown to use combination treatment (van de Kerkhof *et al.* 1998a). An important advantage of combination therapy is the opportunity to enhance efficacy and reduce side-effects.

Of particular interest are combinations of treatments with a different mode of action and/or combinations of treatments with a different profile of side-effects.

In the chapters of Part 3 on therapies the authors have provided an update on combinations of treatments. In this chapter an overview on combination therapy is provided. Table 15.3 summarizes different combinations and indicates whether a combination is contraindicated, recommended or strongly recommended.

The combination of vitamin D_3 analogues with other antipsoriatic treatments is of interest as no single combination is contraindicated. Information on the efficacy and side-effects of combinations with calcipotriol has been studied in depth (Chapter 8). Especially the combination of calcipotriol–acitretin (van de Kerkhof *et al.* 1998b), calcipotriol–cyclosporin (Grossman *et al.* 1994) and calcipotriol–PUVA (Frappaz & Thivolet 1993) proved to have a substantially increased efficacy as compared with the monotherapies. The combination of calcipotriol–UVB (Kragballe 1990; Molin 1995) and calcipotriol–topical corticosteroids (Ortonne 1994; Kragballe *et al.* 1998; Lebwohl *et al.* 1996) proved to have at least some increase of efficacy as compared with monotherapies. These combination therapies resulted in a reduction of the total doses of acitretin, cyclosporin and PUVA, required for a marked improvement or total clearing. The irritation by calcipotriol proved to be markedly reduced by topical corticosteroids.

Topical corticosteroids are frequently combined with various antipsoriatic treatments. Although this addition may contribute to the clearing of some lesions, an increased relapse rate has been reported in patients using the combination of PUVA and topical corticosteroids vs. patients who were treated exclusively with PUVA (Morrison *et al.* 1978).

Tazarotene is a topical retinoid which has been recently introduced in the treatment of psoriasis in some countries (Chapter 13). Combination of tazarotene with phototherapy (UVB) proved to be a very successful combination (Chapter 13).

Dithranol can be combined with all antipsoriatic treatments. The combination with phototherapy is an advantageous combination. However, the additional effect of dithranol on high-dose phototherapy (UVB) does not result in an increased clearing capacity; the advantage of this combination is a prolongation of the remission period (Chapter 10). The addition of topical corticosteroids to dithranol results in shortening of the remission time (Chapter 10).

Table 15.3 Combination of treatments in psoriasis.

	Topical vitamin D$_3$	Topical corticosteroid	Tarazotene	Dithranol	Coal tar	UVB	PUVA	Methotrexate	Cyclosporin
Acitretin	++	+	+	+	+	++	++	-	-/+
Cyclosporin	++	+	+	+/++	+	-	-	-/+	
Methotrexate	+	+	+	+	+	-	-		
PUVA	++	+	+	+/++	-	-			
UVB	+/++	+	++	+/++	-/+				
Coal tar	+	+	+	+/++					
Dithranol	+	-/+	+						
Tarazotene	+	+							
Topical corticosteroid	+/++								

-, not recommended; +, poor; ++, moderate; +++, excellent

Crude coal tar can be combined with most antipsoriatic treatments. Although the combination of crude coal tar and UV radiation is a time-honoured principle (Goeckerman treatment) crude coal tar does not contribute to the efficacy of optimal UV treatment. In view of the potential carcinogenic effect of both treatments the combination of tar–UVB and tar–PUVA is not advised anymore (Chapter 11).

UVB and PUVA should not be combined with cyclosporin and methotrexate. The immunosuppressive actions of both systemic treatments imply a theoretical hazard for the induction of cutaneous malignancies. UVB can be combined efficiently with topical vitamin D$_3$ analogues, crude coal tar and dithranol. The combination of PUVA with calcipotriol has been shown to be highly effective. The combinations UVB–acitretin and PUVA–acitretin have been accepted as highly effective approaches. Following a pretreatment with acitretin over 2 weeks, UVB or PUVA treatment is started. Both combinations provide perhaps the most effective clearing therapy for psoriasis (Lauharanta *et al.* 1981; Lowe *et al.* 1991).

Methotrexate can be combined with all topical treatments. The combination of methotrexate with phototherapy (UVB) and photochemotherapy (PUVA) is not advisable in view of the theoretical risk on tumour promotion by this combination and the delayed photosensitivity which is induced by methotrexate (Chapter 12). The combination of methotrexate and acitretin is contraindicated; this combination has induced in some patients toxic hepatitis (Chapter 12). The combination of cyclosporin and methotrexate has been applied with success (Chapter 12). However, the combination requires intensified supervision as decreased kidney functioning, induced by cyclosporin, will decrease clearing of methotrexate by the kidneys. Further, both treatments are major treatments with potentially serious side-effects.

Cyclosporin can be combined with several antipsoriatic treatments (Chapter 14). The combination is especially effective with calcipotriol and dithranol (Chapters 8 and 10). The combination of cyclosporin with photo(chemo)-therapy (PUVA) is contraindicated, whereas the combination of cyclosporin with methotrexate requires intensified supervision (Chapters 11 and 12).

As indicated above, the combination of acitretin with photo(chemo)-therapy and cyclosporin with calcipotriol are highly effective. Whereas the combination of acitretin with methotrexate is contraindicated. The combination of acitretin and cyclosporin might be advantageous theoretically, as both treatments have a different mode of action. However, retinoids and cyclosporin are metabolized in the liver via a cytochrome P-450-dependent system. Therefore, the combination has the theoretical risk for cumulation of cyclosporin with an increased expression of its side-effects (Webber & Back 1993). Recently, we have treated three patients suffering from severe psoriasis with this combination, without any additional therapeutical effect of cyclosporin treatment to acitretin therapy (Kuijpers, 1997).

15.3 Conclusions

Comparisons between different antipsoriatic treatments reveal that a spectrum of treatment options is available ranging from mild treatments with minimal side-effects to major treatments with more serious side-effects. Treatment management should be individualized resulting in the optimal treatment for an individual patient at the very moment of consultation.

Various combination treatments are possible. Some combinations clearly have an additive efficacy. However, in view of side-effects some combinations are contraindicated.

From a practical point of view every patient has his or her own distinct form of psoriasis.

References

Baker, H. (1976) Methotrexate the conservative treatment for psoriasis. In: *Farber EM* (ed. Cox, A.J.), p. 42, abstract 235. York Medical Books, New York.

Boer, J., Schothorst, A.A. & Suurmond, D. (1980) UV-B phototherapy of psoriasis. *Dermatologica* **161**, 251–258.

Bos, J.D., Meinardi, M.M.H.M., Joost, Th. *et al.* (1989) Use of cyclosporin in psoriasis. *Lancet* **30**, 1900–1902.

Bruse, S., Epinette, W.W., Funicella, T. *et al.* (1994) Comparative study of calcipotriene (MC 903) ointment and fluocinonide ointment in the treatment of psoriasis. *Journal of the American Academy of Dermatology* **31**, 755–759.

Dubertret, L., Wallach, D., Souteyrand, P. *et al.* (1992) Efficacy and safety of calcipotriol (MC903) ointment in psoriasis vulgaris. *Journal of the American Academy of Dermatology* **27**, 983–984.

Frappaz, A. & Thivolet, J. (1993) Calcipotriol in combination with PUVA: a randomized double-blind placebo study in severe psoriasis. *European Journal of Dermatology* **3**, 351–354.

Gollnick, H., Bauer, R., Brindley, C. *et al.* (1988) Acitretin versus etrinate in psoriasis. Clinical and pharmakinetic results of a German multicenter study. *Journal of the American Academy of Dermatology* **19**, 458–469.

Grossman, R.M., Thivolet, J., Claudy, A. *et al.* (1994) A novel therapeutic approach to psoriasis with combination calcipotriol ointment and very low-dose cyclosporin: results of multicenter placebo-controlled study. *Journal of the American Academy of Dermatology* **31**, 68–74.

Henseler, T., Wolff, K., Hönigsmann, H. *et al.* (1981) Oral 8-methoxypsoralen photo-chemotherapy of psoriasis. The European PUVA Study: a cooperative study among 18 European Centres. *Lancet* **1**, 853–857.

Katz, H.I., Hien, N. & Prawer, S.E. (1987) Superpotent topical steroid treatment of psoriasis vulgaris. Clinical efficacy and adrenal function. *Journal of the American Academy of Dermatology* **16**, 804–811.

Kragballe, K. (1990) Combination of topical calcipotriol (MC 903) and UVB radiation for psoriasis vulgaris. *Dermatologica* **181**, 211–214.

Kragballe, K., Barnes, L. & Hamberg, K.J. (1998) Calcipotriol cream with or without concurrent topical corticosteroids in psoriasis: tolerability and efficacy. *British Journal of Dermatology* **139**, 649–654.

Kragballe, K., Giertsen, B.T., de Hoop, D. *et al.* (1991) Double blind, right-left comparison of calcipotriol and betamethasone valerate in treatment of psoriasis vulgaris. *Lancet* **337**, 193–196.

Kuijpers, A.L.A., van Dooren-Greebe, R.J., van de Kerkhof, P.C.M. *et al.* (1997) Failure of combination therapy with acitretin and cyclosporin A in 3 patients with erythrodermic psoriasis. *Dermatology* **194**, 88–90.

Labarte, C., Grossman, R. & Abi-Rached, J. (1994) Efficacy and safety or oral cyclosporin (Cy A; Sadimmun®) for long-term treatment of chronic severe plaque psoriasis. *British Journal of Dermatology* **130**, 366–375.

Lauharanta, J., Juvakoski, T. & Lassus, A. (1981) A clinical evalution of the effects of an aromatic retinoid (tigasus), combination of retinoid and PUVA, and PUVA alone in severe psoriasis. *British Journal of Dermatology* **104**, 325–332.

Lebwohl, M., Siskin, S.B. & Epinette, W.W. (1996) A multicenter trial of calcipotriene ointment and halobetasol ointment compared with either agent alone for the treatment of psoriasis. *Journal of the American Academy of Dermatology* **35**, 268–269.

Levine, M.J. & Parrish, J.A. (1980) Outpatient phototherapy of psoriasis. *Archives of Dermatology* **116**, 552–554.

Lowe, N.J., Prystowsky, J.H. & Bourget, T. (1991) Acitretin plus UVB therapy for psoriasis. Comparison with placebo plus UVB and acitretin alone. *Journal of the American Academy of Dermatology* **24**, 591–594.

Molin, L. (1995) Calcipotriol combined with phototherapy (UVB and PUVA) in the treatment of psoriasis (Abstract). *Journal of the European Academy of Dermatology* **5** (Suppl.), 184.

Morrison, W.L., Parrish, J.A. & Fitzpatrick. T.B. (1978) Controlled study of PUVA and adjunctive topical therapy in the management of psoriasis. *British Journal of Dermatology* **98**, 125–132.

Nyfors, A. (1978) Benefits and adverse drug experiences during long term methotrexate treatment of 248 psoriatics. *Danish Medical Bulletin* **25**, 208–211.

Ortonne, J.P. (1994) Psoriasis: New therapeutic modality by calcipotriol and betamethason dipropionate. *Nouvelle Dermatologique* **13**, 746–751.

van de Kerkhof, P.C.M. (1991) Dithranol treatment for psoriasis: after 75 years, still going strong. *European Journal of Dermatology* **1**, 79–88.

van de Kerkhof, P.C.M., Steegers-Theunissen, R.P.M. & Kuipers, M.V. (1998a) Evaluation of topical drug treatment in psoriasis. *Dermatology* **197**, 31–36.

van de Kerkhof, P.C.M., Cambazard, F., Hutchinson, F. *et al.* (1998b) The effect of the addition of calcipotriol ointment (50 µg/g) to acitretin therapy in psoriasis. *British Journal of Dermatology* **138**, 84–89.

van der Vleuten, C.J.M., de Jong, E.M.G.J., Rulo, E.H.F.C. *et al.* (1995) In-patient treatment with calcipotriol versus dithranol in refractory psoriasis. *European Journal of Dermatology* **5**, 676–679.

Webber, I.R. & Back, D.J. (1993) Effect of etretinate on cyclosporin metabolism *in vitro*. *British Journal of Dermatology* **128**, 42–44.

Weinstein, G.D. & Frost, P. (1971) Methotrexate for psoriasis. A new therapeutic schedule. *Archives of Dermatology* **103**, 33–38.

Wolff, K. & Hönigsmann, H. (1982) Clinical aspects of photochemotherapy. *Pharmacological Therapy* **12**, 381–418.

Young, E. (1970) The external treatment of psoriasis. A controlled investigation of the effects of coal tar. *British Journal of Dermatology* **82**, 510–515.

Index